Drug Interactions in Anesthesia

Drug Interactions
in Anesthesia

N. Ty Smith, M.D.
Department of Anesthesia
Veterans Administration Hospital
Professor of Anesthesia
University of California
San Diego, California

Ronald D. Miller, M.D.
Professor of Anesthesia and Pharmacology
School of Medicine
University of California
San Francisco, California

Aldo N. Corbascio, M.D.
Professor of Pharmacology
University of the Pacific
San Francisco, California

Lea & Febiger • 1981 • Philadelphia

Library of Congress Cataloging in Publication Data

Smith, Norman Ty, 1932–
  Drug interactions in anesthesia.

  Includes index.
  1. Drug interactions. 2. Anesthesiology.
I. Miller, Ronald D., 1939– joint author.
II. Corbascio, Aldo N., joint author. III. Title.
[DNLM: 1. Drug interactions. 2. Anesthesia.
3. Anesthetics. QV38 S655d]
RD82.7.D78S6   615′.781   80-17454
ISBN 0-8121-0683-0

Published in Great Britain by Henry Kimpton Publishers, London

PRINTED IN THE UNITED STATES OF AMERICA

Print No.   4   3   2   1

"To Penelope, Marilyn, and Elise:

The beacons which light our way."

Preface

The practice of anesthesia entails a daring incursion into human pharmacology and pharmacodynamics. The anesthesiologist performs daily a complex experiment in patients, with drugs that profoundly affect essential functions, such as respiratory, cardiovascular, and neuromuscular activity. To achieve anesthesia speedily and effectively often requires many agents (six to ten on the average) in patients who may have been exposed to 20 or even more drugs in the preoperative period. There are few other branches of medicine in which polypharmacy is such a necessity and drug interactions such an inevitable consequence. However, the impressive growth of available drugs witnessed during the past two decades has been troubled by the realization that the pharmacodynamics and pharmacokinetics of one drug may be seriously modified by the presence of other drugs. This leads to numerous interactions, some welcome, some less so. The science of interactions is still in its infancy, but it constitutes an area of explosive development that is bound to affect many traditional therapeutic concepts.

At present, the anesthesiologist faces the problem of drug interactions without any useful guide that is both detailed and clinically oriented. The aim of this book is to provide such guidance and to introduce some logic and method into one of the most persistent problems of anesthetic practice. The book explores at least four facets of the interaction process: mechanism, detection, prevention, and management. The approach is mainly clinical and practical. Thus when confronted with a patient who is receiving diuretics and antihypertensives, for example, the anesthesiologist will be able to refer to a systematized approach, rather than to isolated fragments of pharmacologic knowledge. Although we have stressed the clinically important drug interactions, we do discuss those that are less clinically relevant, but that have been overemphasized elsewhere.

We divided the book into two sections. The first five chapters cover some general principles dealing with drug interactions. This section is particularly useful in understanding the subsequent chapters, which describe specific groups of drugs and their interactions. These initial chapters will help to develop an insight into the mechanisms of drug interactions, and to prepare the reader for the inevitable situation involving a new interaction—real or imagined.

The subsequent chapters are arranged according to classes of drugs. The contributors were asked to follow a plan in the writing of a chapter. To emphasize the clinical orientation of the book, each chapter was to include one or more case reports describing a drug interaction, followed by detailed pharmacology of that particular group, especially the pharmacology pertinent to drug interactions. Then the chapter was to bring together case report(s), pharmacology, and advice to the physician on the management of a patient receiving one or more drugs from that class of agents.

The authors did, by and large, succeed in these deceptively modest requests. Inevitably, the order and manner of presentation have varied among the chapters. How successful our somewhat different approach is, and which chapter arrangement offers the best teaching, must be decided by the reader. Any comments will be welcome.

We decided to divide the clinical chapters according to groups of drugs to provide a handy reference for the evening before an operation, for example. Thus for the patient

receiving antihypertensive and diuretic therapy, the two appropriate chapters can be read to determine the potential problems arising from these drugs during anesthesia. Similarly, the choice of an anesthetic agent or the wisdom of a choice already made can often be appraised by consulting a single chapter.

The format of this book should thus please those who use it as a reference. Those who read it straight through as a text will find some overlap, which is intentional. We did not wish to force the reader to peruse several chapters to discover all the information required about a single agent.

The number of possible drug interactions seems almost limitless. We have restricted ourselves to those that occur during anesthesia and operations, or those that may otherwise be important to the anesthesiologist. The latter group takes into account the anesthesiologist's role in areas outside the operating room, such as in the intensive care unit. Since there have been so many false alarms concerning drug interactions, we have defined, when possible, the incidence and clinical relevance of an interaction. This has not always been easy. Many interactions have been described only with anecdotes. Others have been observed only in animals.

Although this book was designed for the practicing or in-training anesthetist, there is enough general information on drug interactions to satisfy many others: the medical student, the pharmacologist, and the internist, to name but a few.

The carefully chosen authors have been given considerable latitude, even to the point of disagreeing with each other. In drug interaction, as in other medical fields, there are no absolutes, and the state of knowledge is such that disagreement and change are inevitable.

It is routine to thank one's editor. However, special thanks are due to Mr. George Mundorff, who has surely been one of the most patient editors, even through the elephantine conceptional period of this book. We wish to thank our authors, who have been willing to try a different format of presentation. Our gratitude ultimately goes to the many investigators who have pioneered in this complex but vital subject. We hope that others will follow in this critical area of knowledge and trust that this book will provide a guide and an incentive.

N. Ty Smith, M.D.
Ronald D. Miller, M.D.
Aldo N. Corbascio, M.D.

Contributors

MILTON H. ALPER, M.D.
Associate Professor of Anesthesia,
    Harvard Medical School;
    Anesthesiologist-in-Chief,
    Boston Hospital for Women,
    Boston, Massachusetts.

A. H. ANTON, Ph.D.
Professor of Anesthesiology and
    Pharmacology, Case Western Reserve
    University School of Medicine;
    Director, Biogenic Amine Laboratory,
    University Hospitals of Cleveland,
    Cleveland, Ohio.

JOHN L. ATLEE, III, M.D.
Associate Professor of Anesthesiology,
    University of Wisconsin Medical
    School, Madison, Wisconsin.

R. DENNIS BASTRON, M.D.
Associate Professor of Anesthesiology,
    University of Arizona School of
    Medicine;
    Chief of Anesthesiology Service,
    Veterans Administration Medical
    Center,
    Tucson, Arizona.

LEO D. H. J. BOOIJ, M.D.
Visiting Professor of Anesthesia, School of
    Medicine, University of California, San
    Francisco, California.

BURNELL R. BROWN, JR., M.D., Ph.D.
Professor and Head, Department of
    Anesthesiology,
    Professor, Department of
    Pharmacology,
    Arizona Health Sciences Center
    School of Medicine,
    Tucson, Arizona.

HELMUT F. CASCORBI, M.D., Ph.D.
Professor of Anesthesiology, Case Western
Reserve University School of
Medicine, Cleveland, Ohio.

DAVID J. CULLEN, M.D.
Associate Professor of Anesthesia, Harvard
Medical School; Associate Anesthetist,
Director, Recovery Room—Acute
Care Unit, Massachusetts General
Hospital, Boston, Massachusetts.

JOAN W. FLACKE, M.D.
Associate Professor of Anesthesiology,
Center for the Health Sciences,
University of California,
Los Angeles, California.

WERNER E. FLACKE, M.D.
Professor of Anesthesiology,
Center for the Health Sciences,
University of California,
Los Angeles, California.

J. S. GRAVENSTEIN, M.D.
Graduate Research Professor of Anesthesia,
University of Florida School of
Medicine, Gainesville, Florida.

DAVID S. JANOWSKY, M.D.
Professor of Psychiatry, School of
Medicine, University of California at
San Diego, La Jolla, California;
Staff Physician and Chief of
Psychopharmacology, Veterans
Administration Medical Center,
San Diego, California.

ESTHER C. JANOWSKY, M.D.
Assistant Clinical Professor of
Anesthesiology, School of Medicine,
University of California at San Diego;
Attending Anesthesiologist, University
Hospital, San Diego, California.

DAVID E. LONGNECKER, M.D.
Professor of Anesthesiology, University of
Virginia Medical Center,
Charlottesville, Virginia.

EDWARD LOWENSTEIN, M.D.
Anesthetist, Massachusetts General
Hospital, Boston, Massachusetts.

GEORGE E. MCLAIN, JR., M.D.
Research Associate, Department of
Anesthesiology, Arizona Health
Sciences Center College of Medicine,
Tucson, Arizona.

ROBERT G. MERIN, M.D.

Professor of Anesthesiology and Associate
Professor of Pharmacology, University
of Rochester School of Medicine and
Dentistry, Rochester, New York.

RONALD D. MILLER, M.D.
Professor of Anesthesia and Pharmacology,
School of Medicine, University of
California, San Francisco, California.

EDWIN S. MUNSON, M.D.
Professor of Anesthesiology, University of
Florida College of Medicine; Chief,
Anesthesiology Service, Veterans
Administration Medical Center,
Gainesville, Florida.

JOHN L. NEIGH, M.D.
Associate Professor of Anesthesia,
University of Pennsylvania; Director of
Anesthesia, Presbyterian–University
of Pennsylvania Medical Center,
Philadelphia, Pennsylvania.

M. F. RHOTON, Ph.D.
Associate Professor of Education in
Anesthesiology, Case Western Reserve
University School of Medicine,
Cleveland, Ohio.

S. CRAIG RISCH, M.D.
Staff Psychiatrist, Clinical
Neuropharmacology Branch, National
Institute of Mental Health, National
Institutes of Health Clinical Center,
Bethesda, Maryland.

BEN F. RUSY, M.D.
Professor of Anesthesiology, University of
Wisconsin Medical School, Madison,
Wisconsin.

N. TY SMITH, M.D.
Professor of Anesthesia, University of
California, San Diego; Professor of
Anesthesia, Veterans Administration
Hospital, San Diego, California.

ROBERT K. STOELTING, M.D.
Professor and Chairman, Department of
Anesthesia, Indiana University School
of Medicine,
Indianapolis, Indiana.

K. C. WONG, M.D., Ph.D.
Professor and Chairman, Department of
Anesthesiology, Professor of
Pharmacology; University of Utah
College of Medicine, Salt Lake City,
Utah.

Contents

Contents

Chapter 1

Dangers and Opportunities

N. TY SMITH

The first recorded anesthetic death could have been prevented by a knowledge of drug interactions. Mortality and morbidity still continue from our understandable ignorance of the subject. On the other hand, drug interactions have helped to transform the course of anesthetic management, which currently relies on the skilled administration of several drugs to the same patient. Certainly combination therapy and drug interactions are the basis of "balanced" anesthesia. Hence the art lies in the avoidance of hazardous interactions and in the expert application of useful ones. This introductory chapter examines the role of drug interactions in the practice of anesthesia. The emphasis is on the practical side of the subject, including the contributions of research to the clinical understanding of drug interactions.

CASE REPORT

In 1848, 16-year-old Hannah Greener came under the care of Dr. Meggison, a country practitioner near Newcastle, England, for the removal of a great toenail. She was terrified of the impending procedure, and accepted gratefully the offer of the new anesthetic agent, chloroform. This only partially calmed her, and she approached the operation with fear. The story of her sudden death during the first few whiffs of chloroform and of the futile attempts to resuscitate her with brandy is too well known to repeat here. There is now little doubt that her death was a direct result of the interaction between chloroform and the excess epinephrine discharged from her adrenal medullae. Had Dr. Meggison chosen ether, her life probably would have been spared. The clarification of the cause of Hannah's mysterious death had to wait over half a century for the classic studies of Goodman Levy, who demonstrated unequivocally that chloroform sensitizes the myocardium to the dysrhythmic actions of epinephrine.[1,2]

Even today, we in medicine often wait until an interaction has occurred and then determine the cause, rather than anticipate an interaction on theoretical grounds. The major difference is that, because of an expanded pool of pharmacologic knowledge, the time scale has been compressed—from over 60 years in the case of chloroform, to a few hours or days.

A useful drug interaction

Drug interactions have exerted a profound effect on the development of modern anesthesia. Neuromuscular blocking agents are an example. Previously, adequate muscle relaxation could be obtained only with the primary anesthetic agent, usually ether. This relaxation was achieved at the risk of profound central nervous, circulatory, and occasionally respiratory depression. The introduction of muscle relaxants allowed the use of lower concentrations of potent inhalation agents, or even their abandonment in favor of the intravenous agents. The latter led to the implementation of the concept of "balanced" anesthesia, which meant balancing the dosage of drugs with different actions to provide adequate hypnosis, muscle relaxation, analgesia, and attenuation of reflexes.

The safe use of curare was certainly an essential feature of this revolution in anesthetic practice. The changes brought about by curare, however, were not the consequence of the introduction of a single drug, but were due to the skillful exploitation of the interactions among three drugs—curare, neostigmine, and atropine. It is not an overstatement to claim that the rapid expansion of modern surgery is closely connected with the purposeful application of drug interactions.

Dangers and opportunities

The guiding principles, then, of the succeeding chapters are avoiding or at least attenuating undesirable and dangerous drug interactions, using desirable and useful interactions to maximum advantage, and converting ostensibly undesirable interactions into useful ones.

One example should suffice for the last principle. Some 20 years ago, the combination of ether and curare was banned in our training program because of a well-known study by Beecher and Todd,[3] who had demonstrated that the mortality following the combination was 1 in 50. Thus my teacher's suggestion to use ether and curare for a case met with my resistance. He explained that the basis of the ether-curare combination was marked synergism, and the solution was simply to use less of each drug, particularly curare. Today we should take this principle for granted—when there is synergism or addition between two agents, less of one, or preferably of both, should be used. However, one still sees, for example, pancuronium administered on a fixed schedule, irrespective of the anesthetic used. The result can be troublesome, particularly with enflurane. Small increments of pancuronium and low concentrations of the inhalation agent will suffice, with adjustment of muscle relaxation according to the concentration of the inhalation agent. This approach takes advantage of a drug interaction, rather than being controlled or hindered by it.

The "ideal" narcotic

The evolution of narcotic "anesthesia" and the narcotic antagonists illustrates a useful drug interaction, as well as the search for the "ideal" drug interaction. Ideally, an antagonist should (1) have no effect of its own, (2) reverse only the "undesirable" effects of the agonist, and (3) last longer than the agonist. The first is easily attained. The third, a long duration of action, is nebulous, since the narcotics vary considerably in this respect. If the antagonist administered in the recovery room lasts too long, pain relief may be delayed. The second criterion (selective antagonism) is even less well defined. The definition of desirability depends upon the circumstances. (The amphetamines have hypertensive, anorectic, and cortical stimulating properties. Each of these properties may be desirable if the agent is used to elevate blood pressure, decrease the appetite, or elevate the mood; the other two automatically become side-effects.) The narcotics, with their protean effects, are no exception. We often use the usually undesirable effect of ventilatory depression in patients who are resisting the ventilator, and the somnolence produced by some narcotics is considered desirable in patients on long-term ventilation. I believe that specificity of action should be built into the agonists themselves, rather than into the antagonists.

An interaction gone astray

Occasionally, a useful drug combination goes beyond its original intent. The addition of epinephrine to a local anesthetic is an example. Its usefulness in decreasing the toxicity and prolonging the duration of the anesthetic is well documented. In the presence, however, of certain inhalation agents, such as halothane, an additional and undesirable interaction may occur: a decrease in the arrhythmic threshold to epinephrine. We now know that enflurane and isoflurane are the optimal agents to use in the presence of exogenously administered epinephrine, halothane permits limited use, and cyclopropane is unacceptable.

Still another unanticipated interaction is the advance warning that epinephrine may provide against local anesthetic toxicity. If rapid intravascular absorption following injection of the test dose occurs, it may be difficult to detect any manifestations of the anesthetic, whereas those of epinephrine are usually obvious—tachycardia, palpitations, and headache. If these symptoms are present, one should assume that significant amounts of the local anesthetic have also been absorbed and that CNS (central nervous system) toxicity may occur on further injection.

On the other hand, if the epinephrine is absorbed slowly during a peridural anesthetic, as is appropriate, still another type of interaction occurs. Blood pressure and systemic vascular resistance may actually *decrease* more when epinephrine is in the anesthetic solution than when it is not.[4] Why should this happen when the original drug interaction depended on the vasoconstrictive properties of epinephrine? In high concentrations, as present in the epidural space, epinephrine does have an *alpha*-adrenergic (vasoconstrictive) action. In low concentrations—diluted in the blood stream—it acts as a *beta*-adrenergic substance. Presumably this vasodilating action adds to the vasodepressant effects of lidocaine—both direct and indirect from the sympathetic block—to produce noticeably greater hypotension. Thus a drug interaction that began as straightforward has become complex.

RESEARCH INTO DRUG INTERACTIONS

The rest of this chapter will deal with the state of research into drug interactions, and with the impact of this research on daily practice. Research is defined here as any concerted effort that increases our knowledge and allows the useful transfer of that knowledge to the practicing physician.

Definitions

The terminology used to describe drug interactions is in a sad state. That the definitions of the terms are not standard has created a problem in this book, since we must use terms as other authors have used them, and their definitions either vary or are nonexistent. For the sake of completeness, I shall outline below some of the definitions that have been proposed. For the sake of standardization, I shall give my own preferences.

The commonly used terms are addition, antagonism, synergism, and potentiation. Before synergism or antagonism can be defined, there must be some agreement on the definition of *addition,* or the mode of summation of drug effects. Two definitions of addition are generally used: (1) *dose addition*, when one-half the dose of drug A plus one-half an equi-effective dose of drug B evokes the same effect as the entire dose of drug A or drug B alone; (2) *effect addition,* when the intensity of the combined effect equals the sum of the intensities of the effect that each drug evokes when administered alone. Effect addition is certainly additive behavior as it may be expected from a superficial examination; each drug simply brings its own effect into the partnership. I prefer the dose-addition definition, although with dose addition, the combined drug effect is not so obvious. It is more easily understood by considering a simple experiment. Equipotent amounts of drug A and drug B can be established. If one-half of each of these amounts is then administered and the same effect is achieved as from either drug alone in its full amount, then dose addition exists. The same will hold true if we use one-third of drug A and two-thirds of drug B, one-quarter of drug A and three-quarters of drug B, one-fifth of drug A and four-fifths of drug B. Thus the one moiety of the combined drug does not add its own effects to that of the other moiety, but complements the effect of the latter exactly to the intensity that would be achieved by the sum of the fractional doses if both were fractions of either A or B.

Synergism has been defined as a type of interaction in which the effect of a combination of drugs is greater than the effect of (1) any drug given singly, (2) the combined effects of the drugs, or (3) the effect of the sum of the drugs, i.e., greater than addition as defined in the previous paragraph. The third definition might be called dose synergism, and in keeping with our acceptance of dose addition, I prefer this definition.

The first definition seems to be the most popular in case and clinical reports. The rationale given is that synergism literally means "working together," and any combination that gives a greater effect than either drug alone is synergistic. However, it would seem that if the effect of the combination of two drugs is less than the sum of the effects of the drugs, the drugs are actually working against each other. For example, if two lumberjacks can saw down trees at the rate of ten trees each per day, and if together they can saw down only 12 trees, it would seem that somehow they were working against each other, perhaps by getting in each other's way; the relationship is in fact antagonism.

Potentiation has had several definitions, most of them the same as the definitions given for synergism above. I prefer the following definition: the enhancement of action of one drug by a second drug that has no detectable action of its own.

In its simplest form, the definition of *antagonism* is the opposing action of one drug toward another. When drugs exert opposite physiologic actions, as do nitroprusside and methoxamine, or when an inactive drug diminishes the effect of an active drug (naloxone and a narcotic) the use of the word antagonism, physiologic or pharmacologic, is straightforward. However, when two drugs produce a similar effect, they may still antagonize each other if the combined effect is less than that of the sum of the drugs, as defined by dose addition.

We can thus summarize the aforementioned definitions: additive interaction may be represented by $2 + 2 = 4$; synergism by $2 + 2 = 5$; potentiation by $0 + 2 = 3$; and antagonism by $0 + 2 < 2$, $1 + 2 < 3$, or $2 + 2 < 4$.

The present state of drug-interaction research

Quantifying drug interactions. The quantitation of drug interactions is an interesting part of pharmacology in which one goes beyond the stage of saying that, for example, synergism is present, and tries to determine how much. This area, however, is replete with complex notions, large numbers of curves placed together on the same graph, and difficult mathematic calculations. Research is usually done *in vitro*, or in animals, at best. It is therefore beyond the purview of this book. Suffice it to say that research into the quantitation of drug interaction is still in a rudimentary state, and is rarely useful to the clinician.

The extent of knowledge of interactions among more than two drugs is discouraging. Few studies even semiquantitatively examine the interaction among three agents, and none has attempted more than three. The experiments are very long, and the display of data requires a three-dimensional plot. That the simplest technique requires one dimension for each drug[5] has discouraged most investigators.

Even the qualitative description of multiple-drug interactions can be overwhelming. Thus we were unable to find an author willing to write a chapter on this subject. The problem must be faced, however; the large number of drugs used by anesthesiologists and other physicians mandates it. It is not unusual for the anesthetist to use six to ten drugs per patient, including preanesthetic medication. Preoperatively, a patient may receive more than 40 medications concurrently, many of which are multicomponent preparations![6]

This information on multiple-drug interaction is important. One would intuitively expect that the interaction among quinidine, a nondepolarizing neuromuscular blocking agent, and an antibiotic would be more severe than that between any two of these agents.

The incidence of drug interactions. Still another difficulty in drug-interaction research has been in estimating the incidence of drug interactions in hospitalized patients in general and not just in those particular patients undergoing anesthesia and surgical procedures. Some attempts have been made,[6,10] but the results vary considerably. Problems arise from variations in the strictness of criteria for the incidence and the clinical relevance of a drug interaction, from whether a study was prospective or retrospective, from the attitude of physicians toward filling out "yet another form," and from whether an interaction or just a potential interaction was reported. (A potential interaction means that two or more drugs that *might* cause an interaction are administered to the same patient.)

One attempt to estimate the incidence of drug interactions has been to establish the relationship between the number of drug *reactions* and the total number of drugs given. It is assumed that this relationship should be linear; that is, twice as many drugs should produce twice the incidence of reactions. Thus any greater increase in drug reactions would be partly due to drug interactions. According to Table 1-1, the number of drug reactions does increase out of proportion to the increase in the number of drugs consumed. One could argue, however, that a larger number of drugs taken indicates a more severely ill patient, and that reactions are determined partly by the condition of the patient.

Bringing information to the physician. Of more interest to the practicing physician than the methodology and the rigidity of assessing drug interactions is the accumulation and maintenance of an accurate mass of information about well documented drug interactions, and a method for disseminating this information in a clinically useful way. This is even more difficult than it sounds. The widespread circulation of inaccurate, poorly documented, or clinically irrelevant information has retarded the general acceptance of the medical significance of drug interac-

Table 1-1

Number of Drugs Given	Reaction Rate (%)
0-5	4.2
6-10	7.4
11-15	24.2
16-20	40.0
21+	45.0

(From Smith, J. W., Seidl, L. G., and Cluff, L. E.: Studies on the epidemiology of adverse drug reactions. V. Clinical factors influencing susceptibility. Ann. Intern. Med., 65:629, 1966.)

tions. Although certain examples of enhancement of toxicity or antagonism of beneficial effects resulting from the use of specific drug combinations are widely recognized by physicians, in general the substantial number of potential drug interactions and the pharmacologic complexities involved in many of these interactions have made it impractical for most anesthesiologists to have adequate drug-interaction information available when therapy is prescribed, when the patient is evaluated, or when anesthesia is administered.

There are a few reliable sources of information on drug interactions. None of them emphasizes the interactions of interest to the anesthesiologist, although some do provide information for those wishing to explore the problem further. Hansten has written a book that summarizes a large number of interactions in a convenient and easy-to-read format.[11] The American Pharmaceutical and Medical Associations have sponsored a book that goes into more detail.[12] It includes short treatises on groups of drugs and the interactions within these groups, as well as a number of succinct monographs dealing with individual drug-drug interactions. The National Institutes of Health have published three enormous volumes, which cover all of the drug interactions reported or investigated between 1967 and 1974.[13] These volumes are a valuable resource for the serious student of drug interactions, but they are impossible to carry around on preanesthetic rounds. In contrast to these large books is a small drug interaction "wheel" (Medisc, Excerpta Medica Services). Whereas this pocket-sized device is probably of more interest to internists, and whereas it gives no other information than the possibility of an interaction, it does alert the physician as to when to seek more information.

It would not be surprising, however, if the physician were wary of schemes that claim to specify drug interactions, since the history of drug interaction recounts many false alarms. In the case of the antihypertensive

agents, we have successively believed that reserpine, guanethidine, *alpha*-methyl-dopa, and propranolol are all dangerous drugs to the anesthetized patient, and that they should be discontinued before operation if at all possible. We have repeatedly conveyed this information to our colleagues. It is no wonder if they do not believe us any more. Many patients were denied timely operation because of this belief. The attitude toward various antihypertensive agents has changed several times over the past few years: (1) We now believe that many of the initially reported problems were due not to the drugs but to the disease and the resulting propensity to labile arterial pressures. (2) Current opinion suggests that to withdraw some antihypertensive agents (clonidine or propranolol) can be dangerous or even lethal. (3) Perhaps therapy *should be initiated before anesthesia* in patients with uncontrolled hypertension. (4) Finally some have gone so far as to suggest that a *beta*-adrenergic blocking agent should be given prophylactically before induction of anesthesia in any patient in whom it is desirable to avoid hypertensive episodes.

Another consideration in transmitting drug-interaction information properly to the physician is the classification of drug interactions in a way that can provide guidelines for dealing with the interaction effectively. Although drug interactions are often thought of in absolute terms, they represent only one of many factors influencing the clinical response to drugs. Moreover, most interacting drug combinations *can* be given concurrently if the interacting potential is kept in mind by the physician and proper adjustments in dosage or route of administration are made, as demonstrated in the case of ether and curare.

The Stanford MEDIPHOR system and the report class-designation developed by Cohen et al.[6] provides in a convenient manner both necessary information and useful guidelines. A brief description of this report class-designation follows. In general, Class 1 contains interactions having clinically significant effects that would be expected to occur relatively quickly after administering the drug combination. In this case, the patient's physician is informed about the potential interaction, its implication, and some suggestions on how to deal with it before the first dose of the interacting drug is administered. For example, the interaction between monoamine oxidase inhibitors and certain sympathomimetic amines is included in this class.

Class 2 interactions have consequences that may be less immediate, but nonetheless serious. In this case, the first dose of the interacting drug may be administered, but the physician is contacted before the drug combination is continued as prescribed. The interference with the hypotensive effects of guanethidine when a tricyclic antidepressant is given concurrently is an example of a Class 2 interaction.

Class 3 is assigned to interactions that have well-documented clinical significance, but do not ordinarily lead to clinically apparent consequences until the interacting drug combination has been administered repeatedly. Information about such an interaction is placed in a conspicuous location in the patient's chart, but the drugs are administered as prescribed unless the physician changes his order. The interaction between phenobarbital and coumarin anticoagulants is included in this class.

Class 4 contains interactions that are not sufficiently well documented to warrant distributing reports to physicians, and are used for investigational purposes only.

In every instance, the physician retains the prerogative of making all decisions about administration of the interacting drug combination. The drug-interaction report is viewed simply as an item of information about a factor that may influence the patient's response to a drug and must be considered in the context of other available clinical information.

Perhaps this system could be modified for use in anesthesia. The reader, however, can appreciate the magnitude of the task. Does it require the services of a computer? Probably. The drug file used in the Stanford reporting system contains more than 4,000 pharmaceutical preparations.[6] In the case of multicomponent preparations, entries identify each generic component of the preparation, as well as its interaction class. Thus the computer can search for interactions of drugs included in various brand-name compounds and in other multicomponent preparations. The interaction search, which occurs following entry of a new prescription to the patient's medication record, often requires a substantial amount of computing time (occasionally as long as one to two min) when the patient is receiving many other drugs. The computer must search every new prescription for possible interactions with the components of *each* of the previous medications. The task would be more complex for an anesthesia drug interaction search system, since the computer would have to search for possible interactions among the patient's present medications and the proposed anesthesia or ancillary agents each time the anesthesiologist contemplated using a new agent during the anesthetic course. The system would require information terminals both on the wards for preanesthetic rounds and in the operating rooms.

What to do until the computer comes. Once information on a potential drug interaction has been received by the anesthesiologist, the problem is only partially solved. The physician must then know how to minimize the occurrence of drug interactions. There are many ways to accomplish this, some obvious, others not. In the case of the Stanford computerized system, the task is simplified by an educational printout that accompanies each drug-interaction warning. Until such a service is generally available, we must adhere to the old rules, however.

1. Obtain a careful history from each patient. When inquiring about the drug history, whether prescribed or self-administered, use understandable terms, for example, pain, fever, or flu

reliever for aspirin, or blood pressure tablets for antihypertensive drugs. Do not neglect useful information that can be obtained from a history of experiences with drugs.

2. Restrict the number of drugs to the essential minimum. This advice is easier for the anesthesiologist to give than to take. I am aware that multiple-drug use is part of the practice of many anesthesiologists and, as outlined above, that drug interactions can be made useful, rather than harmful, if carefully controlled. On the other hand, the concept that fewer drugs are associated with fewer drug interactions has considerable merit.

3. If multiple-drug therapy is required, avoid those drugs that are likely to cause serious interactions or make control of therapy difficult. Some drug combinations are best avoided. Certainly, drugs (for example, monoamine oxidase inhibitors) that can cause serious reactions should be avoided wherever possible. Substitute drugs that can be more safely given. For example, with oral coumarin anticoagulants, consider indomethacin for phenylbutazone, paracetamol (acetaminophen) for aspirin, diazepam for a barbiturate sedative, flurazepam or nitrazepam for a barbiturate hypnotic. When muscle relaxants or potent inhalation agents are used, consider vancomycin or oleandomycin for neomycin, streptomycin, or any one of the many antibiotics that can increase the neuromuscular blocking properties of our agents (see Chap. 17). If fixed combination drugs must be used, the components must be known.

4. Always keep in mind genetic factors and associated diseases or patho-physiologic conditions that may facilitate an interaction. Pseudocholinesterase deficiency comes to mind immediately. The combination of this condition plus succinylcholine plus peritoneal lavage with certain antibiotics could be disastrous. As outlined in Chapters 11 and 17, the presence of renal pathology can accentuate many drug interactions.

5. Changes of drug therapy should be kept to a minimum. Again this advice may seem gratuitous to the anesthesiologist, who must by definition change the patient's drug regimen many times in order to administer an anesthetic. However, one must also consider the role of the anesthesiologist outside the operating room in the long-term care of the patient, for example in the intensive-care unit. If changes are necessary and involve known interactions, some change in dose can be anticipated, but the time, course, and extent of interaction varies with the drugs and the individual patient. Any dose adjustment should only be made on the basis of results derived from close observation of therapy over a period of time after the change. This is especially important with oral coumarin anticoagulants.

6. Pay special attention to problem drugs. These include oral coumarin anticoagulants, oral sulfonylurea, hypoglycemics, digitalis, anticonvulsants, antihypertensive drugs, CNS-depressant or antipsychotic drugs, or neuromuscular blocking agents.

7. Educate the patient and the patient's attending physician. This implies that the anesthesiologist must be educated first. Warn them of the possible dangers that may arise with changes, cessations, or alterations in medication, whether prescribed or self-administered.

The future of drug-interaction research

What are the future needs, then, of research into drug interactions, as well as the clinical understanding of their complexities? (1) We need better methods for quantifying drug interactions. These methods should be clinically relevant, and the results should be understandable and made available to clinicians, and not just to an elite few. (2) The complexities of interactions among more than two drugs must be solved. The solutions may require new mathematic and statistical methods, or they may be based on available methods, as we attempted to do in our early work.[5] (3) A system must be developed for recording and evaluating drug interactions on a prospective basis. A multihospital cooperative study may be necessary, as is done so well in the Veterans Administration Hospitals. (4) Current information should be available to the physician immediately. Thus any drug-interaction warning system, such as that developed at Stanford, should include a mechanism for a continual updating of the information in its files—with all the complexities that this implies. (5) One set of information could give the probability of a clinically important interaction if two or more drugs are given. The physician, after all, considers various probabilities when making diagnostic and therapeutic decisions.

What is the clinician's responsibility in this problem? The anesthesiologist not only must be well informed about drug interactions, but also must be alert for them, both on preanesthetic rounds and each time a drug is administered in the operating or recovery room. This is not possible unless the proper information is supplied. The research scientist can determine whether the information is clinically useful only by observing and by receiving feedback from the clinician on how it is used, the ease with which it is used, and its comprehensibility.

In summary, we have presented a philosophy of drug interactions as seen from the anesthesiologist's viewpoint. We have shown that some drug interactions can be very hazardous, some can be useful, and others can be useful only if manipulated properly. To avoid troublesome interactions and to take advantage of useful ones properly requires extensive knowledge. Unfortunately, the progress of research into drug interactions and the rate of transfer of knowledge to the clinician is still slow. We need more help in discriminating between relevant and irrelevant interactions, and in gaining access to already accumulated knowledge. Computerized systems for detection of drug interactions may be needed, as well as a system for the continual education of the physician.

REFERENCES

1. Levy, A. G.: Sudden death under light chloroform anaesthesia. J. Physiol., *42*:III, 1911.
2. Levy, A. G.: Chloroform Anaesthesia. London, John Bole & Sons & Danielsson, 1922.
3. Beecher, H. K., and Todd, D. P.: A Study of Deaths Associated with Anesthesia and Surgery. Springfield, Ill., Charles C Thomas, 1954.
4. Bonica, J. J., et al.: Circulatory effects of peridural block: II. Effects of epinephrine. Anesthesiology, *34*:514, 1971.
5. Gershwin, M. E., and Smith, N. Ty: Interaction between drugs using three-dimensional isobolographic interpretation. Arch. Int. Pharmacodyn. Ther., *201*:154, 1973.
6. Cohen, S. N., et al.: A computer-based system for the study and control of drug interactions in hospitalized patients. *In* Drug Interactions. Edited by P. L. Morselli, S. Garattini, and S. N. Cohen. New York, Raven Press Brooks, Ltd., 1974.
7. Borda, L. T., Slone, D., and Jick, H.: Assessment of adverse reactions within a drug surveillance program. J.A.M.A., *205*:645, 1968.
8. Ogilvie, R. I., and Ruedy, J.: Adverse reactions during hospitalization. Can. Med. Assoc. J., *97*:1445, 1967.
9. Seidl, L.G., et al.: Studies on the epidemiology of adverse drug reactions. Bull. Johns Hopkins Hosp., *119*:299, 1966.
10. Stewart, R.B., and Cluff, L. E.: Studies on the epidemiology of adverse drug reactions VI: Utilization and interactions of prescription and nonprescription drugs in outpatients. Johns Hopkins Med. J., *129*:319, 1971.
11. Hansten, P. D.: Drug Interactions. Third Edition. Philadelphia, Lea & Febiger, 1975.
12. Ascione, F.J.: Evaluations of Drug Interactions. Second Edition. Washington, D.C., American Pharmaceutical Association, 1976.
13. Drug Interactions: an annotated bibliography with selected excerpts, 1967–1970. Vol. 1, 1972, HEW publication no. (NIH) 73–322; Vol. 2, 1974, (NIH) 75–322; Vol. 3, 1975, (NIH) 76–3004.

Chapter **2**

Mechanisms:
General Principles

WERNER E. FLACKE
and
JOAN W. FLACKE

Modern anesthesia is based on planned use of the effects and interactions of several, sometimes multiple, drugs. This is a significant departure from earlier times, when a single, ''complete'' anesthetic agent was employed to bring about the conditions required for the conduct of surgical and other diagnostic and therapeutic procedures. Of the several reasons for this change, the first is the recognition that clinical anesthesia combines several different conditions: analgesia, loss of consciousness and memory, skeletal muscle relaxation, and autonomic, especially cardiovascular, stability in the face of major stresses. Next is the increasing realization that general anesthetics are toxic. Finally, the introduction of so-called adjuvant drugs has made it possible to achieve several of the foregoing components of anesthesia by means other than the use of classic general anesthetic agents. Not only can muscle relaxation be produced by intravenous injection of neuromuscular blocking drugs, but almost any degree of analgesia can be achieved by large doses of potent analgesics. We are even beginning to see efforts to bring about clouding of consciousness and inhibition of memory formation by drugs other than general anesthetics.

Although each adjuvant drug needed to produce a part of the total syndrome of clinical anesthesia has its own drawbacks, the disadvantages of single-agent anesthesia are such that the proponents of that practice have all but disappeared. Indeed, a return to it is unlikely unless new agents with properties that would increase their safety considerably become available.

11

These continuing developments place a much greater burden on the anesthesiologist to understand drug interactions. It is not our purpose here to reexamine well-established practices. Although we shall discuss general principles of drug interaction that have a bearing on present-day anesthesia, we wish to focus mainly on unintentional interactions whose mechanisms are often controversial and obscure.

The clinical significance of many drug interactions is often undetermined, and few of the questions posed have been answered definitively.[1,2] For example, the answer to the question whether to discontinue antihypertensive medication before anesthesia and operation was not presumable, but required observation and careful comparative evaluation.[3-5] This answer remains to be documented for the newer antihypertensive agents. The important issue of the optimal use of *beta*-adrenergic antagonists during anesthesia is still unresolved and is the subject of debate.[6] Even such long-established practices as the use of anticholinergic agents in anesthesia are not universally decided.[6a] More careful work is needed to settle these and other questions. This is one reason for including in this chapter not only interactions of unquestioned significance but also those of unknown importance.

There are certain general difficulties and limitations in the discussion of drug interactions. First we have to *recognize* when the effects of a drug are altered by one or several other drugs, that is, whether or not an interaction has taken place. Frequently, finding the answer is not as easy as may appear at first.

Normal variability

Drug responses, like other biological variables, can only be described statistically. Ideally, a drug response centers on a mean with a normal distribution. This is true for both "normal" and "abnormal" responses. A difference is statistically significant only when the mean responses of two compara-

ble groups differ by more than twice the standard error. One must constantly be careful not to be misled by random variations within the norm.[7-9]

Strictly speaking, a drug interaction must be described in statistical terms before it can be accepted as scientifically proven. Often, however, a statistical description is not available in anesthesia, at least not initially. This is the rationale for case reports, which serve to alert the profession and perhaps to solicit confirmations or denials of such observations.

Other factors affecting drug responses

Apart from this "normal biologic variation," many factors that may affect a drug response are potentially recognizable. Perhaps the most important factor is the influence of *underlying disease*. (This is the first question one asks in the face of a possibly altered response. A definite answer is often impossible.) We also know that internal and external *environmental factors* may alter drug responses. For example, the effect of halothane on body temperature depends greatly on room temperature and humidity. Circadian rhythms, seasonal variations, climate, and diet may alter drug responses, but the clinical significance of these factors in anesthesia is unknown. The importance of *genetic factors* has been appreciated by anesthesiologists for some time, particularly in connection with abnormal pseudocholinesterase and the response to succinylcholine, with porphyria, hemoglobinopathies, and malignant hyperpyrexia.[10-13] Although the incidence of each such abnormality is low, the list of recognized genetic factors is growing steadily.

Special aspects of drug interaction in anesthesia

The anesthesiologist's role in medicine is unique because he or she:

(a) predominantly uses rapidly acting drugs;

(b) measures, often very precisely, the response to the drugs administered;

(c) frequently relies on drug antagonism; and

(d) is accustomed to titrating the dose or concentration of a drug.

Individual titration of dose according to the response obtained is important in administering potent drugs with steep dose-response relationships. Unless the variability of the response to a given dose is minimal, titration is the only safe method for dealing with such drugs.

In anesthesia, interactions that result in a minor increase or decrease in responses are of little consequence and are dealt with routinely. The value of understanding and anticipating drug interactions for the anesthesiologist often lies in that this knowledge permits anticipation of the altered response.

Some examples of drug interactions can be found in the Case Reports at the end of this chapter.

TYPES OF DRUG INTERACTIONS

Drug interactions can be divided into three major categories: *in vitro* incompatibilities, physical or chemical, sometimes also called pharmaceutic interactions; interactions resulting from pharmacokinetic factors; and pharmacodynamic interactions.

This categorization is useful for organizing material but does not claim to reflect clinical reality. Actually, some interactions involve all three categories at once, for example, in the case of neuroleptic agents (phenothiazines and butyrophenones). Their antipsychotic effects seem to be related to their ability to block dopamine and/or norepinephrine receptors, and perhaps muscarinic cholinoceptive, histamine, and 5-hydroxytryptamine receptors. They possess local anesthetic activity, and their clinical effects may include sedation or mild stimulation, in addition to the desired antipsychotic effects. These agents also can induce extrapyramidal effects, cholestatic jaundice, dermatitis (both by a photosensi-

tive and an allergic mechanism), and blood dyscrasias. They may depress hepatic metabolism and act as inducers of hepatic microsomal enzymes. They inhibit the amine pump and thus reduce uptake of norepinephrine into adrenergic neurons as well as uptake of drugs that are substrates for the same transport mechanism. Neuroleptic drugs are bound to plasma proteins and may compete there for binding sites with other drugs. Thus these agents possess an enormous potential for interactions that involve every type of known pharmacokinetic and pharmacodynamic mechanism. Obviously, under these circumstances the analysis of a given interaction is difficult or sometimes impossible; nevertheless, an attempt to dissect the mechanisms is essential for prediction and prevention of other pharmacologic hazards. Fortunately, few other drugs are as prone to interaction as the antipsychotic agents.

In vitro incompatibilities

This type of interaction occurs before a drug is absorbed systemically or administered parenterally.[14,15] It includes interactions between drugs in solution as well as in the gastrointestinal tract prior to absorption. The anesthesiologist is concerned with both problems. Premedication is often given by mouth. The most potent drugs used in anesthesia are administered intravenously, often into an infusion line along with drugs that are not inherent to the anesthetic procedure, for example, antibiotics. One should never mix any drugs unless one is absolutely sure that no undesirable interaction can occur. In view of the long list of incompatibilities, it is sound policy to refer to the hospital pharmacist for this type of information. It must also be noted that the same generic drug may be formulated in different ways by different manufacturers, and that its formulation may affect compatibility with other agents. Table 2–1 is an example of the incompatibilities of a number of antibiotic agents frequently given by infusion.

Table 2–1

Incompatibilities of some antibiotics in infusion solutions

Drug	Incompatible with:	Drug	Incompatible with:
Amphotericin B	Penicillin G Tetracyclines Diphenhydramine	Erythromycin gluceptate	Cephalothin Chloramphenicol Colistimethate Tetracyclines Aminophylline Barbiturates Phenytoin Heparin Vitamin B
Cephalothin (Keflin)	Chloramphenicol Erythromycin Kanamycin Polymyxin B Tetracyclines Vancomycin Aminophylline Barbiturates Calcium salts Phenytoin Heparin Norepinephrine Phenothiazines	Kanamycin sulfate	Cephalothin Methicillin Barbiturates Calcium gluconate Phenytoin Heparin
Chloramphenicol	Cephalothin Erythromycin Polymixin B Tetracyclines Vancomycin Aminophylline Barbiturates Diphenhydramine Phenytoin Hydrocortisone	Penicillin G	Amphotericin B Lincomycin Chlorpheniramine Chlorpromazine Dexamethasone Phenytoin Ephedrine Heparin Metaraminol Phenylephrine
Colistimethate	Cephalothin Erythromycin Hydrocortisone		

Drugs compounded in tablet and capsule form may interact after oral administration.[16,17] Chelation and inactivation of tetracyclines by antacids containing polyvalent cations, such as Ca^{++}, Mg^{++}, or Al^{+++} are a typical case. Agents such as kaolin, pectins, charcoal, or hydrated aluminum silicate, which are used in the treatment of diarrhea because of their adsorbent properties, will also adsorb and inactivate many drugs and thus prevent their systemic uptake.[18] Cholestyramine interferes with absorption of warfarin, digitoxin, thyroid preparations, and thiazide diuretics.[19] The effect of changes in pH on the gastrointestinal absorption of aspirin is known even to television viewers. Drugs that affect gastrointestinal motility such as narcotic analgesic and anticholinergic drugs can modify or delay the absorption of orally administered preparations.[20–22]

Pharmacokinetic interactions

A good definition of pharmacokinetics is: "everything that happens to the drug in the organism." (Pharmacodynamics, on the other hand, is: "everything the drug does to the organism.") Thus pharmacokinetics includes processes of drug absorption (unless the drug is injected directly into the bloodstream), distribution, including the influence of plasma protein binding, and elimination, by excretion through the bile or kidney or by metabolic inactivation.

Hemodynamic conditions. Since the intravenous route provides the fastest and most direct access to sites of drug action, it is essentially the only route used during anesthesia. The onset and duration of action of most drugs administered intravenously are more profoundly affected by distribution processes than by excretion and metabolism.[23] Intravenous induction agents like thiopental and thiamylal are typical examples. The concentration of the drug leaving the heart is a function of the rate of injection and the volume into which the drug is injected, that is, the venous return over the period of injection. The rate of delivery to the tissues is determined by the concentration in the arterial blood and the tissue blood flow. Any drug that affects either cardiac output or flow distribution will affect the rate of drug delivery and the total amount delivered, especially to the brain and the myocardium, the two organs most closely involved both in the anesthesia desired and in the most serious potential adverse effect, myocardial depression. For a given rate of injection, the concentration of a drug in the arterial blood is a function of cardiac output. Although this is rarely determined before induction, one can make an educated guess as to the cardiovascular status of the patient and the likely changes that may be produced by the drug injected. For example, if thiopental is given to a patient with low cardiac output, a ''normal'' rate of injection will result in the delivery of a higher-than-normal drug concentration to the brain and the myocardium, where most of the output is being distributed. There, the high concentration may further compromise cardiac function, if the low output is secondary to reduced cardiac competence. Another example is propranolol, or any other *beta*-adrenergic antagonist. In doses that are now used intravenously in anesthesia, propranolol acts entirely by attenuating or blocking adrenergic influences on the heart, influences either neurogenic or resulting from circulating catecholamines. Such deprivation does not affect the output of a heart with normal contractility, which is capable of accommodating venous return without adrenergic support. It may, however, decrease the output of a marginally competent heart dependent on neurogenic support to maintain output. It also reduces output elevated by abnormal sympathetic activity secondary to, for example, anxiety or pain. Of course, propranolol will blunt the normal sympathetic reflex response to any drug-induced decrease in cardiac output and blood pressure.

With inhalation anesthetic agents, the rate of rise of the anesthetic's concentration in the alveolar gas and the cardiac output (or pulmonary flow) are the important parameters for rate of uptake. The relative importance of these two processes with agents of low and high blood-gas solubility coefficients are too well known to be reviewed here.[24] It should be noted, however, that the processes can be influenced by prior drug therapy and preanesthetic medication, as discussed in the examples concerning cardiac output. Bronchodilator drugs decrease airway resistance and may improve the ventilation/perfusion ratio in patients with obstructive disease and hence accelerate the mean rate of rise of the anesthetic's concentration in the alveolar gas. The opposite occurs with drugs that cause an increase in airway resistance. The most common example of the latter may again be propranolol, which permits unopposed bronchoconstriction by blocking the bronchodilator effect of sympathetic innervation mediated by *beta*-adrenergic receptors.

The retarding effect of epinephrine on the rate of absorption of local anesthetics exemplifies the general rule that perfusion determines the rate of absorption and mobilization of any drug from its tissue depot when other factors are equal.[25] The influence, however, of systemic changes in cardiovascular function on drug absorption after local administration is not as familiar. Such changes may be dramatic after intramuscular or subcutaneous administration of certain drugs to patients in shock or impending shock. In these cases, correction of cardiovascular failure leads to an improvement of tissue blood flow and mobilization of a previously stagnant tissue drug depot. Rebound respiratory depression from excessive morphine injected intramuscularly under combat conditions is well known; equally instructive are cases of subcutaneous epinephrine overdosage during acute circulatory failure. These problems are avoided by the IV route.

Protein binding. Displacement from plasma protein binding of one drug by another is an important possible cause of drug interaction.[26] However, most examples of clinical significance have involved long-acting drugs. Perhaps the most debated example is the displacement of warfarin by phenylbutazone with an increase in free warfarin concentration and consequent slow increase in clotting time.[27] Although the importance of this example for anesthesiologists is limited, many drugs used in anesthesia have steep dose-response curves, are given in near-toxic doses, and are highly protein bound. Hence the potential for this type of interaction in anesthesia is strong. Displacement of quinidine and of phenytoin (diphenylhydantoin) has been reported and could represent an example of this type of interaction. The high protein binding of propranolol and its potential as a cause of myocardial depression makes this drug another candidate for displacement with harmful consequences.[19a] Unfortunately, no documentation for such consequences has been presented, probably because the situation in clinical anesthesia is so complex that the distinction of possible causes is difficult. Wardell has listed the requirements for demonstrating a displacement reaction:[28]

(a) *in vitro* demonstration of displacement,
(b) demonstration of displacement *in vivo,*
(c) demonstration that the time course of the toxic symptoms parallels the rise and subsequent fall in free drug concentrations, and
(d) elimination of other possible causes for the symptoms.

In anesthesiology one must also consider protein binding in connection with other circumstances. Plasma protein and drug concentrations may change massively and quickly during infusion of crystalloid solutions or infusion of whole blood and plasma preparations. Thus the concentration of free, that is, pharmacologically active, drug may change as the binding percentage rises and falls. This is likely to be of practical importance only with potent drugs that are highly protein bound.

Biotransformation. The majority of metabolic transformations of drugs occurs in the liver. Since these processes will be reviewed in Chapter 3, only a few general points will be made here.

Both inhibition and stimulation of metabolism of one drug by another can occur. The first is due to the acute interaction of two drugs competing for the same metabolic pathway; the second may be the consequence of previous prolonged administration of a drug followed by enzyme induction. Although the usual result of metabolization of a drug is detoxification, that is, inactivation and increased renal excretion, there are also examples of the transformation of a drug to a more active form, for example, parathion, chloral hydrate, and cyclophosphamide. In anesthesia, metabolism is important in the formation of toxic metabolites. Hepatic metabolism may be influenced also by changes in liver blood flow produced by another drug.[23,36]

Some drugs are not metabolized in the liver. The best-known example in anesthesia is, of course, the hydrolysis of succinyldicholine by plasma cholinesterase. Clinical doses of anticholinesterase drugs prolong the effect of the muscle relaxant.[29] Inadvertent inhibition of cholinesterases is probably most common today as the result of exposure to organophosphates used as pesticides. Fortunately, clinical signs of plasma cholinesterase inhibition are seen only when enzyme activity is severely depressed.[29]

Another important example of extrahepatic enzyme inhibition is the inhibitors of monoamine oxidases (known as MAO inhibitors or MAOI). These drugs were widely used in the treatment of depressive disorders but fortunately they have been largely displaced by tricyclic antidepressants. MAO are widely distributed, especially in adrenergic nerve terminals, and metabolize monoamines like norepinephrine, dopamine, and 5-hydroxytryptamine. Because the main mechanism for termination of norepinephrine is reuptake into the nerve ending, MAOI do not prolong the effect of exogenously administered norepinephrine. However, the effect of indirectly acting sympathomimetics, of which tyramine is the prototype, is greatly potentiated, especially if the sympathomimetics themselves are substrates for MAO. This is the basis of the well-known "cheese reaction" elicited by foodstuffs containing tyramine.[30,31] For the anesthesiologist it is more important to know that sympathomimetics such as phenylephrine and dopamine are potentiated in patients on MAOI.[32,33]

Another significant effect of these drugs is the potentiation and alteration of the effect of meperidine.[34] The exact mechanism of the interaction is not clear, although inhibition of N-dimethylation by MAOI has been demonstrated.[35] However, the effect of meperidine is not simply increased and prolonged; it is altered in character. This may be because MAOI are not specific for MAO alone, and their administration results in an increase in brain monoamines other than norepinephrine.[34] The interaction of different monoamines in the CNS (central nervous system) is far from fully understood.

Renal excretion. Renal excretion is the route of elimination for drugs metabolized either slowly or not at all. The kidneys also excrete the products of drug metabolism after they have become polar or water soluble, hence more suitable for renal excretion. Because the role of the kidney is discussed in more detail in Chapter 11, we outline here some general principles only.

Renal excretion proceeds by: (1) glomerular filtration (passive), with and without reabsorption, and (2) active tubular secretion. Substances filtered but not reabsorbed are those unable to cross cell-membrane barriers. Such polar substances, for example, quaternary ammonium compounds, are restricted to the extracellular space, and permeate the gastrointestinal-tract mucosa or the blood-brain barrier poorly, if at all. Therefore, the calculation of their excretion rate is a simple matter. The extracellular volume is cleared by glomerular filtration. In the normal case the glomerular filtration volume per minute is about one-one hundredth of the extracellular volume, so the extracellular fluid should be cleared in about 100 minutes. Since the process is not linear but exponential, the half-time of excretion is not 50 but about 70 minutes.

Other approximations follow from this basic premise. Tubular secretion, clearing total renal plasma flow, is about five times the glomerular filtration rate; hence a drug restricted to the extracellular space but secreted by the kidney has a half-time of one-fifth of the above, that is, about 14 minutes.

Conversely, a highly lipid soluble drug (not metabolized) that crosses all membranes easily would be distributed in the total body water at least and be fully reabsorbed in the tubules. Thus its concentration in the final urine is only equal to that in the plasma, which is equal to that in the total body water. The half-time of excretion is about 20 days. If, as expected, the drug is also bound to tissue macromolecules or dissolved in body fats, its virtual volume of distribution can be many times the total body water volume and excretion would be accordingly prolonged. Such drugs cannot be excreted unless they are metabolized to a more polar derivative.

These examples define the periods of time involved and give an approximation of the orders of magnitude of renal excretion for different drugs. Drugs secreted by the tubules and nonlipid-soluble (polar) drugs are subject to modification of excretion by other drugs within the perioperative period.

In order to predict renal handling of a drug, it is necessary to know its physicochemical properties and its metabolic fate. Unfortunately, this information is not easily available. With it one can make useful predictions of the changes in renal excretion that will result from administration of other drugs that may produce changes in renal blood flow and filtration rate.[36] In drugs actively secreted, one must also consider interactions resulting from competition for the secretory process. However, the number of those interactions is small, and such information should be provided routinely by manufacturers.

The case of partially ionized weak acids and weak bases and the influence of the pH of urine on their excretion is often discussed, but its importance is limited because most of these drugs are metabolized in the liver.[37] (See Chap. 4).

Pharmacodynamic interactions

These are the most important from an anesthesiologic standpoint. Since drug selectivity is never absolute, and since every drug usually produces several effects, the variety of possible interactions almost defies organization. Any attempt to categorize must remain artificial and simplistic. The effect of a given combination should never be ascribed to a single type of interaction, unless there is solid evidence for excluding multiple mechanisms.

It is best to use different methods of organization that overlap and are not mutually exclusive. Even so, there are cases that cannot be definitively grouped, because of our limited understanding of the exact mechanism of action of drugs. Categorization only helps to improve our thinking about general principles, which, in turn, may help to anticipate unknown and prospective interactions.

It is generally accepted that many drugs exert their effects by combining with specific "receptors." Hence we can distinguish among drug interactions at the same receptor, drug interactions involving different receptors, and drug interactions not mediated by receptors.

Drugs acting on the same receptor. It is becoming clearer that pharmacologic receptors, i.e., molecular structures of high specificity, exist only for agents that occur physiologically, that is, neurotransmitters and hormones: acetylcholine (ACh), norepinephrine (NE), epinephrine (EPI), dopamine, 5-hydroxytryptamine, histamine, endorphins/enkephalins, angiotensin, pituitary hormones, corticosteroids, for example. Only drugs that in chemical structure sufficiently resemble these physiologic agents can be expected to interact specifically with these receptors. Yet the number of these drugs is large, both agonists and antagonists: it includes analogs of acetylcholine such as carbachol or succinylcholine, sympathomimetics, morphine and related agents, and analogs of corticosteroids and of sex hormones. There is also the long list of drugs that do not mimic but block the effects of physiologically occurring agonists: atropine, curare-like agents, hexamethonium, *beta*-adrenergic antagonists, *alpha*-adrenergic antagonists, naloxone, aldosterone antagonists, and antiestrogens, for example.

Drugs interacting with the same receptor can only elicit or block the same effects as the normal physiologic agonist, albeit of different magnitude and duration. However, a given receptor may activate different effector systems: for example, ACh relaxes smooth muscle in the vascular bed but constricts airway and gastrointestinal smooth muscle. It depolarizes the end-plate of skeletal muscle and of ganglionic and CNS postsynaptic membranes; it slows the rate of cardiac pacemakers and the rate of atrioventricular conduction. Nature uses the same neurotransmitter because it has developed "delivery systems" that permit exquisite localization. Unfortunately, we have developed nothing like it, and in our crude hands receptor-specific agonists and antagonists produce a variety of effects. Thus atropine, given intravenously, will block all muscarinic cholinergic receptors wherever they are located. In addition to preventing bradycardia and conduction block, it may cause urinary retention and precipitate glaucoma. Furthermore, atropine is not alone in causing this type of effect. Many other drugs that are not used primarily for the purpose of blocking muscarinic receptors, such as antihistaminics, tricyclic antidepressants, some phenothiazines, benzodiazepines, pancuronium, gallamine, and meperidine have properties similar to those of atropine. In a whole organism, or patient, many possibilities for drug interaction with agents of this type exist, even though we would like to think of such drugs as "receptor-specific."

As previously mentioned, interaction with a receptor may result in activation or block, i.e., *agonistic* or *antagonistic* activity. In principle, receptor-active compounds have two properties: *affinity* for the receptor and *intrinsic activity* (or *efficacy*) once the drug-receptor complex has been formed.[38,39] Affinity determines the potency of the drug; intrinsic activity can vary between maximal and zero. If a compound has sufficient affinity but no intrinsic activity it is an antagonist. With intermediate levels of intrinsic activity, compounds are partial agonists; in the presence of a full agonist, such compounds behave as partial antagonists.[40,41]

Paton has proposed a hypothesis that accounts for the differences in efficacy or intrinsic activity of drugs.[42,43] Though the hypothesis lacks proof, it deserves discussion, because it provides some intuitive framework for phenomena whose relation is not easily seen. Paton postulates that the magnitude of the drug response is related not to the concentration of the existing drug-receptor complexes (occupation theory) but to the rate of formation of complexes (rate theory). When the rate of drug-receptor interaction is sufficiently high, the drug elicits a response, that is, it is an agonist. When the rate is low, no response occurs, and the drug is an antagonist. Partial agonists show an intermediate behavior.

The hypothesis accounts for some well-known facts: the onset of action of agonists is faster than that of antagonists, for example, the response to ACh as opposed to the response to atropine, or the response to succinylcholine as opposed to that to curare-like agents. The difference between agonistic and antagonistic activity becomes a quantitative rather than a qualitative difference. Thus some compounds that are typical antagonists may behave like partial agonists under some conditions and in some tissues: this may account for the agonist activity of atropine, slowing heart rate and conduction and producing vasodilation in certain skin areas (atropine blush).

In accordance with Paton's rate theory, antagonists dissociate from the receptor much more slowly than do agonists, as witnessed in every-day experience. The action of curare-like agents lasts longer than the action of depolarizing neuromuscular blocking agents; propranolol has a longer action than NE; the actions of atropine are prolonged (hours to days), whereas ACh is evanescent (even if its rapid destruction is prevented).

Surmountable and nonsurmountable antagonists. The rate theory reduces the difference between agonist and antagonist drugs to the difference in their rate of association (and dissociation) with the receptor; hence the difference between surmountable and nonsurmountable drugs may also be viewed as an expression of the actions of time constants. An antagonist is considered surmountable if its rate of dissociation from the receptor during the presence of an agonist is sufficiently fast that equilibration between the two occurs during the presence of the agonist. However, several typical surmountable antagonists may behave as though nonsurmountable when they are tested in sufficiently high concentrations against agonists released by nerve activity.[44] For example, propranolol will cause a parallel shift to the right of the dose-response curve of an adrenergic agonist (for instance, NE) when the agonist is given by continuous infusion (or present in the bath fluid in an *in vitro* experiment). However, if the same agonistic response is produced by nerve stimulation, that is, by NE released from the nerve terminal, the antagonism appears nonsurmountable (Fig. 2–1). Presumably, the nerve is not capable of releasing the con-

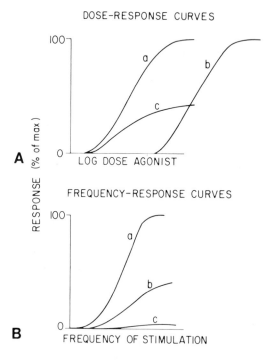

Fig. 2–1. *A*, Curve a is a typical dose-response curve to an agonist drug. Curve b shows the response to the same agonist in the presence of a surmountable, competitive antagonist. Curve c shows the response to the same agonist in the presence of a nonsurmountable antagonist. This example depicts the situation that occurs when there is complete equilibrium between the agonist and the antagonist molecules competing for the receptor. When the antagonist is surmountable and competitive, the maximum response (curve b) depends only on the ratio of agonist/antagonist and the agonist concentration can be increased at will by the experimenter. A nonsurmountable antagonist reduces the number of receptors available regardless of the concentration of agonist present, i.e., the maximum response is reduced (curve c).
B, Curve a describes the response to increasing frequency of nerve stimulation under control conditions. Even in the presence of a surmountable antagonist the maximal response is decreased (curves b and c). In this situation the concentration of agonist available cannot be increased at will, but depends on the ability of the nerve endings to release transmitter. Since this capacity is limited, the response will decrease above a certain concentration of antagonist, although the antagonist is surmountable in principle.

centration of the transmitter needed to restore the equilibrium in favor of the agonist (transmitter) when the antagonist concentration exceeds a certain limit. Functionally, when the agonist is a nerve-derived transmitter, a "surmountable" antagonist may produce a "nonsurmountable" block. The frequency-response curve shift is skewed rather than parallel, and the ceiling of the response is decreased. The antagonist ultimately can produce a complete nerve-effector block, that is, a pharmacologic denervation. This occurs with propranolol and may occur with atropine, although the doses of atropine used clinically are not sufficient to cause this type of block.

True *nonsurmountable antagonists* are characterized by a very slow rate of dissociation or none at all. This is the case with phenoxybenzamine and Dibenamine (*alpha*-adrenergic antagonists) for which no significant reversal of the drug-receptor bond occurs during the lifetime of the receptor.[45] This means that a response can be elicited again only after the regeneration of the receptor, that is, after two or three weeks. With this type of drug the rate of administration is unimportant, as long as successive doses are given while the effect of the previous dose is still present. The drugs are highly cumulative. Other examples of this irreversible type of antagonism are the organophosphate anticholinesterases and the monoamine oxidase inhibitors discussed previously. Echothiophate and isoflurophate are the only anticholinesterase organophosphates used clinically (as miotics), but exposure to insecticide organophosphates is common, especially among agricultural workers.

Drugs acting on different receptors. Drugs may act on different receptors to produce the same or opposing effects. The receptors may be located on the same or on different cells in the same organ or in different organs or systems, but they must affect the same function.

Drugs acting on different receptors and exerting the same effect are said to be *addi-*

tive. (The terminology is often confusing, because the terms addition, summation, synergism, potentiation do not always have the same meaning [See Chap. 1].) What is important about such a drug interaction is that different drugs that share the same type of desired activity may possess different toxic properties. In this case the desired effects will be additive, whereas the toxic effects, one hopes, would not.

If one drug exerts no effect by itself but increases the effect of another drug, the interaction is called *potentiation*. An example of this type is the effect of cocaine and cocaine-like drugs in potentiating the effects of NE. Cocaine inhibits uptake of NE into adrenergic nerve terminals, the major mechanism of dissipation of free NE, and thus increases and prolongs the NE concentration near the receptor sites. When cocaine is given to a patient, its effect depends upon the presence or absence of free NE.

In the case of drugs that exert opposite effects, the result of the interaction is *antagonism*. In contrast to the *pharmacologic antagonism* (on the same receptor) previously described, this type of antagonism is usually called *"functional"* or *"physiologic" antagonism*.[47] The latter is thus named because all physiologically occurring antagonisms are of this type. This applies to the well-known antagonism between sympathetic and parasympathetic innervation (or of sympathomimetic and parasympathomimetic drugs) in the heart, in the airways, and in the gastrointestinal tract, as well as to the antagonism between two nerve endings impinging on the same postsynaptic membrane (called in this case "postsynaptic inhibition"). Nature does not seem to have developed the idea of a pharmacologic interaction, although there is no *a priori* reason why this should be so.

Clinical examples of functional antagonism are few. One example is the case in which histamine and other vasodilator agents are released during an anaphylactic reaction or by a histamine releasing agent

and are "antagonized" by epinephrine or another vasoconstrictor. In this case, the antagonism is not between the drug causing the anaphylactic reaction (or the histamine release) and the vasoconstrictor directly, but between the released vasodilators and the constrictor.

More common and more important is the situation in which a drug or several drugs influence an existing physiologic antagonism, for example, when atropine or propranolol are used to influence heart rate or impulse conduction. In this case, the effect of the antagonist is not only a function of its dose (or rate of administration) but also of the magnitude of the existing tone of sympathetic or parasympathetic nerve activity, as well as of the magnitude of the physiologically opposing innervation. For example, the increase in heart rate after a given dose of atropine differs depending on the type of anesthesia, because sympathetic cardiac tone is variably affected by general anesthesia (and also by other conditions, such as surgical stimulation).

If both atropine and propranolol are used, the effect of the first will influence that of the second. Atropine tachycardia is not as marked in a patient treated with propranolol or other *beta* blockers. Patients treated with a *beta* blocker or a reserpine-type drug are more likely to develop reflex bronchospasm in response to mechanical stimulation or after anticholinesterase administration.[48] In this case, the existence of a physiologic sympathetic bronchodilator tone was initially realized only after the introduction of *beta*-adrenergic drugs.

Recently, the function of sympathetic nerves has been found to be regulated by a peripheral negative feedback mechanism involving *alpha* receptors, and, perhaps, by muscarinic receptors and interaction with parasympathetic nerves.[49-51] Administration of an *alpha*-adrenergic antagonist increases the release of norepinephrine and the effect of sympathetic nerve activity. Under normal conditions the transmitter, NE, may exert an inhibitory effect on its own release (negative feedback). Thus, the tachycardia seen after phentolamine is due not only to the activation of baroreceptor reflexes and to an intrinsic positive chronotropic effect of the drug, but also to the increased release of NE resulting from the block of *alpha* receptors in the adrenergic terminal. Atropine also increases the release of NE, and some of the effects of atropine on the heart may be caused by increased sympathetic transmitter release.[52] Of course, this interaction occurs only where sympathetic and parasympathetic nerves are present simultaneously, such as in the heart.

Interactions at different receptors occur following inhibition of the amine pump that transports NE back into adrenergic nerve terminals. Cocaine produces its cardiovascular toxicity by this mechanism, as do the tricyclic antidepressants.[53,54] This type of drug action results in potentiation of NE, and to a lesser extent EPI. (Isoproterenol is not taken up into adrenergic neurons and thus is not potentiated.) NE may be administered externally or released endogenously. Cocaine toxicity is the subject of the first case report in this chapter.

A consequence of the cocaine-like action of tricyclic antidepressants is their antagonism to antihypertensive agents of the adrenergic neuron-blocking type such as reserpine, guanethidine, and bethanidine. These drugs are substrates of the amine pump and exert their blocking effect on the adrenergic neuron after being concentrated in adrenergic nerve endings. The administration of tricyclic antidepressant results in loss of blood-pressure control by adrenergic neuron-blocking drugs.[55,56]

Recently, tricyclic antidepressants were found to jeopardize blood-pressure control in patients treated with clonidine.[57] The mechanism has not been elucidated, but it is possible that the increased level of free norepinephrine that results from the action of the antidepressants antagonizes the effect of clonidine on central *alpha* receptors, where clonidine is thought to exert its antihypertensive effect.

Drug interactions not mediated by pharmacologic receptors. The main drugs used in anesthesia, general and local anesthetic agents, do not act on specific receptors but produce their effects by physicochemical interactions and cause conformational changes of biologic macromolecules, proteins, and lipids, especially those in excitable membranes. This has now been demonstrated directly,[58-62] but the lack of receptor-specificity had been postulated long ago, because there are no specific structural requirements for anesthetic activity and no pharmacologic antagonists. In fact, physicochemical rather than chemical properties provide the best correlation with anesthetic potency, for example, lipid solubility.[62]

Because of this, the effects of general anesthetics are roughly additive. Moreover, the effects of drugs used for premedication are additive with general anesthetics. The addition of nitrous oxide reduces the anesthetic concentration of halothane and other inhalation agents required to achieve MAC (minimum alveolar concentration),[63,64] but the toxic dose is also lowered. Hence there is no significant increase in the therapeutic index (lethal dose 50/therapeutic dose 50).[65,66] The use of premedication, such as barbiturates and benzodiazepines, also reduces the required concentration of the general anesthetic, but in these cases the therapeutic index has not been determined.[67] Although the "sparing" effect of narcotic analgesics is clear, their effect on the therapeutic index depends on the parameter chosen.[63,64] They produce respiratory depression and a condition of complete analgesia by a receptor-specific effect.[68] Thus the combination of narcotic analgesics and general anesthetics represents an interaction between two types of drugs.

These two types of central nervous system (CNS) drugs must be distinguished. The first consists of general anesthetic agents, alcohol, sedative-hypnotics, the so-called minor tranquilizers, and antiepileptic agents. For these agents there is no evidence for a specific receptor site.[26] This and the similar behavior of these drugs in certain *in vitro* test systems are evidence that they share a similar mechanism of action.[69] Shanes has coined for them the term: "membrane stabilizers."[70] As expected, they have additive effects, both therapeutic and toxic. The second group of CNS drugs are known to affect receptor mechanisms. Morphine and other narcotic analgesics, the major tranquilizers, and the antidepressants belong to this group.

Agents of the first group are capable of inducing tolerance, dependence, and withdrawal symptoms, and there is a high degree of cross-tolerance among them. Of the agents in the second group, only the narcotics cause addiction. Narcotic addiction and dependence on sedative-hypnotics are different entities, and there is no real cross-tolerance. In spite of the important differences between the CNS effects of the different drugs of the first group and various general anesthetics, their toxic actions are roughly additive.

General anesthetics act in principle on all cells and tissues of the body. As discussed previously, even receptor-specific drugs lack selectivity when given systemically, because appropriate receptors may occur in many tissues and organs. However, anesthetic agents can affect almost all tissues and organs because the macromolecules that are the target of their action are ubiquitous. Relative selectivity may result from differences both in the concentration of lipids in different tissues and in the functional importance of affected macromolecules. This, and the functional complexity of the central nervous system, is what makes these agents suitable for clinical anesthesia.

A good example of the degree of parallelism between central and peripheral effects of general anesthetics is the strong correlation between direct myocardial depressant activity and anesthetic potency over a variety of absolute potencies.[71,72] (The extent of autonomic compensation for the direct myocardial depressant effect determines the overall cardiac depression under clinical conditions.) Other examples of the peripheral effects of general anesthetics are: effects on neuromuscular and ganglionic transmission, on airway and vascular smooth muscle, on liver function, and on cardiac electrical events.[73,74]

Antiarrhythmic agents such as quinidine and procainamide are drugs used for their peripheral effects but known to possess CNS side effects. These agents are close to local anesthetics and overlap with them in clinical use. The peripheral effects of local anesthetics (from myocardial depression, to smooth muscle relaxation, to potentiation of neuromuscular block) are well known.

Depression of nerve function does not necessarily manifest itself in a general progressive and systematic decrease of all CNS activity. Inhibitory neurons and synaptic processes are important for overall function. Inhibition of such inhibitory processes by depressant drugs may lead to transient neuronal activation, which may even lead to convulsions, but overall depression ultimately supervenes.[75]

Time sequence and drug interaction. The time course of action of a CNS drug is not related to the blood or tissue level in a simple fashion. With intravenous anesthetic agents, the blood level at the time of recovery from anesthesia is higher than the level at which anesthesia begins. This is known as "acute tolerance." On the other hand, the "calming" effect of a moderate, or sedative, dose of a sedative-hypnotic or the "antianxiety" effect of a tranquilizer often lasts longer than the plasma or tissue concentration. Preanesthetic medication should be given at the appropriate time, so that the blood level of the drug is past its peak at the time of induction. In this way the drug effect is greater than proportional to the blood level, and toxic or side effects of premedicant and anesthetic are less than arithmetically additive.

Recently cocaine was reported not to cause cardiac arrhythmias during halothane anesthesia.[76] This is obviously at variance with our experience (see Case Report) and that of others.[87] The difference lies in the sequence of administration. In our case, the patient had absorbed cocaine and was undergoing a difficult operation, accompanied by considerable excitement and anxiety with sympathetic activation, when general anesthesia with halothane was induced. This sympathetic activity was potentiated by cocaine with disastrous consequences. In the study quoted,[76] cocaine was administered to patients already under halothane anesthesia. Sympathetic activity *during* halothane anesthesia is low. Hence there was little NE to be potentiated.

A special situation exists in patients with drug dependence resulting from chronic or subchronic administration of either the sedative-hypnotic or the narcotic-analgesic class.[77] It is common practice to maintain the state of dependence during anesthesia, since that is not the time to bring about withdrawal. This requires that the appropriate dose of the appropriate drug be given at the proper rate, which in the clinical situation is often not simple. The diagnosis of the type of drug required and the determination of the correct dose can usually be made only on the basis of the patient's history. As mentioned, any sedative-hypnotic agent can be used to substitute for any drug of the "general CNS-depressant" class, including alcohol. Pentobarbital is the usual sedative-hypnotic used. Any narcotic can be used to substitute for any other narcotic, but the severity of withdrawal symptoms seems to be related to the rate of elimination of the narcotic. Methadone may offer an advantage because of its longer duration of action.

The administration of a narcotic antagonist, for example, naloxone, is dangerous in the case of a narcotic addict because the displacement of the narcotic from receptor sites is rapid, and an acute withdrawal syndrome is precipitated, the severity of which depends on the naloxone dose and on the intensity of the existing addiction. On the other hand, in the nonaddict, the *acute* effects of even a high dose of a narcotic may be terminated without risk. No recognizable withdrawal syndrome is thereby precipitated, except for the reappearance of pain, which may elicit a typical autonomic response.[78]

Other drug interactions. The classifications used cannot encompass all forms of drug interactions. Two of special importance to the anesthesiologists are discussed briefly.

It is well documented that several antibiotics, especially aminoglycosides and polymyxin B, may depress neuromuscular transmission and cause prolongation of the action of nondepolarizing neuromuscular blocking drugs.[79] The major site of action is on prejunctional nerve terminals. The antibiotics interfere with the synthesis and function of the bacterial cell wall. This action may extend as well to the motor nerve terminals and the end-plate, and may account for other toxic effects of the same antibiotics, especially their ototoxicity and nephrotoxic effect.

Another serious complication of anesthesia is malignant hyperpyrexia or hyperthermia.[81-84] There is evidence that different clinical and pathogenic forms of malignant hyperthermia occur, but the common denominator is the role of general anesthetic agents and the contribution of neuromuscular blocking drugs in triggering the syndrome. There is also good evidence for a genetic predisposition. The most dangerous form of the syndrome is due to dysfunction of the release and reuptake mechanisms of calcium in skeletal muscle. In view of the multiple roles of calcium in many enzymatic and membrane processes, it is possible that other functions involving calcium are also affected.

Biological effects produced by altered concentrations of the ionic milieu are also hard to categorize. These alterations may occur as a result of drugs such as diuretics, which mobilize tissue fluids and electrolytes and promote their renal excretion, or they could be due to the direct injection of parenteral fluids and ion solutions, for example, calcium and potassium.

Combination of factors in pharmacodynamic drug interactions. There are important clinical entities of drug interactions that cannot be readily discussed in the framework we have chosen, because they involve the intricate interaction of nondrug factors and of drugs belonging to different classes. We shall discuss the precipitation of cardiac arrhythmias as an example of this type of situation.

The following are presently considered to be causally related to the occurrence of cardiac arrhythmias:[85,86] (1) the basic propensity of myocardial cells to discharge spontaneously; (2) the influence of autonomic transmitters or endogenous humoral agents, which may either directly affect the "automaticity" of aberrant foci or create the conditions for discharge by reducing the rate of the normal pacemaker and by slowing or blocking normal impulse conduction; (3) the influence of hypoxia and hypercarbia and of hypokalemia and hypercalcemia; (4) the role of ventricular wall tension, determined in turn by arterial pressure (afterload), diastolic filling (preload), and the contractility of the myocardium; and finally, (5) the direct effects of drugs, such as the sensitizing effects of some general anesthetics, the actions of digitalis, and the effects of antiarrhythmic drugs.

These factors and their combinations can be influenced in many ways by drugs, even those without a direct effect on the heart. For example, diuretics may cause hypokalemia and affect total circulating fluid volume. Apart from its possible sensitizing effect, a general anesthetic in interaction with surgical stimulation affects cardiac autonomic nerve activity, arterial and venous pressures, myocardial contractile force, and secondarily, ventricular volumes. Digitalis increases the susceptibility of the heart to arrhythmias, especially in the presence of hypokalemia or hypercalcemia, though its positive inotropic actions may prevent ventricular dilatation or cardiac failure with secondary catastrophic decrease of myocardial perfusion. Many more examples could be given, but the point is clear: in preventing or treating cardiac arrhythmias it is important to remember the variety of possible contributing factors and the ways in which they may be influenced by drug action. Arrhythmias are more frequent during the induction period. This is partly due to events such as afferent stimulation during laryngoscopy and intubation, injection of succinylcholine, and skin incision, but a contributing factor is the exposure of the heart to high concentrations of the anesthetic at a time when CNS depression is still insufficient to suppress autonomic reflex activity.

No one can be aware of every possible drug interaction. The volume of literature on drug interactions has greatly increased in recent years. Some reports are based on single case observations that do not fit into any logical framework. Other suggestions are simply extrapolations from *in vitro* experiments or animal observations that may or may not have relevance to clinical situations.

We feel that it is necessary to distinguish carefully between general observations of factors underlying drug interactions, which can be and must be verified and quantified, and the virtually limitless potential for juxtaposition and combination of factors that may be encountered in the individual clinical case. For example, the effect of cocaine and of tricyclic antidepressants on the amine pump that transports endogenous catecholamines and antihypertensive drugs of the adrenergic neuron blocking type is a verifiable observation. However, whether this interaction will lead to a clinical manifestation in a specific case, that is, a hypertensive episode or loss of blood-pressure control, depends on the circumstances of that particular situation. The observation must be known, but for the evaluation of the individual case an understanding of the many potentially contributing factors is required.

We have tried to show on one hand the enormous complexity of drug interactions, and on the other the possibility of reducing the variety of potential interactions to a more manageable framework. The unavoidable corollary of this undertaking, the occasional oversimplification of complex entities, seems justified to us by the advantage of a more comprehensive perspective.

CASE REPORT

A 25-year-old, 70-kg man underwent an operation for correction of a deviated nasal septum. The operation was begun under local anesthesia. Four milliliters of 5% cocaine were used topically to anesthetize the nostrils, and the area of operation was infiltrated with 2% lidocaine, 5 ml, without epinephrine. After about 30 minutes, the patient became restless and complained of pain. Therefore, it was decided to administer general anesthesia. The anesthetist elected to use halothane with 50% nitrous oxide for both induction and maintenance of anesthesia. No atropine was given. During induction, about five minutes after the start of halothane 2 to 2.5%, the patient experienced severe cardiac arrhythmias: first bradycardia, then multifocal ventricular extrasystoles, and finally ventricular fibrillation. In spite of strenuous efforts at resuscitation and defibrillation, the patient died in the operating room.

Comment. The cocaine used for local anesthesia was absorbed with time. Even if only a part of the total dose of 200 mg was absorbed, it was sufficient to decrease reuptake of norepinephrine into the adrenergic nerve terminals. In the absence of high sympathetic activity there might not have been any manifestation of this pharmacologic condition. However, with the development of pain, causing an increase in sympathetic nervous activity, and the subsequent inhalation of halothane, there were additional factors: sensitization of the heart to catecholamines by halothane's reaching the heart in a high concentration, and pain, which further increased sympathetic cardiac-nerve activity. In the presence of previously administered cocaine, these conditions combined were sufficient to elicit severe and irreversible arrhythmias. It is not clear whether vagal activity (initial bradycardia) contributed to the result. The choice of halothane, administered after cocaine in the presence of pain, was tragic.

CASE REPORT

A 70-year-old, 70-kg man with angina pectoris and mild congestive heart failure was scheduled to undergo an open heart operation for replacement of the mitral valve and placement of bypass grafts to the left anterior descending and right coronary arteries. He was taking digoxin, 0.25 mg/day, and propranolol, 100 mg four times a day, with the last dose given three hours before the operation. Anesthesia was induced with morphine, 2 mg/kg, and diazepam, 10 mg. Nitrous oxide, 50%, was added to the oxygen after intubation, which was facilitated by intravenous curare, 24 mg. About two minutes after intubation, the patient's blood pressure fell to 80/50 torr, his heart rate fell to 50/minute, and the central venous pressure remained low at about 4 to 5 torr. (A Swan-Ganz cathether had not been placed and left heart filling pressures were not known.) He was given ephedrine intravenously in 5-mg increments until his pressure and pulse returned to acceptable levels without elevation of central venous pressure; the total dose of ephedrine was 50 mg. The operation proceeded satisfactorily and the patient was "put on the pump" without further difficulty.

Comment. Ephedrine acts directly as a pressor agent, and indirectly by the release of norepinephrine (NE) from the adrenergic nerve endings. Hence the improvement in blood pressure could have been caused by two kinds of drug interactions: (1) ephedrine constricted the peripheral, especially the venous, vascular bed, dilated as a result of histamine release by morphine. The action of ephedrine (and the NE it released) was on the adrenergic, not the histaminergic, receptors, that is, the antagonism was physiologic; (2) the improvement in heart rate and in myocardial contractility represented the action of the drug on the *beta*-adrenergic receptors in the heart, the same receptors in the vicinity of which an unknown concentration of propranolol was present. This was a pharmacologic drug antagonism. The presence of both physiologic and pharmacologic antagonists explains the need for such a large dose of the agonist (ephedrine) to surmount it. The dose required could only have been determined by titration.

Case Report Continued. The period of extracorporeal perfusion proceeded in a satisfactory manner. At the conclusion of the operation, the heart did not pump adequately and an isoproterenol infusion was necessary to allow the discontinuance of bypass. However, shortly after protamine was given (to reverse the residual heparin), cardiac performance improved and the isoproterenol was no longer needed.

Comment. At the time heparin was given prior to insertion of the cannulae there was a large increase in free (as opposed to bound) propranolol because of the interference by the heparin (probably mediated by free fatty acids[19a]) with the protein binding of propranolol. The concentration of free propranolol decreased again at the time protamine was given, and more protein became available again for binding. This represents a change in drug effect secondary to a change in protein binding and accounts for the apparent cardiotonic effects of the protamine.

Case Report Continued. The patient was taken to the intensive care unit in good hemodynamic condition with a blood pressure of 110/80, cardiac output of 6 liters per minute, a pulse of 80, a temperature of 36.5°C, and central venous pressure of 9 torr. His chest was clear and blood gases were normal on controlled ventilation with oxygen, 40%. His peripheral circulation was good, as evidenced by pink, warm skin and strong pedal pulses. As he was still unconscious, he was given a dose of 0.2 mg naloxone IV (intravenously) with disastrous consequences: sudden awakening, apprehension, excitement, hypertension (but no tachycardia), and onset of severe pulmonary edema (rales, foam from endotracheal tube, deterioration of arterial blood gases). This was treated satisfactorily with morphine (required total dose 40 mg IV) and positive pressure ventilation with oxygen, 100%. The patient recovered uneventfully.

Comment. This course of events after the administration of naloxone represents once more two kinds of drug interactions: (1) the reversal of the morphine-induced central-nervous-system (CNS) depression by naloxone is an example of drug interaction on the same receptor; (2) however, the resultant awakening, accompanied by pain and excitement, in turn led to a generalized sympathetic nervous system discharge, causing release of endogenous norepinephrine with its vasoconstrictor *(alpha-*adrenergic) as well as cardiac *(beta-*adrenergic) effects. The result was the autotransfusion of large amounts of fluid from the dilated capacitance vessels of the peripheral vasculature into the central vascular compartment, which the recently traumatized left heart, still under the influence of the *beta*-adrenergic antagonist, was unable to handle. This combination of factors resulted in pulmonary edema. When analgesia, histaminergic peripheral vasodilation, and CNS sedation were again provided by means of more morphine, the situation reversed itself once more.

REFERENCES

1. Koch-Wester, J., and Greenblatt, D.J.: Drug interactions in clinical perspective. Eur. J. Clin. Pharmacol., *11*:405, 1977.
2. Avery, G. S.: Drug interactions that really matter: A guide to major important drug interactions. Drugs, *14*:132, 1977.
3. Alper, M. H., Flacke, W. E., and Krayer, O.: Pharmacology of reserpine and its implications for anesthesia. Anesthesiology, *24*:524, 1963.
4. Ominsky, A. J., and Wollman, H.: Hazards of general anesthesia in the reserpinized patient. Anesthesiology, *30*:443, 1969.
5. Prys-Roberts, C., Meloche, R., and Foex, P.: Studies of anesthesia in relation to hypertension I: Cardiovascular responses of treated and untreated patients. Br. J. Anaesth., *43*:122, 1971.
6. Prys-Roberts, C.: Beta-receptor blockade and anaesthesia. *In* Drug Interactions. Edited by D. G. Grahame-Smith. Baltimore, University Park Press, 1977.
6a. Eikard, B., and Andersen, J. R.: Arrhythmias during halothane anesthesia II: The influence of atropine. Acta Anaesthesiol. Scand., *21*:245, 1977.
6b. Eikard, B., and Sørensen, B.: Arrhythmias during halothane anesthesia. I: The influence of atropine during induction with intubation. Acta Anaesthesiol. Scand., *20*:296, 1976.
7. Smith, S. E., and Rawlins, M.: Variability in Human Drug Response. London, Butterworth, 1973.
8. Sjöqvist, F.: The role of drug interactions in interindividual variability of drug metabolism in man. Arch. Pharm., *297*:S35, 1977.
9. Gilette, J.R.: Individually different responses to drugs according to age, sex, functional and pathological state. *In* Drug Responses in Man. Edited by G. Wolstenholme and R. Porter. London, Ciba Foundation, Churchill, 1967.
10. Vesell, E. S., and Page, J. G.: Genetic control of drug levels in man: Antipyrine. Science, *161*:72, 1968.
11. Alexanderson, B., Price Evans, D. A., and Sjöqvist, F.: Steady state plasma levels of nortriptyline in twins: Influence of genetic factors and drug therapy. Br. Med. J., *4*:764, 1969.
12. Bertler, A., and Smith, S. E.: Genetic influences in drug responses of the eye and the heart. Clin. Sci. Mol. Med., *40*:403, 1971.
13. Kalow, W.: Genetic factors in relation to drugs. Annu. Rev. Pharmacol., *5*:9, 1965.
14. Cadwallader, D. E.: Biopharmaceutics and Drug Interactions. Montclair, N. J., Rocom Press, 1974.
15. Griffin, J. P., and D'Arcy, P. F.: A Manual of Adverse Drug Interactions. Bristol, John Wright & Sons, 1975.
16. Prescott, L. F.: Drug interaction during absorption. Arch. Pharm., *297*:S29, 1977.
17. Nimmo, W. S.: Drugs, diseases and altered gastric emptying. Clin. Pharmacokinet., *1*:189, 1976.
18. Brown, D. D., and Juhl, R. P.: Decreased bioavailability of digoxin due to antacids and Kaolin-Pectin. N. Engl. J. Med., *295*:1034, 1976.

19. Benjamin, D., Robinson, D. S., and McCormack, J.: Cholestyramine binding of warfarin in man and *in vitro*. Clin. Res., *18*:336, 1970.

19a.Wood, M., Shand, D. G., and Wood, A. J. J.: The Effect of Cardiopulmonary Bypass on the Binding of Propranolol in Man. Abstr., A.S.A. meeting, Chicago, 1978, p. 515.

20. Prescott, L. F.: Gastric emptying and drug absorption. Br. J. Clin. Pharmacol., *1*:189, 1974.

21. Adjopon-Yamoah, K. K., Scott, D. B., and Prescott, L. F.: The effect of atropine on the oral absorption of lidocaine in man. Eur. J. Clin. Pharmacol., *7*:397, 1974.

22. Nimmo, W. S., et al.: Inhibition of gastric emptying and drug absorption by narcotic analgesics. Br. J. Clin. Pharmacol., *2*:509, 1975.

23. Nies, A. S.: The effects of hemodynamic alterations on drug disposition. Hemodynamic drug interactions. Neth. J. Med., *20*:46, 1977.

24. Eger, E. I.: Anesthetic Uptake and Action. Baltimore, Williams & Wilkins, 1974.

25. Evans, E. F., et al.: Blood flow in muscle groups and drug absorption. Clin. Pharmacol. Ther., *17*:44, 1975.

26. Goldstein, A., Aranow, L., and Kalman, S. M.: Principles of Drug Action. The Basis of Pharmacology. 2nd Edition. New York, John Wiley & Sons, 1974.

27. Aggeler, P. M., et al.: Potentiation of anticoagulant effect of warfarin by phenylbutazone. N. Engl. J. Med., *276*:496, 1967.

28. Wardell, W. M.: Redistributional drug interactions: a critical examination of putative clinical examples. *In* Drug Interactions. Edited by P. L. Marselli, S. Garratini, and S. N. Cohen. New York, Raven Press, 1974.

29. Sunew, K. Y., and Hicks, R. G.: Effects of neostigmine and pyridostigmine on duration of succinylcholine action and pseudocholinesterase activity. Anesthesiology, *49*:188, 1978.

30. Blackwell, B., and Marley, E.: Interaction between cheese and monoamine oxidase inhibitors in rats and cats. Lancet, *1*:530, 1964.

31. Blackwell, B., et al.: Hypertensive interactions between monoamine oxidase inhibitors and foodstuffs. Br. J. Psychiatry, *113*:349, 1967.

32. Barar, F. S. K., et al.: Interactions between catecholamines and tricyclic monoamine oxidase inhibitor antidepressive agents in man. Br. J. Pharmacol., *43*:472P, 1971.

33. Cocco, G., and Ague, C.: Interactions between cardioactive drugs and antidepressants. Eur. J. Clin. Pharmacol., *11*:389, 1977.

34. Evans-Prosser, C. D. G.: The use of pethidine and morphine in the presence of monoamine oxidase inhibitors. Br. J. Anaesth., *40*:279, 1968.

35. Clark, B., and Thompson, J. W.: Analysis of the inhibition of pethidine. N-demethylation by monoamine oxidase inhibitors and some other drugs with special reference to drug interactions in man. Br. J. Pharmacol., *44*:89, 1972.

36. Freeman, J.: The renal and hepatic circulation in anaesthesia. Ann. R. Coll. Surg. Engl., *46*:141, 1970.

37. Prescott, L. F.: Clinically important drug interactions. *In* Drug Treatment. Edited by G. S. Avery. Sidney, Adis Press, 1976.

38. Stephenson, R. P.: A modification of receptor theory. Br. J. Pharmacol., *11*:379, 1956.

39. Ariens, E. J., van Rossum, J. M., and Simons, A. M.: Affinity, intrinsic activity and drug interaction. Pharmacol. Rev., *9*:218, 1957.

40. Furchgott, R. F.: Receptor mechanisms. Annu. Rev. Pharmacol., *4*:21, 1964.

41. Waud, D. R.: Pharmacological receptors. Pharmacol. Rev., *20*:49, 1968.

42. Paton, W. D. M.: A theory of drug action based upon the rate of drug receptor combination. Proc. R. Soc., Lond. [Biol.] *154*:21, 1961.

43. Paton, W. D. M. and Rang, H. P.: A kinetic approach to the mechanism of drug action. *In* Advances in Drug Research. Edited by H. J. Harper and A. B. Simmonds. New York–London, Academic Press, 1966.

44. Flacke, W. and Flacke, J. W.: Effects of surmountable antagonists on cardiac responses to nerve stimulation. Proc. VII. Internat. Congress Pharmacol., Paris, July, 1978.

45. Nickerson, M.: Nonequilibrium drug antagonism. Pharmacol. Rev., *9*:246, 1957.

46. Reference 46 has been deleted.

47. Ariens, E. J., Simonis, A. M., with van Rossum, J. M.: Drug receptor interaction: Interaction of one or more drugs with different receptor systems. *In* Molecular Pharmacology. Edited by E. J. Ariens. New York-London, Academic Press, 1964, Vol. I.

48. MacDonald, A. G., and McNeill, R. S.: A comparison of the effect on airway resistance of a new beta blocking drug ICI 50,172. Br. J. Anaesth., *40*:508, 1968.

49. Langer, S. Z.: Presynaptic regulation of catecholamine release. Biochem. Pharmacol., *23*:1793, 1974.

50. Stjärne, L.: Basic mechanisms and local feedback control of secretion of adrenergic and cholinergic neurotransmitters. *In* Handbook of Psychopharmacology. Edited by L. L. Iversen, S. D. Iversen, and S. H. Snyder. New York–London, Plenum Press, 1975, Vol. 6.

51. Starke, K.: Regulation of noradrenaline release by presynaptic receptor systems. Rev. Physiol. Biochem. Pharmacol., *77*:2, 1977.

52. Löeffelholz, K., and Muscholl, E.: Inhibition by parasympathetic nerve stimulation of the release of the adrenergic transmitter. Naunyn Schmiedebergs Arch. Pharmacol., *267*:181, 1970.

53. Trendelenburg, U.: Supersensitivity and subsensitivity to sympathomimetic amines. Pharmacol. Rev., *15*:225, 1963.

54. Iversen, L. L.: Inhibition of noradrenaline uptake by drugs. J. Pharm. Pharmacol., *17*:62, 1965.

55. Mitchell, J. R., et al.: Guanethidine and related agents. III. Antagonism by drugs which inhibit the norepinephrine pump in man. J. Clin. Invest., *49*:1596, 1970.

56. Boakes, A. J., et al.: Interactions between sympathomimetic amines and antidepressant agents in man. Br. Med. J., *1*:311, 1973.

57. Briant, R. H., Reid, J. L., and Dollery, C. T.: Interaction between clonidine and desipramine in man. Br. Med. J., *1*:522, 1973.
58. Hubbell, W. L., et al.: The interaction of small molecules with spin labeled erythrocyte membranes. Biochim. Biophys. Acta, *219*:415, 1970.
59. Koehler, L. S., Curley, W., and Koehler, K. A.: Solvent effects on halothane 19 Fe nuclear magnetic resonance in solvents and artificial membranes. Mol. Pharmacol., *13*:113, 1977.
60. Eyring, H., Woodbury, J. W., and D'Arrigo, J. S.: A molecular mechanism of general anesthesia. Anesthesiology, *38*:415, 1973.
61. Halsey, M. J.: Mechanisms of general anesthesia. *In* Anesthetic Uptake and Action. Edited by E. I. Eger, II. Baltimore, Williams & Wilkins, 1974.
62. Cuthbert, A. W.: Membrane lipids and drug action. Pharmacol. Rev., *19*:59, 1967.
63. Saidman, L. J., and Eger, E. I., II: Effect of nitrous oxide and of narcotic premedication on the alveolar concentration of halothane required for anesthesia. Anesthesiology, *25*:302, 1964.
64. Munson, E. S., Saidman, L. J., and Eger, E. I., II: Effect of nitrous oxide and morphine on the minimum anesthetic concentration of fluroxene. Anesthesiology, *26*:134, 1965.
65. Wolfson, B., Keilar, C. M., and Lake, C. L.: Anesthetic index, a new approach. Anesthesiology, *38*:583, 1973.
66. Wolfson, B., et al.: Anesthetic Indices—Further data. Anesthesiology, *48*:187, 1978.
67. Perisho, J. A., Buechel, D. R., and Miller, R. D.: The effect of diazepam (Valium^R) on minimum alveolar anesthetic requirement (MAC) in man. Can. Anaesth. Soc. J., *18*:536, 1971.
68. Lowenstein, E., Hallowell, P., and Levine, F.: Cardiovascular response to large doses of intravenous morphine in man. N. Engl. J. Med., *281*:1389, 1969.
69. Seeman, P.: The membrane actions of anesthetics and tranquilizers. Pharmacol. Rev., *24*:583, 1972.
70. Shanes, A. M.: Electrochemical aspects of physiologic and pharmacologic action in excitable cells. Pharmacol. Rev., *10*:59, 1958.
71. Price, H. L., and Helrich, M.: The effect of cyclopropane, diethyl ether, nitrous oxide, thiopental, and hydrogen ion concentration on the myocardial function of the dog heart-lung preparation. J. Pharmacol. Exp. Ther., *115*:206, 1955.
72. Brown, B. R., and Crout, J. R.: A comparative study of the effects of five general anesthetics on myocardial contractility. Anesthesiology, *34*:236, 1971.
73. Richter, J., Landau, E.M., and Cohen, S.: The action of volatile anesthetics and convulsants on synaptic transmission: a unified concept. Mol. Pharmacol., *13*:548, 1977.
74. Garfield, J. M., et al.: A pharmacological analysis of ganglionic actions of some general anesthetics. Anesthesiology, *29*:79, 1968.
75. Mori, K., and Winters, W.: Neural background of sleep and anesthesia. Int. Anesthesiol. Clin., *12*:76, 1975.
76. Chung, B., Naraghi, M., and Adriani, J.: Sympathomimetic effects of cocaine and their influence on halothane and enflurane anesthesia. Anesthesiology Rev., *5*:16, 1978.
77. Dundee, J. W., and McCaughey, W.: Interaction of drugs associated with anesthesia. *In* Recent Advances in Anesthesia and Analgesia. Edited by C. L. Hewer. Boston, Little Brown, 1973.
78. Flacke, J. W., Flacke, W. E., and Williams, G. D.: Acute pulmonary edema following naloxone reversal of high-dose morphine anesthesia. Anesthesiology, *47*:376, 1977.
79. Pittinger, C., and Adamson, R.: Antibiotic blockade of neuromuscular function. Annu. Rev. Pharmacol., *12*:169, 1972.
80. Fogdall, R., and Miller, R. D.: Prolongation of a pancuronium-induced neuromuscular blockade by polymyxin B. Anesthesiology, *40*:84, 1974.
81. Denborough, M. A., and Lovell, R. R. H.: Anesthetic deaths in a family. Lancet, *2*:45, 1960.
82. Britt, B. A., and Kalow, W.: Malignant hyperthermia: A statistical review. Can. Anaesth. Soc. J., *17*:293, 1970.
83. Isaach, H., and Barlow, M. B.: Malignant hyperpyrexia. J. Neurol. Neurosurg. Psychiatry, *36*:228, 1973.
84. Editorial: New causes for malignant hyperpyrexia. Br. Med. J., *4*:488, 1974.
85. Katz, R. L., and Epstein, R. A.: The interaction of anesthetic agents and adrenergic drugs to produce cardiac arrhythmias. Anesthesiology, *29*:763, 1968.
86. Hoffman, B. F.: The genesis of cardiac arrhythmias. *In* Mechanisms and Therapy of Cardiac Arrhythmias. Edited by L. S. Dreifus and W. Likoff. New York, Grune and Stratton, 1966.
87. Adriani, J., and Campbell, D.: Fatalities following topical application of local anesthetics to mucous membranes. J.A.M.A., *162*:1527, 1956.

Chapter 3

The Role of the Liver

BURNELL R. BROWN, JR.
and
GEORGE E. McLAIN, JR.

Within the last two decades, clinical pharmacology has been complicated by the realization that the pharmacodynamics of one drug can rarely be considered independent from that of other drugs. In practice, the surgical patient is frequently administered several drugs, each given for a particular therapeutic purpose. When these drugs are combined, the possibilities of various mechanisms of interaction become astronomic. The science of drug interactions is new, and knowledge in the area is outstripped by the pragmatics of vogues of current therapy. It is the purpose of this chapter to present in brief format some of the classic drug interactions mediated specifically by the liver.

DRUG BIOTRANSFORMATION IN THE LIVER

The liver is the largest organ of the body and has manifold functions. It is unique because the hepatocyte, the major cell type, is histologically consistent but is functionally inconsistent, capable of undergoing a variety of biochemical reactions. From a strictly pharmacologic point of view, one of the major tasks of the liver is the biotransformation of drugs. Within the framework of this goal, numerous drug interactions may occur.

Although the lung and the kidney actively participate in the biotransformation of xenobiotics, the bulk and degree of activity of the liver dictate that it be considered the primary organ involved in this function. The reason for biotransformation is simple. Many drugs, particularly CNS (central nervous system)-active ones administered during the course of anesthesia, are lipophilic, because of their intrinsic physicochemical structure. Penetration of the blood-brain barrier by a drug is predicated on its lipid-soluble characteristics. Thus inhalation anesthetics, barbiturates, tranquilizers, sedatives, and analgesics must be able to penetrate into the brain to produce the desired pharmacologic result. Except for inhalation anesthetics, which are eliminated primarily through the lungs, excretion of drugs is entirely by the renal route. The tubular epithelium of the nephron is essentially a lipid layer. Thus centrally active drugs are secreted by the glomeruli of the nephron unit but rapidly reenter the systemic circulation because they are taken up by the tubular epithelium. It has been estimated that the half-life of an extremely lipophilic "fixed" (nonvolatile) drug, such as thiopental, would be approximately 20 years if no biotransformation occurred. The essence of drug biotransformation is: the conversion of a lipid-soluble compound into one of increased polarity, or water solubility, so that it may be easily eliminated by the kidneys.

Electron microscopy of the hepatocyte reveals loose sheets of contiguous membranes and channels within the cytoplasm, termed the endoplasmic reticulum.[3] The endoplasmic reticulum is rich in lipids, particularly unsaturated ones such as arachidonic acid, coupled as esters to phosphatidylcholine and phosphatidylethanolamine. Such a biochemical structure mandates that lipid-soluble drugs will be found in high concentrations in the endoplasmic reticulum once entry into the hepatocyte occurs. Most of the enzymes of biotransformation are located within this organelle.[1] If the endoplasmic reticulum is extracted from the hepatocyte by cell disruption and ultracentrifugation, the endoplasmic reticulum can be isolated for *in vitro* studies. This process, however, converts the endoplasmic reticulum from contiguous sheets into membrane fragments that coalesce into spheres, the so-called microsomes. Thus the enzymes of biotransformation may appropri-

ately be termed microsomal enzymes, although microsomes are artifacts, which do not exist *in vivo*.

There are four chemical reactions by which lipophilic drugs are converted into water-soluble, or polar ones: (1) *Oxidation*, (2) *Conjugation*, (3) *Hydrolysis*, and (4) *Reduction*. The most commonly employed processes are oxidation and conjugation. Hydrolysis is uncommon and is dependent on the drug substrate's possession of an ester group. Reduction is a rare form of biotransformation. In an attempt to increase polarity, a drug may undergo several sequential reactions, such as oxidation followed by conjugation. A classic example of this is found in the biotransformation of pentobarbital. Initially, aliphatic hydroxylation occurs. This is followed by conjugation with glucuronic acid, a highly polar derivative of glucose. In addition to facilitating excretion, biotransformation usually results in the termination of pharmacologic activity of the drug. This is not universally the case, however. Drug metabolites may be as active as, and sometimes more active than, the parent compound.

Strictly speaking, oxidation is defined not only as the addition of molecular oxygen, but also as the removal of an electron, or relative diminution of electronegativity. A variety of reactions occurs under the general heading of oxidation, such as (1) *Hydroxylation (OH group addition)*, (2) *Dealkylation (CH$_3$ and C$_2$H$_5$ group removal)*, (3) *N-oxidation (N to N–O), O-dealkylation (C$_2$H$_5$O to OH)*, and (5) *Dehalogenation*. Oxidative biotransformation is accomplished in the endoplasmic reticulum of the hepatocyte by a series of enzymes termed the *mixed-function oxygenases*. This enzymatic system is particularly adapted to metabolism of foreign drugs, pollutants, and carcinogens (xenobiotics). A few naturally occurring endogenous compounds are metabolized by the system (for example, steroids) but in general it acts only on xenobiotics.[2]

The prominent features of the drug-metabolizing enzymes are: (1) *Lack of sub-*

strate specificity, (2) Low turnover number, and (3) Ability to be induced. A unique property, which differentiates this system from other enzymatic reactions of the body, is the low order of substrate specificity. This means that the same series of enzymes can biotransform many structurally unrelated compounds. Drugs of different structures, such as general inhalation anesthetics, acetaminophen, meperidine, barbiturates, benzodiazepines, and phenothiazines are biotransformed by a single group of enzymes. The disadvantage of this apparently simple arrangement is that the reactions proceed slowly, defined biochemically as a low-turnover number. Thus the metabolic half-time of drugs is measured in terms of hours rather than milliseconds as is common in many enzymatic reactions such as the acetylcholine-acetylcholinesterase system.

In order to compensate for the low-turnover number, the microsomal enzymes have the capacity to increase drug metabolic rates by the process of induction.[4-6] This sometimes misunderstood concept is really straightforward and teleologically appealing: when the enzymes are chronically stimulated by certain drugs or environmental pollutants, the content and hence the activity of the enzymes increase. There are at least 300 drugs and chemicals known to produce microsomal enzyme induction. Chronology is important in assessing induction status. The inducing agents work both by causing increases in synthesis of new enzymatic protein and by decreasing catabolic rates; thus, the content of enzyme increases. This phenomenon takes time. A good example of a clinically employed drug that induces biotransformation enzymes is phenobarbital. Although a single dose of the barbiturate produces clinically insignificant induction, maximal induction does not occur until the drug has been administered for four to five days. When the drug is discontinued, microsomal enzyme levels fall to normal in approximately 48 to 72 hours. Since the microsomal enzyme systems are not substrate-specific, induction of them by one drug usually results in an increased rate of biotransformation of many other drugs. Induction would seem to be nature's defense mechanism to prevent pharmacologic overdosage when the body is assailed chronically by foreign substances.

The following changes are seen following drug induction: (1) decreased pharmacologic activity and half-life of other drugs; and (2) increased enzyme and protein content of the endoplasmic reticulum of the hepatocytes, as seen by electron microscopy.[7]

Figure 3–1 illustrates the enzymes of oxidative biotransformation.[8] Cytochrome P-450 is the terminal enzyme of the system. The overall reaction involves a combination of drug and molecular oxygen with cytochrome P-450. Reducing equivalents (electrons) derived from reduced nicotinamide-adenine dinucleotide (NADPH) are transferred to this enzyme-O_2-substrate complex by means of the enzyme NADPH cytochrome C reductase. After activation of diatomic, molecular oxygen to the monatomic species, one oxygen atom is reduced to water, the other incorporated into the drug.

A concept that must be discussed is the description of induction and its effects on the enzymes of biotransformation as an entirely quantitative phenomenon. This is not true—qualitative changes also occur. Cytochrome P-450 is not a single entity but a mixture of enzymes, many of which have not yet been identified. Thus one inducing drug may stimulate one subset of cytochrome P-450 enzymes and not another. As an example, phenobarbital treatment of animals not only increases the rate and amount of biotransformation of methoxyflurane, but also qualitatively stimulates metabolism toward the pathway of free fluoride production. Qualitative differences explain why some inducing drugs are more selective than others, and why some inducers such as 3-methylcholanthrene stimulate such a narrow spectrum of biotransformation of other drugs. A corollary of this fact has to do with the genetics of drug bio-

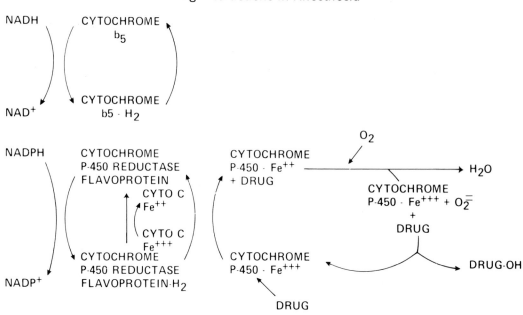

Fig. 3–1. The microsomal oxidation electron transfer system.

transformation, since there are variations in the rates and quality of biotransformation in different persons.[9] Perhaps this is explained by genetic differences in the quality and quantity of the isoenzymes contained in cytochrome P-450.

HEPATIC DRUG INTERACTIONS

Several mechanisms of drug interactions occurring in the liver can be explained by alterations in the drug-metabolizing enzyme sequence.

Inhalation anesthetics

Any inhibition of one drug biotransformation by another would result in prolongation of the half-life and the potentiation of one or both of the drugs. The inhalation anesthetics in common use (for example, halothane) are lipophilic substances. The cytochrome P-450 system is imbedded in the matrix of the endoplasmic reticulum, mentioned as being a lipid-rich area. Following an accumulation of inhalation anesthetics, there

is inhibition of biotransformation of the barbiturate.[10,11] This inhibition is noncompetitive, leading to the speculation that the effect is allosteric. Glucuronide conjugation reactions are also inhibited by anesthetics, but not to the same degree as oxidative drug metabolism.[12] If drugs with a short metabolic half-life, such as pentazocine, lidocaine, and hexobarbital, are injected into animals equilibrated with anesthetic concentrations of halothane, the half-life is prolonged. However, this is not entirely due to enzymatic inhibition. Most inhalation anesthetics decrease splanchnic blood flow, so that the distribution of fixed drugs to the liver is impaired. The prolonged half-life is thus a resultant both of reduced enzymatic biotransformation and of decreased hepatic bioavailability. This is seen in man with the combination of halothane and pentobarbital. The net clinical effect is a prolongation and intensification of the pharmacologic action of fixed drugs given during the course of inhalation anesthesia. The general implications have not been studied in great detail in man.

Combinations of fixed agents

Because of the nature of cytochrome P-450, with its intrinsic low substrate specificity, any particular drug is liable to inhibit the biotransformation of another, and thus increase its potency. This has been repeatedly demonstrated *in vitro* with many fixed drugs, including barbiturates, narcotics, and tranquilizers.[13] There are reasons to believe that fixed drugs act competitively to inhibit metabolism, but the exact enzyme kinetics in a complex system such as this are unknown. Also unknown is the precise clinical relevance of this type of interaction. The terms used by clinicians to describe this mechanism are "potentiation," "synergism," and "addition" (see Chap. 1).

Induction

A partial list of drugs capable of inducing liver microsomal enzymes is: *(1) Barbiturates, (2) Glutethimide, (3) Phenylbutazone, (4) Chloral hydrate, (5) Meprobamate, (6) Chlordiazepoxide, (7) Phenytoin (Diphenylhydantoin) (8) Cortisone, (9) Ethanol, (10) Diphenylhydramine, (11) Polychlorobiphenyls, (12) DDT, Lindane, (13) Cigarette smoke, and (14) Cannabis.* It must be remembered that all inducing substances do not produce identical increases in cytochrome P-450, because of the variability and multiplicity of the isoenzymes of that system. For example, ethanol is not only a quantitatively weaker inducing drug than phenobarbital, but qualitatively it induces a narrower spectrum of enhanced biotransformation of other drugs. In clinical practice, a careful history is perhaps the best way to determine whether drug induction is present, but this is not absolute since genetic factors may either inhibit or enhance induction.

The classic drug interaction in the induced patient results in decreased effectiveness of a drug given simultaneously with the inducer. In the clinical situation, this would be defined as tolerance. A typical example is the barbiturate user, who requires increasing amounts of the drug to achieve a euphoric state. Repeated ingestion of the barbiturate leads within days to enzyme induction, consequent increased biotransformation rate, and shortened half-life. In anesthetics, tolerance to preoperative medications may be noted, as well as an increased requirement for intravenous barbiturates and sedatives. Narcotics are not considered inducing drugs, and tolerance to these addictive drugs is not predicated on this mechanism, although on the other hand, the inducing drugs can enhance biotransformation of certain narcotics.

There are times when abrupt reduction of the induced state can lead to problems, as illustrated by the following example.[14] Patients suffering from myocardial infarction may simultaneously receive sodium warfarin as an anticoagulant and a sedative, such as phenobarbital. The phenobarbital acts as a potent enzyme-inducer, stimulating the rapid biotransformation of sodium warfarin. Thus while on this regimen, the patient requires a larger dose of sodium warfarin than normal to maintain desired prothrombin levels. When the inducing drug, phenobarbital, is discontinued, microsomal enzyme levels fall abruptly. Now the same dose of sodium warfarin becomes an overdose since biotransformation has returned to a normal rate. Prothrombin time is prolonged and bleeding occurs with a possible fatal outcome (see Chap. 14).

Abnormal shunting of biotransformation

This category of hepatic drug interaction is rare. A clinical example is observed when a monoamine oxidase (MAO) inhibitor and meperidine are combined. There have been numerous case reports to the effect that when patients on chronic MAO-inhibitor therapy receive conventional amounts of parenteral meperidine (50 to 100 mg), a sudden reaction consisting of hypertension, convulsions, and hyperthermia is frequently produced. Although the mechanism is not proven, it has been hypothesized that MAO inhibitors block the normal route of meperidine biotransformation to meperidinic acid, and that this causes meperidine to form normeperidine, a convulsant.[15]

VISCEROTOXICITY AND ANESTHETIC DRUG INTERACTIONS

An unusual drug reaction encountered in clinical anesthesia is postanesthetic hepatic necrosis. Whether this represents a true drug interaction in human beings is speculative, although there are abundant animal data to support the hypothesis. Halothane is used as an example in the following discussion, since more work has been done with it in this regard than with any other anesthetic.

It is now recognized that enzyme-inducing drugs cause increased rates and amounts of biotransformation of volatile inhaled anesthetics.[16] Obviously, volatile anesthetics differ from fixed drugs in that the former are primarily eliminated by the lungs, whereas the latter require biotransformation to decrease activity and to facilitate renal elimination. In general, biotransformation, whether induced or not, is helpful, since it shortens a prolonged pharmacologic action and provides a defensive compensatory mechanism against chronic drug accumulation. In halogenated volatile anesthetics, this may not always be so, as in the case of methoxyflurane. It is established that the biotransformation of methoxyflurane leads to the formation of a free fluoride ion, which can damage the renal tubule, and produce renal impairment of the high-output failure type.[17] Less well known is that inducing drugs enhance biotransformation both qualitatively and quantitatively. Thus extrapolating from animal data, the use of this anesthetic in a patient with a drug history conducive to the induced state may be hazardous regardless of dose.

That hepatotoxicity is a manifestation of drug interaction is not certain. Animals pretreated with phenobarbital are more susceptible to carbon tetrachloride and chloroform

hepatotoxicity than are untreated animals.[18] Free radicals and reactive intermediates produced in quantity from these halogenated alkanes by the induced enzymes attack liver macromolecules, with a result of centrolobular necrosis. Ordinarily, the oxidative biotransformation of halothane is benign. The products formed are trifluoroacetic acid and bromide and chloride ions, all innocuous.[19] However, metabolites of great potential reactivity have been observed in the urine and exhaled air of both persons and animals following a conventional exposure to halothane.[20,21] There is strong experimental evidence to indict an abnormal, reductive pathway of halothane that may produce reactive intermediates leading to hepatic necrosis. Two animal models of "halothane hepatotoxicity" have been produced.[22-24] In the first, a single dose of a mixture of polychlorobiphenyls is given to the animals. These compounds greatly induce both oxygen- and nonoxygen-dependent subunits of cytochrome P-450. When these animals are subsequently anesthetized with 1% halothane in 99% oxygen, classic centrolobular necrosis occurs. The second model involves pretreatment with phenobarbital followed by anesthesia with 1% halothane in a hypoxic environment ($F_IO_2 = 0.14$). Again, centrolobular necrosis results. Another factor contributing to the nonoxygen-dependent or "reductive" biotransformation of halothane is the known propensity of the anesthetic to decrease liver blood flow variably by direct action on the splanchnic flow, primarily by the constriction of the hepatic artery.

Although unproved, "halothane hepatitis" could be envisioned as a possible drug interaction. In the following hypothetical example, an obese 40-year-old woman is scheduled for an elective hysterectomy. Halothane is used satisfactorily as the primary anesthetic. However, within a few days, the patient develops the symptoms of a vaginal cuff abscess. The gynecologist gives antibiotics as therapy. Because of apprehension on the patient's part, he also prescribes sedatives and hypnotics—inducing drugs—for several days. We shall assume that this patient initially possessed a genetically determined small quantity of a cytochrome P-450 isoenzyme variant that biotransforms halothane through reductive pathways to reactive products.[25] However, the amount of this particular enzyme and hence the amount of reactive metabolites produced are small during the first administration of halothane. Therefore, no overt liver damage is noted. Owing to the failure of antibiotic therapy for the abscess, the patient needs a second operation. At this time, however, the inducing drugs have changed her pharmacologic environment. The enzyme responsible for biotransformation of halothane to reactive metabolites was of low concentration and a low order of activity initially. Now it has been activated and increased by the inducing drugs. A short reexposure to halothane for drainage of the abscess may lead to the production of sufficient reactive metabolites so that autocatalytic destruction of liver macromolecules occurs, leading to centrolobular necrosis and jaundice. We repeat, the existence of this drug interaction has not been proven in man, but animal data corroborate the phenomenon. Such speculation does not imply that a patient with a history of ingestion of a known inducing drug should not receive halothane. Induction of halothane through normal metabolic pathways is apparently harmless. The difference is that this theoretic patient initially had a genetically abnormal cytochrome P-450 variant that could be induced. It must be reiterated that induction of normal cytochrome P-450 does not ordinarily lead to such a catastrophic event.

In summary, the liver is the primary site of a multiplicity of drug interactions. In our drug-oriented society, most of these interactions go unnoticed during clinical anesthesia. We lack sufficiently sophisticated monitoring to detect these events at the molecular level. The anesthesiologist thus perceives them grossly in the form of patient tolerance to drugs or prolonged effects of drugs, but the intelligent practitioner should be aware of the possibilities of these events. Viscerotoxicity following halogenated anesthetics, particularly hepatic necrosis, may be a rare, unpredictable form of subtle drug interaction. If this is true, it will require intensive study for its detection and prevention.

REFERENCES

1. Gillette, J. R., Brodie, B. B., and LaDu, B. N.: The oxidation of drugs by liver microsomes: on the role of TPNH and oxygen. J. Pharmacol. Exp. Ther., *119*:532, 1957.
2. Cooper, D. Y., et al.: Photochemical action spectrum of the terminal oxidase of mixed function oxidase systems. Science, *147*:400, 1965.
3. Claude, A.: Microsomes, endoplasmic reticulum and interaction of cytoplasmic membranes. *In* Microsomes and Drug Oxidation. Edited by J. R. Gillette, et al. New York, Academic Press, 1969.
4. Conney, A. H.: Pharmacological implications of microsomal enzyme induction. Pharmacol. Rev., *19*:317, 1967.
5. Remmer, H., and Merker, H.J.: Effects of drugs on the formation of smooth endoplasmic reticulum and drug metabolizing enzymes. Ann. N.Y. Acad. Sci., *123*:79, 1965.
6. Brown, B. R., Jr.: Hepatic microsomal enzyme induction. Anesthesiology, *39*:178, 1973.
7. Fouts, J. R., and Rogers, L. A.: Morphologic changes in stimulation of microsomal drug metabolizing enzyme activity of phenobarbital, chlordane, benzpyrene, or methylcholanthrene in rats. J. Pharmacol. Exp. Ther., *147*:112, 1965.
8. Gillette, J. R., Davis, D. C., and Sasame, H. C.: Cytochrome P-450 and its role in drug metabolism. Annu. Rev. Pharmacol., *12*:51, 1972.
9. Vesell, E. S., et al.: Genetic control of drug levels and of the induction of drug-metabolizing enzymes in man. Individual variability in the extent of allopurinol and nortryptiline drug metabolism. Ann. N. Y. Acad. Sci., *179*:152, 1971.
10. Baekeland, F., and Greene, N. M.: Effect of diethyl ether on tissue distribution and metabolism of pentobarbital in rats. Anesthesiology, *19*:724, 1958.
11. Brown, B. R., Jr.: The diphasic action of halothane on the oxidation metabolism of drugs by the liver: An in vitro study in the rat. Anesthesiology, *35*:241, 1971.
12. Brown, B. R., Jr.: Effects of inhalation anesthetics on hepatic glucuronide conjugation: A study of the rat in vitro. Anesthesiology, *37*:483, 1972.
13. Rubin, A., Tephly, T. R., and Mannering, G. J.: Kinetics of drug metabolism by hepatic microsomes. Biochem. Pharmacol., *13*:1007, 1964.
14. Goss, J. E., and Dickhaus, D. W.: Increased bishydroxy coumarin requirements in patients re-

ceiving phenobarbital. N. Engl. J. Med., *273*:1094, 1965.

15. Rogers, K. J., and Thornton, J. A.: The interaction between monoamine oxidase inhibitors and narcotic analgesics in mice. Br. J. Pharmacol., *36*:470, 1969.

16. Van Dyke, R. A.: Metabolism of volatile anesthetics, II. Induction of microsomal dechlorinating and ether-clearing enzymes. J. Pharmacol. Exp. Ther., *154*:364, 1966.

17. Mazze, R. I., Trudell, J. R., and Cousins, M. J.: Methoxyflurane metabolism and renal dysfunction: Clinical correlation in Man. Anesthesiology, *35*:247, 1971.

18. Brown, B. R., Jr., Sipes, I. G., and Sagalyn, A. M.: Mechanisms of acute hepatotoxicity: chloroform, halothane, and glutathione. Anesthesiology, *41*:554, 1974.

19. Rehder, K., et al.: Halothane biotransformation in man: A quantitative study. Anesthesiology, *28*:711, 1967.

20. Cohen, E. N., et al.: Urinary metabolites of halothane in man. Anesthesiology, *43*:392, 1975.

21. Mukai, S., et al.: Volatile metabolites of halothane in the rabbit. Anesthesiology, *47*:248, 1977.

22. Sipes, I. G., and Brown, B. R., Jr.: An animal model of hepatotoxicity associated with halothane anesthesia. Anesthesiology, *45*:622, 1976.

23. Sipes, I. G., Brown, B. R., Jr., and McLain, G. E.: Unpublished observations.

24. Widger, L. A., Gandolfi, A. J., and Van Dyke, R. A.: Hypoxia and halothane metabolism in vivo. Anesthesiology, *44*:197, 1976.

25. Brown, B. R., Jr., Sipes, I. G., and Baker, R. K.: Halothane hepatotoxicity and the reduced derivative 1,1,1—trifluoro-2-chloroethane. Environ. Health Perspect., *21*:185, 1977.

4

The Preoperative Visit

J. S. GRAVENSTEIN,
M. F. RHOTON,
and
HELMUT F. CASCORBI

Recently, in consultation with an internist, we performed a careful preoperative assessment and developed a special plan for anesthesia for a patient with sickle cell anemia. This extra effort was questioned by the internist on the grounds that our obligations were the same for all patients regardless of concomitant diseases and that good anesthetic management is supposed to prevent hypoxia, acidosis, stasis, and cooling.

We were unable to counter these arguments satisfactorily. Our colleague was right. All patients deserve the same meticulous anesthesia care, with avoidance of hypoxia and acidosis, as do patients with sickle cell disease. Theoretically, therefore, an extra effort in detecting preoperative problems should not be necessary since, again theoretically, everybody should receive the best possible anesthetic management.

In reality, however, not all patients do receive the best possible anesthetic care. Hypotension, bouts of hypoxemia, and acidosis do occur occasionally and special efforts to prevent such occurrences are in order for patients who cannot tolerate even small deviations from normal. A good preoperative screen is therefore necessary to detect the patients who require these special efforts. Such careful preoperative analysis, unfortunately, is not universal, and thousands of patients each year receive anesthesia and undergo operations without the benefits of a thorough and complete preoperative evaluation. These patients receive little more than a rapid review of the record before induction, because of the time constraints of anesthetic practice. Nonetheless, this perfunctory procedure does identify the occasional patient with a family history of unusual problems (for example, malignant hyperpyrexia) that might have eluded the examination of family physician, internist, or surgeon. Moreover, when combined with good anesthetic management, a brief preinduction assessment does seem to lower morbidity and mortality levels.

In light of these arguments, why do we insist on a complete preoperative workup? First, we believe that the encounter with the anesthesiologist before an operation is psychologically beneficial to the patient. Here the anesthesiologist has an opportunity to answer questions, allay unfounded fears, provide support, and instill confidence.

Second, there is a small group of patients (in our hospital, probably less than 1%) for whom a complete anesthetic history and an examination of the drug regimen for potential drug-interaction problems requires postponement of the anesthesia and the operation. For these selected patients, a complete anesthetic evaluation is lifesaving. Since they cannot be identified in advance, it is mandatory to screen *all* patients for the benefit of these few. Hence the routine preoperative workup is an obligation we cannot escape.

What happens during a preanesthetic visit? The physician meets the patient, seeks to establish rapport and inspire confidence, in short, develops the elements of a patient-physician relationship. Simultaneously, the anesthesiologist seeks the special information (history of disease, drug intake, previous anesthetics) that will influence his choice of anesthesia for this particular patient. We find that the experienced clinician seems to employ intuition, which is difficult to define and impossible to teach. Analysis of "intuition," however, reveals a structure that can be identified and taught. We call this the *key-words* structure. At first glance, many key words might appear to be common, informational medical terms. Indeed, these words only become special when the anesthesiologist recognizes them as signals

to be translated into a *category*. These categories then invite a clear exposition of the therapeutic issues under the heading *problems*, which makes it easier to outline options or *actions*. Given the *key word* "crush injury" we think of the *category* "muscle damage." The *problem* is potassium release with succinylcholine and the logical *action* is avoidance of depolarizing drugs.

Let us take a more complex but common anesthetic problem.

CASE REPORT

Mrs. S., a 40-year-old white housewife, was plump, but not grossly overweight. She was seeing a surgeon because of repeated attacks of biliary colic. Scheduled for elective cholecystectomy, she was examined preoperatively by the anesthesiologist. During the interview, the patient related nothing unusual except a history of asthma. The patient also revealed that she was taking steroids, phenobarbital, and that she used an isoproterenol inhaler whenever she felt tightness in the chest. The last serious attack of asthma had occurred fifteen months before.

Some experienced anesthesiologists might have decided to premedicate her with 20 mg of diazepam intramuscularly 1 hour before anesthesia, to add intravenous atropine prior to induction of anesthesia with thiopental, and to maintain anesthesia with halothane, 60% N_2O, and oxygen, without an endotracheal tube. Others might have used a different approach. In any case, all should have been able to present a rationale for their choice.

How is the rationale for a given anesthetic management developed? We extract several *key words*; cholecystectomy, phenobarbital, and asthma, as shown in Table 4–1.

The reasoning for a somewhat unusual management, that is, no intubation for an upper abdominal incision and halothane for a juxtahepatic operation, becomes clear with this analysis.

There are other key words in this history, for instance, 40-year-old woman.

As in the case of phenobarbital, this key word itself can have several categories (see Table 4–2, which has two of the many possible subcategories for phenobarbital):

Table 4–1
Key Word–Analysis–Actions

Key Word	Category	Problem	Actions
Asthma	Airway management	Bronchospasm (Laryngeal irritation-intubation, extubation, suctioning)	Avoid intubation; deep anesthesia; use halothane; have *beta*-2 stimulators available; avoid neostigmine
Cholecystectomy	Upper abdominal incision	Muscle relaxation; postoperative splinting	Don't use balanced anesthesia. Use intermittent succinylcholine?
Phenobarbital	Chronic use of sedatives	Tolerance	Large dose of premedication

The same *key word* can lead to another action:

Phenobarbital	Enzyme inducers	Increased drug metabolism	Avoid methoxy-flurane

Table 4–2
Key Word—Analysis—Actions
Multiple Subcategories for Phenobarbital

Key Word	Category	Problem	Actions
40-year-old woman	Pregnancy	Malformation, abortion	Pregnancy test, delay surgery?
40-year-old woman	Birth-control pills	Thrombosis, embolism	Low-dose heparin? Early ambulation

The *key-word* system leads to rational, teachable plans of action, development of alternatives, and assignment of priorities to therapeutic issues. For instance, a gynecologic history is needed regarding possible pregnancy and the use of contraceptive pills. The use of *beta*-2-adrenergic stimulating drugs reduces the likelihood of arrhythmias when halothane is employed because of its bronchodilating effects. Methoxyflurane is excluded because the history of phenobarbital intake suggests the activation of microsomal enzymes and consequently the excessive biotransformation of methoxyflurane into toxic breakdown products. As a result of these considerations of drug interaction, a third drug (for example, enflurane) may be chosen.

In the search for drug interactions and by the use of this approach, we can record a drug history using the familiar *review of systems*. There are many different ways to organize such an approach. It makes little difference which one adopts as long as one adheres to a method, which is the only way to minimize the chance of forgetting a system, a drug, or a problem.

Table 4–3 shows the "review of systems" approach and important drugs with their most frequent perianesthetic problems.

Table 4–3

Review of Systems: Drugs and Problems

System	Drugs	Perianesthetic Problems	Chapter
CNS (central nervous)	Antipsychotic	Cardiovascular instability	13
CNS	Sedatives	Enzyme induction	14
CNS	Antiparkinson drugs	Stiff chest	13
CV (cardiovascular)	*Beta*-adrenergic blockers	Congestive heart failure	7
CV	Antihypertensives	CV instability	8
CV	Diuretics	Arrhythmias	11
CV	Digitalis	Arrhythmias	10
CV	Quinidine	Arrhythmias (muscle relaxation)	12
Blood	Anticoagulants	Hematomas	14

Those drugs involved in interactions important to the anesthesiologist are discussed in the chapters listed in the right-hand column of the table.

The *key-word* system and the *review-of-systems* approaches are by no means complete. They are open systems that allow the clinicians to organize and analyze clinical problems and to structure a review of the enormous amount of information that must be processed whenever a medical decision is made.

Chapter 5

The Effect of pH

J. S. GRAVENSTEIN
and
A. H. ANTON

In the following pages we present an example of how a shift in pH can alter the pharmacologic effectiveness of drugs that are weak acids or weak bases. A pH shift can affect the (1) pharmacologic effectiveness, (2) absorption, (3) distribution, (4) renal excretion, and (5) metabolism of drugs. Although these categories are interrelated, it is helpful to discuss them separately.

CASE REPORT

A 20-year-old man was admitted to the hospital emergency ward in a coma. He had ingested an unknown quantity of tablets and capsules. It was known that the drugs included phenobarbital, meperidine, and amphetamine. After tracheal intubation, controlled ventilation, and an intravenous infusion were established, an arterial blood-gas analysis showed a mixed metabolic-respiratory acidosis, with pH 7.00 and P_{CO_2} 60 torr. The patient's arterial pressure was low (65/40 torr) and his heart rate was fast (115 beats/min).

The following questions are now raised: (a) Will gastric absorption of the drugs have progressed at an equal rate? (b) Is the acidemia equally beneficial (or detrimental) to a patient with barbiturate, opioid, and amphetamine intoxication? (c) Can renal excretion of these drugs be enhanced by therapeutic maneuvers?

PHARMACOLOGIC EFFECTIVENESS OF SHIFTS IN pH

In order to examine these questions and to consider the therapeutic consequences, it is necessary to review how pH changes are expressed and what such changes do to weak acids (such as barbiturates) and to weak bases (such as opioid and amphetamine).

The central issue is that these substances dissociate, the degree of dissociation being H-dependent. For phenobarbital, the products of this dissociation would be the ionized form of the drug,

and H$^+$

and the un-ionized form:

Better known are the products of dissociation of carbonic acid:

un-ionized   ionized
H_2CO_3 HCO_3^- and H$^+$

As a general rule, the un-ionized form is more lipid-soluble than the ionized form.[1–3] The un-ionized species, therefore, can cross cellular membranes and is more likely to reach across the blood-brain barrier to the brain, and in pregnancy to reach across the placenta to the fetus. While the un-ionized state favors the diffusion across cellular membranes, other factors are also important. There are, for example, differences in lipid-solubility among un-ionized drugs. For example, un-ionized phenobarbital is less lipid-soluble than un-ionized thiopental.

To express or calculate the degree of ionization, the anesthesiologist can use formulas that relate the concentration of hydronium ions to the proportion of the ionized and un-ionized species of any given weak acid or weak base. Instead of H_3O^+ (hydronium ion) we use, for the sake of convenience, the concentration of [H$^+$] (hydrogen ion).

The [H$^+$] in water—we are dealing with aqueous systems—is temperature-dependent. Water dissociates into [H$^+$] and [OH$^-$]. At 25° C, pure water has an equal amount of both ions. The pKa is 7 and at the pH of 7 neutrality exists. As the temperature is raised in aqueous solutions, the equilibrium shifts and the pH falls.[4] In the ensuing discussion we ignore the temperature effect on pKa, since it is small and for the purpose of clinical decisions can be overlooked. Many pKa values reported in the literature refer to measurements at room temperature (usually 25° C). However, since we are not discussing precise physicochemical changes, it is enough to be aware of our imprecision. The following is our shorthand notation for the substances to be discussed:

ionized phenobarbital   = PL$^-$
un-ionized phenobarbital = PL
ionized meperidine   = ME$^+$
un-ionized meperidine   = ME
hydrogen ion   = H$^+$
ionized lidocaine   = LI$^+$
un-ionized lidocaine   = LI
ionized amphetamine   = AM$^+$
un-ionized amphetamine   = AM

Since the degree of ionization is dependent on the [H$^+$] in the aqueous system in which the drugs are dissolved, we utilize Henderson's equation, the simplest formulation that describes this relationship. For phenobarbital it reads:

$$[H^+] = K_a \cdot \frac{PL}{PL^-}$$

This formula states that a doubling of [H$^+$] leads to a change of the ratio $\frac{PL}{PL^-}$ by a factor of 2. K_a is a constant. The value of K_a can be determined by assuming a 50% ionization at which point $\frac{PL}{PL^-}$ becomes 1. Thus K_a is the hydrogen ion concentration at which 50% of a weak acid is ionized. For phenobarbital, $K_a = 63$, that is, when a liter of aqueous solution has 63 nmol (nanomoles) $[H^+]$, there is as much PL as PL^-. At that $[H^+]$, half of the present phenobarbital is available in the form that easily penetrates membranes. Reducing $[H^+]$ by half would also reduce $\frac{PL}{PL^-}$ by half.

It is easy to convert this simple relationship into familiar pH values as follows:

pH	4	5	6	7	8	9	10
$[H^+]$nmol	100000	10000	1000	100	10	1	.1

In the upper scale we have shown pH units and in the lower scale the hydrogen ion concentration in nanomoles per liter. As with any logarithmic scale, each full step on the scale (for example, from 6 to 7, or from 9 to 8) results in a tenfold change in the hydrogen ion concentration. A patient with a pH of 7.2 has ten times as many hydrogen ions in his blood as he would at a pH of 8.2.

The hydrogen ion concentration $[H^+]$ shown in this example is expressed in nanomoles (1 nmol = 10^{-9} mol). At a physiologic pH of 7.4, we have 40 nanomoles, hence at pH 8.4 we have 4 nanomoles and at 6.4 we would count 400 nanomoles/liter of blood.

Since pH 7.4 is not shown on this scale, we have prepared an enlargement of the scale from pH 6.7 to 8.0.

pH	6.7	6.8	6.9	7.0	7.1	7.2	7.3	7.4	7.5	7.6	7.7	7.8	7.9	8.0
$[H^+]$nmol	200	160	128	100	80	64	50	40	32	25	20	16	12.5	10

This scale shows us that with each 0.3 unit shift in the pH scale (or any such logarithmic scale) we must multiply or divide by a factor of 2 on the scale for the hydrogen ion concentration. Thus if we move from pH 7.40 (40 nanomoles) to 7.1 (80 nanomoles), we shift by 0.3 pH units and increase the hydrogen concentration by a factor of 2.

Or, if we start with 55 nanomoles H^+ and increase to 110, the pH must shift by 0.3 units, that is, from pH 7.26 to 6.96. In order to enter data between 7.3 and 7.4 (or between any other units), we need to expand the scale further (see Table 5–1).

From these scales it is possible to approximate other values not shown. Since our ability to make precise pH measurements is limited and since in clinical practice a pH difference between, say, 7.29 and 7.31 rarely matters, we can conclude that without log table, slide rule, or calculator a conversion of H^+ into pH and vice versa is easy and sufficiently accurate to be clinically adequate. For intervals other than from 7.0 to 7.1, 7.3 to 7.4, and 7.7 to 7.8, we have to estimate to obtain fair approximations.

For interesting mathematical reasons, many researchers and clinicians in the field prefer to use logarithmic scales and expressions, and they use Hasselbalch's version of Henderson's equation, the so-called Henderson-Hasselbalch equation:

$$pH = pK + \log \frac{\text{ionized weak acid}}{\text{un-ionized weak acid}}$$

Where $pH = -\log[H^+]$

$pK_a = -\log K_a$

We observe that in the Henderson-Hasselbalch equation used for weak acids the relation of ionized to un-ionized now shows as

$$\log \frac{\text{ionized weak acid}}{\text{un-ionized weak acid}}$$

Any increase in hydrogen ion concentration (= decrease in pH) results in an increase in the un-ionized fraction. What is true for the relation of $[H^+]$ to pH is also true for the other side of the equation, where $\frac{PL}{PL^-}$ is converted into $\log \frac{PL^-}{PL}$. From this information we can prepare a table by following these steps: (1) by determining what the pK_a of the weak acid is (here phenobarbital) (equal to a K_a of 63) = pK_a = 7.2, and (2) by filling in the figures following the numbered steps on the left (Table 5–2).

RELATION OF SHIFT IN pH TO DRUG ABSORPTION

We can now return to our patient and make certain statements. Theoretically the

Drug Interactions in Anesthesia

Table 5–1

pH values and the calculated values of hydrogen ion concentration (actual) as well as suggested approximations.

pH	7.30	7.31	7.32	7.33	7.34	7.35	7.36	7.37	7.38	7.39	7.40	
[H$^+$] nmol	50 (50.12)	49 (48.98)	48 (47.86)	47 (46.77)	46 (45.71)	45 (44.67)	44 (43.65)	43 (42.66)	42 (41.68)	41 (40.7)	40 (39.8)	(approximate) (actual)

From here it is easy to go up or down by 0.3 units:

Up pH

pH	7.60		7.62		7.64		7.66		7.68		7.7
[H$^+$] nmol	25		24		23		22		21		20

Down pH

pH	7.0	7.01	7.02	7.03	7.04	7.05	7.06	7.07	7.08	7.09	7.1
[H$^+$] nmol	100	98	96	94	92	90	88	86	84	82	80

Table 5–2

The impact of a pH change on the ionization of a drug. *

$$pH = pk_a + \log \frac{\text{ionized weak acid}}{\text{un-ionized weak acid}}$$

Step	Instruction	Prepare in Advance	Result
4	up 0.3 pH units doubles PL$^-$/PL ratio	$8.1 = 7.2 + \log$	$\frac{8\ PL^-}{1\ PL}$
8	up 0.3 pH units doubles PL$^-$/PL ratio	$8.0 = 7.2 + \log$	$\frac{6.4\ PL^-}{1\ PL}$
12	up 0.3 pH units doubles PL$^-$/PL ratio	$7.9 = 7.2 + \log$	$\frac{5\ PL^-}{1\ PL}$
3	up 0.3 pH units doubles PL$^-$/PL ratio	$7.8 = 7.2 + \log$	$\frac{4\ PL^-}{1\ PL}$
7	up 0.3 pH units doubles PL$^-$/PL ratio	$7.7 = 7.2 + \log$	$\frac{3.2PL^-}{1\ PL}$
11	up 0.3 pH units doubles PL$^-$/PL ratio	$7.6 = 7.2 + \log$	$\frac{2.5\ PL^-}{1\ PL}$
2	up 0.3 pH units doubles PL$^-$/PL ratio	$7.5 = 7.2 + \log$	$\frac{2\ PL^-}{1\ PL}$
6	up 0.3 pH units doubles PL$^-$/PL ratio	$7.4 = 7.2 + \log$	$\frac{1.6\ PL^-}{1\ PL}$
10	up 0.3 pH units doubles PL$^-$/PL ratio	$7.3 = 7.2 + \log$	$\frac{1.25\ PL^-}{1\ PL}$
1	Start with pK of substance. Ratio PL$^-$/PL = 1	$7.2 = 7.2 + \log$	$\frac{1\ PL^-}{1\ PL}$
5	Down 1 pH unit 1/10 of PL$^-$/PL ratio	$7.1 = 7.2 + \log$	$\frac{.8\ PL^-}{1\ PL}$
9	Down 1 pH unit 1/10 of PL$^-$/PL ratio	$7.0 = 7.2 + \log$	$\frac{.64\ PL^-}{1\ PL}$

*To estimate the impact of a pH change on the ionization of a drug, follow the steps outlined. First prepare the list of pH and pK$_a$ values. Then go to Step 1, i.e. the pK$_a$ of the drug in question (phenobarbital) and write in the ratio of ionized to un-ionized, which at this point is $\frac{1}{1}$. Then follow the steps numbered on the left.

absorption of PL from the acid medium of the stomach should be rapid (provided the drug is sufficiently lipid-soluble) if gastric pH is low.[5,6] At a gastric pH of 7.2, the PL$^-$/PL ratio is 1, at 6.2 it is .1/1, at 5.2 it is .01/1, at 4.2 it is .001/1, and at 3.2 it is .0001/1. At the assumed gastric pH 3.2 the drug is almost completely un-ionized, which facilitates absorption of weak acids, such as PL. If PL is absorbed, gastric lavage may not yield much PL.

The rules for dissociation of weak bases are essentially the same, except that in Henderson-Hasselbalch's equation the position of ionized to un-ionized is reversed.

$$pH = pK_a + \log \frac{\text{un-ionized weak base}}{\text{ionized weak base}}$$

Since ME has a pK$_a$ of 8.5 and AM 9.8, we can estimate that in an acid pH of the stomach practically all ME and AM are in ionized form. Little may be absorbed and gastric lavage may yield more of these bases than of phenobarbital if both are taken in equal amounts at the same time. Of course, gastric activity may propel the drugs into a more akaline small intestine where the pH is closer to the pK$_a$ values of these drugs, and absorption may progress more rapidly.

There is evidence that the un-ionized part of the barbiturates is pharmacologically active, with respect to both its CNS and its cardiac effects.[7,8] Now we can say that an elevation of pH is beneficial because it reduces PL while it increases PL$^-$. Theoretically, the patient's ratio at pH 7.0 should be about .64 PL$^-$/1PL, that is, about 39% ionized. By raising pH to 7.4 the ratio should rise to 1.6 PL$^-$/1PL or about 62% ionized. That rise should produce a noticeable lessening of the barbiturate-induced depression.

How is this pH shift accomplished? If we bring it about by hyperventilation alone, a rough estimate suggests that we have to double ventilation in order to reduce P_{CO_2} by a factor of 2, which in turn increases pH by about 0.3 units. This makes a few untrue suppositions, for example, it presupposes that HCO_3^- does not change when P_{CO_2} is altered. However, for a quick estimate our system works in this case as well (Table 5–3) and offers useful clinical approximations. H_2CO_3 is obtained by converting P_{CO_2} torr into meq/L by multiplying it by .03. Thus 60 torr P_{CO_2} converts into 1.8 meq/L H_2CO_3. At pH 7.0 the bicarbonate must be 14.4 meq/L. Lowering P_{CO_2} to 30 torr without changing the HCO_3^- (unlikely in real life) brings the pH to 7.3.

The advantage of correcting the acidosis with hyperventilation is that the intracellular pH experiences about the same shift in pH, since CO_2 readily diffuses across cell membranes.

The toxicity of some local anesthetics can also be reduced in this way[9,10] even though these drugs are weak bases. Their active form appears to be, perhaps exclusively, the ionized form.[11] Elevating intracellular pH therefore would cause these anesthetics to become less ionized and hence less toxic.

DRUG DISTRIBUTION IN RELATION TO SHIFT IN pH

There is a disadvantage in relying on P_{CO_2} alone for the pH shift. A simple three-compartment model of our patient's heart, blood, and urine illustrates the point (Fig. 5–1). The model assumes that the intracellular pH of the myocardium is 0.1 pH unit lower than that of the blood. That of the urine is even lower. Using the prepared format we can fill in the spaces. We need to assume a definite quantity of phenobarbital in the blood (ignoring protein binding).

The figure shows that the most alkaline

Table 5–3

The effect of the ratio of bicarbonate (HCO_3^-)
to P_{CO_2} ($P_{CO_2} \times 0.03$) on pH

$$pH = pK_a + \log \frac{\text{ionized weak acid}}{\text{un-ionized weak acid}}$$

3	up 0.3 pH units doubles HCO_3^-/H_2CO_3 ratio	$7.4 = 6.1 + \log$ 7.3 7.2	$\dfrac{20\ HCO_3^-}{1\ H_2CO_3}$
2	up by 1 pH unit tenfold increase in HCO_3^-/H_2CO_3 ratio	$7.1 = 6.1 + \log$	$\dfrac{10\ HCO_3^-}{1\ H_2CO_3}$
6	up by 0.3 pH units doubles HCO_3^-/H_2CO_3	$7.0 = 6.1 + \log$	$\dfrac{8\ HCO_3^-}{1\ H_2CO_3}$
5	up by 0.3 pH units doubles HCO_3^-/H_2CO_3 ratio	$6.7 = 6.1 + \log$	$\dfrac{4\ HCO_3^-}{1\ H_2CO_3}$
4	down 1 pH unit 1/10 of HCO_3^-/H_2CO_3	$6.4 \times 6.1 + \log$	$\dfrac{2\ HCO_3^-}{1\ H_2CO_3}$
1	enter pH at pK of carbonic acid	$6.1 = 6.1 + \log$	$\dfrac{1\ HCO_3^-}{1\ H_2CO_3}$

compartment has the greatest amount of phenobarbital. The reason is that it has the greatest concentration of ionized weak acid. The un-ionized fraction can equilibrate across the membranes and is therefore the same in all compartments. For a weak base the situation is inverse. The most acidic compartment has the highest concentration of the ionized weak base and therefore has the greatest concentration of the drug (for example, meperidine and amphetamine here concentrate in the urine compartment). To look at it in another way, un-ionized material passively distributes itself, seeking an equilibrium. The pH in the different compartments then establishes how much total drug the compartment holds by forcing a certain

amount (satisfying the Henderson-Hasselbalch equation) into the ionized form. Whatever is taken away from the un-ionized species in this process reestablishes a gradient, and more un-ionized drug flows into the compartment until equilibrium is established, as shown in Figure 5–1.

Now we decrease P_{CO_2} so that the pH in all compartments rises by 0.3 units (Fig. 5–2).

The total phenobarbital in these three compartments now is $88 + 100 + 72 = 260$. At the lower pH it was $91.5 + 100 + 80.5 = 272$. Therefore, we have reduced the cardiac PL total.

We repeat the treatment, but this time with $NaHCO_3$ (Fig. 5–3). It is ionized to a

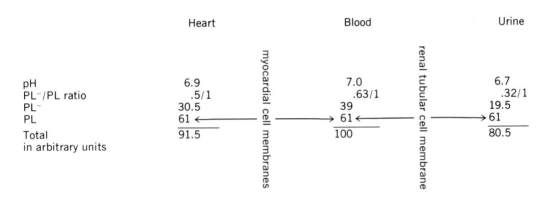

	Heart		Blood		Urine
pH	6.9		7.0		6.7
PL⁻/PL ratio	.5/1		.63/1		.32/1
PL⁻	30.5		39		19.5
PL	61 ←	myocardial cell membranes	→ 61 ←	renal tubular cell membrane	→ 61
Total	91.5		100		80.5
in arbitrary units					

Fig. 5–1. A simplified model showing a "heart," a "blood," and a "urine" compartment. The un-ionized species of phenobarbital (PL) equilibrates across the membranes separating the compartments. The ionized species does not cross.

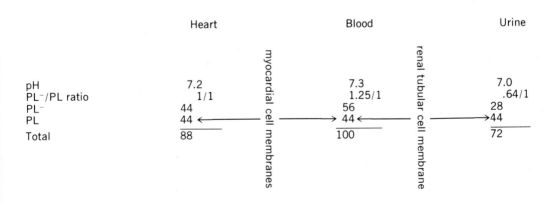

	Heart		Blood		Urine
pH	7.2		7.3		7.0
PL⁻/PL ratio	1/1		1.25/1		.64/1
PL⁻	44		56		28
PL	44 ←	myocardial cell membranes	→ 44 ←	renal tubular cell membrane	→ 44
Total	88		100		72

Fig. 5–2. As in Fig. 5–1, but after decreasing P_{CO_2}.

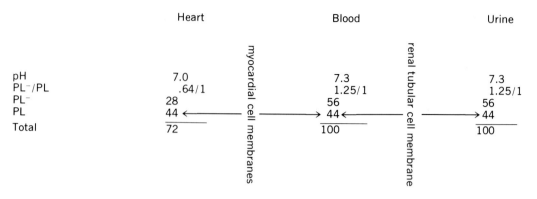

Fig. 5–3. As in Fig. 5–1 after treatment with bicarbonate.

great degree and therefore does not penetrate rapidly intracellularly. Nonetheless, it is subject to glomerular filtration, and urine pH rises. The assumption is that we injected enough $NaHCO_3$ intravenously to obtain the result shown in the figure without changing P_{CO_2}.

THE EFFECT OF SHIFT IN pH ON RENAL EXCRETION

Total phenobarbital is again 272, but in this case urine concentration is high. If we alkalinize the urine further, more of the drug is trapped in the urine and carried away.[12,13] Alkalinization of urine and active diuresis are therefore important therapeutic goals.[14] The heart has less phenobarbital than in the example where P_{CO_2} was lowered, even though the PL, the most active form pharmacologically, is the same in both instances. We argue, then, that adequate ventilation with normalization of P_{CO_2} is desirable but that alkalinization should be accomplished with $NaHCO_3$.

We have omitted several features in order to simplify the presentation of the principles involved. For one, the pK_a of weak acids and bases needs to be close to physiologic pH values in order to realize clinically noticeable effects when pH is changed. For instance, a measurable effect of pH on the CNS (central nervous system) toxicity of local anesthetics was described by Engleson and Grevsten for a series of local anesthetics,[9,10] among them:

	pK_a
lidocaine	7.9
prilocaine	7.9
procaine	9.1
mepivacaine	7.7
bupivacaine	8.1

All of these have pK values not far removed from 7.4. For a drug such as benzocaine (pK_a = 2.8) a pH effect would probably not become noticeable because benzocaine is almost completely un-ionized whether the pH is 6.8 (un-ionized to ionized $\frac{10000}{1}$) or 7.8 $\left(\frac{100000}{1}\right)$.

Recently Benson and co-workers tested the pH effect *in vitro* in a series of opiates and their antagonists.[15] These drugs—all weak bases—have pK_a values between 7.59 (nalorphine) and 9.38 (cyclazocine). In all instances the drugs became more soluble as pH was increased (more un-ionized) and this has clinical implications. However, the progression of changes in the distribution coefficient was not as predictable as we have presented it, possibly because of differences in lipid-solubility (independent of ionization). For meperidine, pK_a 8.5, however, the distribution coefficient rose from 20.2 at pH 7.1 to 38.2 when the pH was raised to 7.4, that is, almost by the predicted factor of 2 with a 0.3 unit pH shift.

The protein binding of drugs may be affected by pH, but these effects are usually small in the physiologic pH range. For example, some barbiturates and muscle relaxants become more protein bound as pH rises within physiologic limits.[3,16,17] We are not aware, however, of any observation where this mild effect was shown to be clinically noticeable.

Amphetamine, as well as related ephedrines, are weak bases. Their excretion rate can be influenced by urine pH, as expected for drugs of that category.[18] Similar relationships have been demonstrated for local anesthetics and procainamide.[19,20]

RELATION OF SHIFT IN pH TO DRUG METABOLISM

If we alkalinize the blood and urine of our patients and thereby delay the excretion of the drugs that are weak bases, do we thereby increase the metabolism of these drugs?

Metabolism needs to be considered when it produces a pH-induced change in the relative ratio of the ionized and un-ionized fractions of a drug. Metabolism is a slow process, and we think more in terms of enzyme induction and inhibition. Depending on the drug, however, a shift in the pH can significantly influence not only a drug's urinary excretion rate but also its metabolic inactivation if its passage through the body is prolonged. This is due to a close relationship between the lipid-solubility of a drug and its metabolism by the hepatic microsomal enzyme system.[21] As described earlier, the un-ionized fraction is more lipid-soluble and therefore can reach the major drug-metabolizing machinery housed in the endoplasmic reticulum of the liver.

For example, we consider what happens to amphetamine as the pH of plasma and urine is changed. It is well known that the urinary excretion of amphetamine and other weak organic bases can be increased significantly in man under conditions that lead to the production of an acid urine.[22–25] Decreasing the pH of urine from 7 to 5 with only a minor change in plasma pH, for example,

decreases the un-ionized fraction of amphetamine in urine one hundredfold and thereby favors a shift of drug from plasma into the flowing urine, even though it is already more than 99.9% ionized at pH 7.0. This is referred to as the ion-trapping mechanism and is effective in removing such drugs from the body. Thus, under conditions leading to an acid urine, Beckett et al. found that approximately 60% of ingested amphetamine is excreted within the first 16 to 48 hours, whereas in an alkaline urine only about 5% is excreted during the same interval.[22,23] The metabolic consequences of such pH-induced changes in the rate of excretion of amphetamine were recently studied by Davis et al. in four subjects either on an acid diet (urine pH 5.5 to 6.0) or after the administration of sodium bicarbonate (urine pH 7.5 to 8.0) (blood pH and gases were not measured).[25] The plasma half-life of amphetamine averaged seven hours in metabolic acidosis and increased almost threefold to 20 hours with the administration of sodium bicarbonate. Since more amphetamine remained in the body under alkaline conditions, one might have expected more opportunity for metabolism. That is what happened. During acid urine production, with an increase in the ionized fraction, less un-ionized amphetamine was available for metabolism, so that most of the administered drug was excreted unchanged, in about four times the amount of the deaminated product. Conversely, during metabolic alkalosis, more un-ionized amphetamine was metabolized and the excretion of the deaminated metabolite approximated that of the unchanged parent compound. Thus the longer amphetamine remains in the body, that is, the higher the urinary pH, the more it is metabolized. In addition, the greater are its pharmacologic effects, since metabolism is slow.[22]

We can speculate on the clinical implications of this relationship. If the effects of weak acidic or basic drugs are mainly terminated by metabolism, a shift in the acid-base status or a depression of renal or liver function by pathologic condition or by anesthesia could make more drug available than could be metabolized. This could result in an increased amount of active drug in the body and possible toxicity. Since enzymes function optimally at a certain pH, to what extent would an altered (pathologic or iatrogenic) acid-base status modify the efficiency with which an enzyme inactivates a drug? How many incidents of drug toxicity attributed to "biologic variation" may be due to an increase in bioavailability because of a change in acid-base status?

Although the number of such incidents is small, the results described above with amphetamine suggest that the relationship of toxicity, drug metabolism, and acid-base status deserves closer attention. A candidate for such pH-mediated differences in metabolism is meperidine with its pK_a of 8.5, close to physiologic values. Since some meperidine is demethylated into a toxic normeperidine in man, a patient with active enzyme systems and delayed meperidine excretion may show unexpected signs of toxicity.[26]

Our patient raises many issues related to the pH effect on drugs, their action, and their disposition. In our example, treatment with bicarbonate and artificial ventilation is in order. It hastens the renal elimination of phenobarbital and helps to reduce its effects on the brain and the heart. At the same time we inhibit, through alkalinization, the elimination of meperidine and amphetamine. Both drugs may become subject to more metabolic biotransformation, a slow process at best. Nevertheless, the undesirable effects of meperidine and amphetamine are more acceptable and are more readily treated than those of the barbiturates.

REFERENCES

1. Goldstein, A., Aronow, L., and Kalman, S.M.: Principles of Drug Action. 2nd Ed. New York, John Wiley & Sons, 1974.
2. Goodman, L. S., and Gilman, A.: The Pharmacological Basis of Therapeutics. 5th Ed. New York, Macmillan, 1975.
3. Eger, E. I., II: Anesthetic Uptake and Action. Baltimore, Williams & Wilkins, 1974.
4. Hills, A. G.: Acid Base Balance, Chemistry, Physiology, Pathophysiology. Baltimore, Williams & Wilkins, 1973.
5. Schanker, L. S.: On the mechanism of absorption of drugs from the gastrointestinal tract (a review). J. Med. Pharm. Chem., 2:343, 1960.
6. Hogben, C. A. M., et al.: Absorption of drugs from the stomach. II. The human. J. Pharmacol. Exp. Ther., 120:540, 1957.
7. Waddell, W. J., and Butler, T. C.: The distribution and excretion of phenobarbital. J. Clin. Invest., 36:1217, 1957.
8. Hardman, H. F., Moore, J. I., and Lum, B. K. B.: A method for analyzing the effect of pH and the ionization of drugs upon cardiac tissue with special reference to pentobarbital. J. Pharmacol. Exp. Ther., 126:136, 1959.
9. Englesson, S.: The influence of acid-base changes on central nervous system toxicity of local anaesthetic agents. I. Acta Anaesthesiol. Scand., 18:79, 1974.
10. Englesson, S., and Grevsten, S.: The influence of acid-base changes on central nervous system toxicity of local anesthetic agents. II. Acta Anaesthesiol. Scand., 18:88, 1974.
11. Ritchie, J. M., and Greengard, P.: On the active structure of local anesthetics. J. Pharmacol. Exp. Ther., 133:241, 1961.
12. Milne, M. D., Scribner, B. H., and Crawford, M. A.: Non-ionic diffusion and the excretion of weak acids and bases. Am. J. Med., 24:709, 1958.
13. Weiner, I.M., and Mudge, G.H.: Renal tubular mechanisms for excretion of organic acids and bases. Am. J. Med., 36:743, 1964.
14. Lassen, N. A.: Treatment of severe acute barbiturate poisoning by forced diuresis and alkalinisation of the urine. Lancet, 2:338, 1960.
15. Benson, D. W., Kaufman, J. J., and Koski, W. S.: Theoretic significance of pH dependence of narcotics and narcotic antagonists in clinical anesthesia. Anesth. Analg. (Cleve.), 55:253, 1976.
16. Cohen, E. N., Corbascio, A., and Fleischli, G.: The distribution and fate of d-tubocurarine. J. Pharmacol. Exp. Ther., 147:120, 1965.
17. Hughes, R.: The influence of changes in acid-base balance on neuromuscular blockade in cats. Br. J. Anaesth., 42:658, 1970.
18. Wilkinson, G. R., and Beckett, A. H.: Absorption, metabolism and excretion of the ephedrines in man. I. The influence of urinary pH and urine volume output. J. Pharmacol. Exp. Ther., 162:139, 1968.
19. Eriksson, E., and Granberg, P.O.: Studies on the renal excretion of Citanest[R] and Xylocaine.[R] Acta Anaesthesiol. Scand. [Suppl.], XVI:79, 1965.
20. Weily, H. S., and Genton, E.: Pharmacokinetics of procainamide. Arch. Intern. Med., 130:366, 1972.
21. Conney, A. H.: Pharmacological implications of microsomal enzyme induction. Pharmacol. Rev., 19:317, 1967.
22. Beckett, A. H., Rowland, M., and Turner, P.: Influence of urinary pH on excretion of amphetamine. Lancet, 1:303, 1965.

23. Beckett, A. H., and Rowland, M.: Urinary excretion kinetics of amphetamine in man. J. Pharm. Pharmacol., *17*:628, 1965.

24. Astatoor, A. M., et al.: The excretion of dextroamphetamine and its derivatives. Br. J. Pharmacol., *24*:293, 1965.

25. Davis, J. M., et al.: Effects of urinary pH on amphetamine metabolism. Ann. N. Y. Acad. Sci., *179*:493, 1971.

26. Stambaugh, J.E., et al.: A potentially toxic drug interaction between pethidine (meperidine) and phenobarbitone. Lancet, *1*:398, 1977.

Chapter 6

Sympathomimetic Drugs

K. C. WONG

The integrity of the sympathetic nervous system is essential for the optimal homeostatic control of the cardiovascular system. Anesthesiologists rely on routine monitoring of the arterial blood pressure as an expression of adequate perfusion of vital organs. This fundamental concept is clinically useful. However, adequate pressure does not always reflect adequate blood flow, since the arterial blood pressure is the product of cardiac output and peripheral vascular resistance, and since cardiac output is the product of stroke volume and heart rate. Stimulation of the sympathetic nervous system can be induced by (1) reflex or direct stimulation of sympathetic nerves to cause a release of norepinephrine from adrenergic nerve terminals, (2) endogenous release of catecholamines (epinephrine and norepinephrine) from the adrenal medulla, or (3) exogenous administration of sympathomimetic drugs. Regardless of the mode of sympathetic stimulation, the caliber of blood vessels, the strength of cardiac contraction, and the heart rate or rhythm are usually affected. Thus arterial blood pressure is regulated by sympathetic activities.

Anesthesiologists are not infrequently called on to anesthetize a patient who has been exposed to drugs that alter the normal physiology of the sympathetic nervous system. Furthermore, all anesthetics and other drugs used by the anesthesiologist affect the sympathetic system to varying degrees. Interactions between these drugs and anesthetics constitute a complex problem for optimal patient care. Rational use of sympathomimetic agents is made only after proper appreciation of the normal physiology of the adrenergic nervous system and of the drugs and anesthetics that alter normal adrenergic responses.

This chapter deals with adrenergic mechanisms, agents that influence normal adrenergic mechanisms, the influence of anesthetics on sympathomimetic drugs, and sympathomimetic drugs in hypotension or shock.

ADRENERGIC MECHANISMS

CASE REPORT

A healthy 22-year-old man was anesthetized with halothane–N$_2$O–O$_2$ for an operation on maxillofacial injuries from a motorcycle accident. The only relevant history was a habitual use of cocaine by inhalation. An uneventful induction and oral tracheal intubation were performed following the intravenous injection of thiopental and succinylcholine. Anesthesia was maintained with halothane and N$_2$O–O$_2$. During the operation cocaine (10%) was applied topically on the nasal mucosa to minimize bleeding. Prior to the application of cocaine the patient had stable vital signs except for transient periods of junctional rhythm (formerly nodal) observed on the electrocardiogram (ECG). However, after cocaine was applied, he developed tachycardia, hypertension, and ventricular extrasystoles. Frequent measurements of arterial blood pressure by an arm cuff showed a systolic blood pressure of between 150 and 200 torr. The 3-liter flow of N$_2$O, 60% of the inspired gas mixture, was replaced by an equal-volume flow of O$_2$. Three divided doses of propranolol totaling 3 mg were administered over a period of 15 minutes. The blood pressure and cardiac rhythm gradually returned to normal within five minutes.

The first question is why the patient developed episodes of junctional rhythm following the administration of halothane-N$_2$O and prior to the topical application of cocaine on the nasal mucosa. Halothane anesthesia induces cardiac junctional rhythm both in man and in experimental animals.[1-6] Halothane has been shown to depress the sinoatrial node and the atrial conduction *in vitro* and to enhance nodal activity *in vivo*;[1,2,4-6] both mechanisms can promote the development of junctional rhythms.[7-9] Moreover, the heart is more susceptible to circulating or exogenously administered catecholamines during halothane.[10-12]

Tachycardia and hypertension frequently occur immediately following the induction of anesthesia and endotracheal intubation. This response represents a reflex increase in sympathetic tone due to the endotracheal intubation. With the further deepening of anesthesia, the sympathetic response usually subsides. Thus junctional rhythm is frequently seen following the induction and endotracheal intubation of the patient anesthetized with halothane and during periods in which anesthetic depth may be inadequate to suppress sympathetic responses. Normally, junctional rhythms do not require treatment unless they induce hypotension and ventricular dysrhythmias. Repeated cocaine intake may change the disposition of catecholamines. This change may account for the development of junctional rhythms.

It is unclear whether N$_2$O augments the dysrhythmic effects of halothane in man. Nitrous oxide alone is known to possess an inherent adrenergic stimulatory effect.[13] The addition of N$_2$O to halothane, ether, and morphine in man also produces a predominant *alpha*-adrenergic stimulatory response.[14-16] However, the interaction of N$_2$O with fluroxene produced a mixed *alpha* and *beta* response.[17] In dogs, the addition of 50% N$_2$O to halothane, enflurane, or methoxyflurane significantly reduces the dose of epinephrine required to induce ventricular dysrhythmias in comparison with similar studies, in which N$_2$O was not added.[17a]

The second question is why the topical application of cocaine caused hypertension, tachycardia, and ventricular dysrhythmias in this patient. A discussion of the normal disposition of catecholamines in the body is necessary for a better understanding of the interaction of cocaine and halothane.

Disposition of catecholamines (Fig. 6–1)

Uptake by Adrenergic Nerve Terminals. Norepinephrine and epinephrine are re-

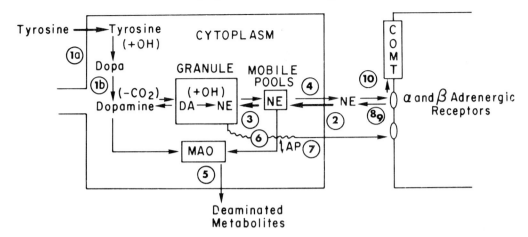

Fig. 6–1. Synthesis, uptake, release and actions of norepinephrine (NE) at adrenergic nerve terminals. Dopamine (DA) nerve action potential (AP).

1. a. Synthesis blocked (*alpha*-methyl-p-tyrosine) b. Synthesis of false transmitters (*alpha*-methyldopa → methylnorepinephrine).

2. Active transport (extracellular fluid → cytoplasm) blocked by cocaine, imipramine, chlorpromazine, ouabain, ketamine.

3. Blockade of transport system of storage granule membrane (reserpine). Destruction of NE by mitochondrial MAO.

4. Displacement of transmitter from axonal terminal (amphetamine, tyramine, ephedrine).

5. Inhibition of enzymatic breakdown of transmitter (pargyline, nialamide, tranylcypromine).

6. Depletion of norepinephrine from granule (guanethidine).

7. Prevention of release of transmitter (bretylium).

8. Transmitter interaction with postsynaptic receptor (phenylephrine, isoproterenol).

9. Blockade of endogenous transmitter at postsynaptic receptor [phenoxybenzamine *(alpha)*; propranolol *(beta)*; practolol *(beta* 1); butoxamine *(beta* 2)].

10. Inhibition of COMT (pyrogallol). (Adapted from Goodman, L. S., and Gilman, A.: *The Pharmacological Basis of Therapeutics.* New York, Macmillan, 1975.)

leased from the adrenergic nerve terminals and the adrenal medulla, respectively. The released catecholamines interact with receptor sites to elicit adrenergic responses. The catecholamine is removed in part by reuptake into the nerve terminal. This active transport (reuptake) of the catecholamines from the extracellular fluid into the intraneuronal (cytoplasmic) sites is the most important way of terminating adrenergic responses.[18,19] Other sympathomimetics to be discussed may also depend on this mechanism for terminating their adrenergic actions.

Catechol-O-Methyl Transferase (COMT). Catechol-O-methyl transferase is an enzyme that is widely distributed in the soluble cytoplasmic fraction of cells and plasma and that has no selective localization within ad-

renergic nerves. This enzyme transfers a methyl group to the 3-hydroxy position of the catechol nucleus (Fig. 6–2). The methoxy derivative of the catecholamine has only a fraction of the pharmacologic activity of its parent structure.[19,20] COMT is a slow mechanism for terminating catecholamine response.

Monoamine Oxidase (MAO). Monoamine oxidase is mainly an intramitochondrial enzyme present in all sympathetic nerve terminals. MAO cleaves the amino group of catecholamines and oxidizes the terminal carbon to an acid (mandelic acid) that is pharmacologically inactive (Figs. 6–1, 6–2). MAO is believed to be important in maintaining proper levels of catecholamine in sympathetic nerve terminals. Inhibition of MAO leads to some accumulation of

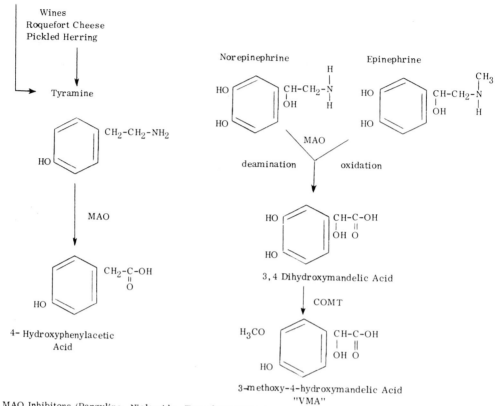

Fig. 6–2. Disposition of monoamines.

norepinephrine in the terminals, which has a clinical implication in the anesthetic management of patients taking MAO inhibitors (sometimes known as MAOI).[18,19,21,22]

Catecholamine-induced cardiac dysrhythmias

There are three important components to catecholamine-induced dysrhythmias: (1) *alpha*-adrenergic stimulation to produce peripheral vascular constriction, (2) vagal stimulation to suppress the rate of spontaneous depolarization of the sinoatrial node and of atrioventricular (AV) conduction,

and (3) myocardial *beta*-adrenergic stimulation to produce tachycardia and to increase automaticity of excitable cardiac cells. Cardiac dysrhythmias can develop without the simultaneous presence of all three components, especially in patients with preexisting myocardial ischemia (for example, myocardial infarction, congestive heart failure, hypotension or hypertension, congenital or acquired heart disease, or cardiac trauma). Rational treatment of cardiac dysrhythmias during anesthesia requires the correct diagnosis of its cause. Before making the diagnosis, the physician should focus immediate attention on oxygen delivery to the patient and adequate maintenance of blood pressure. Most supraventricular dysrhythmias with acceptable blood pressures are self-limiting, provided the anesthetic depth, oxygen delivery, and tissue perfusion are satisfactory. Bradycardia with junctional rhythm frequently responds to intravenous atropine, 0.2 to 0.4 mg, whereas junctional rhythm without bradycardia may respond to intravenous succinylcholine, 20 mg/70 kg.[5] Intravenous lidocaine (4 mg/ml; 4 mg/min) or 1 to 2 mg/kg bolus is an effective treatment for ventricular extrasystoles.[23,24] Catecholamine-induced ventricular extrasystoles may be more specifically antagonized by propranolol administered in 1-mg doses.[25,26]

Factors (nondrug-induced) that increase sympathetic activity

1. *Carbon dioxide*. Hypercapnia induces adrenal medullary release of epinephrine directly.[27-29]
2. *Pheochromocytoma*. Large amounts of catecholamines are released by this adrenal medullary tumor.[30,31]
3. *Hyperthyroidism*. Thyroid hormone potentiates the cardiovascular responses to catecholamines.[32-34]

4. *Congestive heart failure*. Patients with uncompensated myocardial failure have elevated blood levels of circulating catecholamines with a simultaneous reduction in myocardial catecholamine content.[35-38]
5. *Sympathectomy*. Denervated sympathetic organs are hypersensitive to exogenously administered catecholamines.[39]
6. *Spinal cord transection*. The sympathetic nervous system is hyperactive in response to certain stimuli (for example, cold and bladder distension).[40]

Since discussion of these factors is beyond the scope of this chapter, the indicated references should be consulted for detailed information.

AGENTS THAT INFLUENCE NORMAL ADRENERGIC MECHANISMS

The biosynthesis of catecholamines and some enzyme inhibitors is summarized in Table 6–1. *Alpha*-methyldopa, MAO inhibitors, and disulfiram are enzyme inhibitors with important clinical anesthetic implications.

Table 6–1
Biosynthesis and metabolism of catecholamines

		Enzyme	Enzyme Inhibitors
Phenylalanine ↓	←	hydroxylase	
Tyrosine ↓	←	hydroxylase ←	*alpha*-methyl-p-tyrosine
DOPA ↓	rate limiting ←	decarboxylase ←	*alpha*-methyldopa (Aldomet)
Dopamine ↓	←	*beta*-hydroxylase ←	disulfiram (Antabuse)
Norepinephrine ↓	rate limiting ←	N-methyltransferase	
Epinephrine ↓	←	COMT ←	Pyrogallol, Tropolone
Metanephrine ↓	←	MAO ←	MAO Inhibitor (Pargyline)
Vanillylmandelic acid			

Agents that decrease sympathetic activity

Disulfiram (Antabuse). Disulfiram is used to treat chronic alcoholism.[41] Treatment of the alcoholic patient with disulfiram causes an accumulation of acetaldehyde in the body following ingestion of alcohol. Acetaldehyde is produced by the initial oxidation of ethanol by alcohol dehydrogenase in the liver and is further oxidized to acetic acid. Disulfiram not only inhibits the rate of oxidation of acetaldehyde, but also inhibits dopamine *beta*-hydroxylase, which is needed for the synthesis of norepinephrine from dopamine.[42,43] Hypotension could develop, especially in the anesthetized patient.

Alpha-*methyldopa (Aldomet).* Alpha-methyldopa is a decarboxylase inhibitor that interferes with the formation of dopamine (Fig. 6–1). More important, its structural similarity with DOPA allows *alpha*-methyldopa to act as a false transmitter. The decarboxylated *alpha*-methyldopa (*alpha*-methylnorepinephrine) is stored in the adrenergic nerve terminal and is released by neural stimulation. However, *alpha*-methylnorepinephrine has only a fraction of the potency of normally synthesized catecholamines. *Alpha*-methyldopa is commonly used to treat patients with moderate hypertension (diastolic pressure 100 to 120 torr) and can theoretically exert a hypotensive effect during general or regional anesthesia.[44] However, there are no published data to indicate the incidence of alarming hypotension in the anesthetized patient who has been taking *alpha*-methyldopa. Adequate volume replacement with balanced electrolyte solution and/or blood or blood products prevents hypotension. *Alpha*-methyldopa does not significantly inhibit the synthesis of norepinephrine, as demonstrated by normal urinary vanillylmandelic acid excretion during *alpha*-methyldopa therapy.[45] Moderate hypotension caused by *alpha*-methyldopa is characterized by a decline in cardiac output, whereas peripheral vascular resistance is significantly reduced.[46–49] Preoperative interruption of *alpha*-methyldopa therapy is unnecessary, although careful intraoperative monitoring is essential.

Reserpine (Serpasil). Reserpine is an alkaloid of rauwolfia serpentina that is believed to exert its antihypertensive effect by depletion of catecholamine storage granules in the adrenergic nerve terminals of the brain, the heart, and the blood vessels (Fig. 6–1).[50–53] Depletion is slower and less complete in the adrenal medulla. It is commonly used to treat patients with mild hypertension (diastolic pressure of 90 to 100 torr), for which reserpine's sedative and bradycardic effects are desirable.[44] The latency of onset of orally administered reserpine is about one week; a full effect is achieved in three to four weeks. Likewise, reserpine's cardiovascular and other effects may persist for two to four weeks following its withdrawal. The parenteral injection of reserpine exerts a hypotensive effect in 15 to 30 minutes, with a maximal response in two to four hours.

Earlier reports indicated the need for the discontinuance of reserpine therapy two weeks prior to the administration of anesthesia. The reasons given for the withdrawal of rauwolfia therapy are (1) that the depletion of catecholamine stores can produce profound hypotension during general anesthesia,[54,55] (2) that the cardiovascular response to exogenous administration of sympathomimetic drugs may be unpredictable,[54–58] and (3) that reserpine may exert a neurodepressant action on reflex baroreceptor mechanisms.[54–58]

Munson and Jenicek observed no significant decrease in the incidence or severity of hypotension during anesthesia of patients whose rauwolfia therapy was continued up to the day of anesthesia in comparison with patients whose therapy was discontinued 10 to 14 days before elective surgical procedures.[59] Therefore, they concluded that rauwolfia therapy need not be discontinued before anesthesia and surgical procedures, but that it is important for the anesthesiologist to be aware of the patient's drug intake and to consider this in anesthetic management.[59] Katz et al. drew similar conclusions from observations in 100 patients undergoing rauwolfia therapy.

Hypertensive patients are frequently hypovolemic.[60,61,62] All general anesthetics produce a direct depressant effect on the cardiovascular system. Therefore, an anesthetic that causes the least cardiovascular depression when compared with others of equal potency is the best choice. Methoxyflurane or narcotic-N_2O-O_2 ("balanced" anesthesia) produces less hypotension than halothane or enflurane. In my experience, patients who are adequately controlled by the oral administration of reserpine alone require no interruption of therapy. Hypotension may be minimized by intravascular replacement prior to and during anesthetic induction.[58–60,63,64] Suggested guidelines are the infusion of 15 ml/kg of balanced crystalloid solution during the night before an operation and 7 to 10 ml/kg of crystalloid solution during induction of anesthesia. Patients with total serum protein of less than 5 gm% (normal = 6 to 9 gm%) are also benefited by the infusion of 5% Purified Protein Fraction (that is, 12.5 gm albumin/250 ml) to reduce intravascular fluid shift to the interstitial space. Vasopressors should be used only for temporary support of arterial blood pressure, and the vasopressor chosen should not entirely depend on the endogenous release of stored catecholamines.[65–68]

A percutaneous arterial catheter for continuous pressure monitoring and ECG observations are useful for the optimal care of any patient with a labile cardiovascular system.

Guanethidine (Ismelin). Guanethidine is one of the most potent antihypertensive drugs used today. Thus its use has been generally limited to patients with a diastolic pressure in excess of 120 torr.[44] Its potent hypotensive effect is the result of several pharmacologic actions on the sympathetic nervous system: (1) blockade of postganglionic adrenergic nerve transmission and (2) displacement of norepinephrine from granular storage (Fig. 6–1).[69–71] Guanethidine has little effect on the catecholamine content of the adrenal medulla and penetrates the central nervous system (CNS) poorly following systemic administration. The hypotensive effects of guanethidine reach a maximum in 10 to 14 days. Similarly, its hypotensive effects persist for several days after its withdrawal. The therapeutic benefit of guanethidine can be antagonized by tricyclic antidepressants.[72]

Important anesthetic considerations for the management of patients undergoing prolonged guanethidine therapy are related to the drug's pharmacologic actions. Hypotension is accentuated by CNS depressants. The induced chemical sympathectomy may result in increased fluid accumulation in the body and decreased myocardial performance, leading to overt heart failure. However, withdrawal of guanethidine in a severely hypertensive patient may result in undesirable rebound hypertension.

Clonidine (Catapres). Clonidine is a potent antihypertensive drug that is gaining popularity in the treatment of moderate to severe hypertension. Clonidine is structurally similar to tolazoline (Priscoline) and likewise has been shown to have some *alpha*-adrenergic blocking activity.[73] Clonidine's antihypertensive effect is attributed to the inhibition of the bulbar sympathetic cardiovascular and sympathetic vasoconstrictor centers.[74,75] Severe rebound hypertension has been reported when clonidine therapy is terminated abruptly.[76] This rebound hypertension may also occur following the patient's emergence from general anesthesia.[77] Gradual replacement of clonidine with another antihypertensive agent several days before an operation may be helpful.[77] However, continued clonidine therapy without interruption, including the day of an operation, is also recommended.

Propranolol (Inderal). The *beta*-adrenergic receptors were first described by Ahlquist in 1948 and have been further differentiated pharmacologically into *beta* 1 and *beta* 2 receptors.[78,79,80] Stimulation of *beta* 1 receptors produces positive inotropic and chronotropic effects on the heart, whereas stimulation of *beta* 2 receptors results in vasodilation of pulmonary and peripheral vasculature. Propranolol blocks both *beta* 1- and *beta* 2-adrenergic receptors. Blockade of these receptors results in reduced inotropy and chronotropy, decreased velocity of mechanical systole, prolonged AV conduction, and hypotension.[25,26,81] In the presence of preexisting partial heart block, administration of propranolol may cause complete AV dissociation and cardiac arrest. Peripheral resistance is increased by the reflex compensatory mechanism, and blood flow to all tissues except the brain is reduced.[82] Propranolol is used in the treatment of cardiac arrhythmias, angina pectoris, and the cardiovascular manifestations of thyrotoxicosis.[83] Although propranolol is used as an adjunct to other antihypertensive agents, its myocardial depressant effects may preclude its long-term use in the continuous treatment of essential hypertension.[81]

Anesthetic management of the patient with cardiac disease who requires propranolol for control of angina pectoris is still subject to debate. Should this drug be discontinued before operation? If so, when? The plasma half-life in man is approximately three hours.[84] No plasma level or atrial depressant effect from propranolol can be found 48 hours after discontinuation.[85] Propranolol and its active metabolite, 4-hydroxypropranolol, are primarily excreted in the urine.

Sudden withdrawal of propranolol is associated with recurrence of angina, dysrhythmias, and even myocardial infarction.[86–88] Kaplan et al. show that propranolol can be given safely to within 24 to 48 hours of a coronary artery bypass operation and then discontinued under close medical supervision without an increase in prebypass or postbypass complications.[89] If pain recurs, propranolol can be resumed and administered to within 12 hours of an operation. Others recommend a gradual withdrawal of propranolol over several days.[87] Patients requiring coronary artery revascu-

larization are suffering from a myocardial oxygen debt manifested by pain and inadequate cardiac function. Some return of sympathetic integrity to the myocardium may allow the heart to function more effectively during anesthesia and the postoperative period.

Drug Interactions with Propranolol. The positive inotropic effect of digitalis is not antagonized by propranolol, although both drugs can depress AV conduction. Propranolol is considered effective in treating digitalis-induced arrhythmias.[25] However, caution should be exercised when these two drugs are used concurrently, because their additive effect on AV conduction may lead to complete heart block.

Large doses of morphine are known to release histamine and increase airway resistance in man.[16,90] *Beta*-adrenergic blockade also increases airway resistance. There is potential danger of an additive effect when morphine and propranolol are used concurrently. Propranolol should not be administered to patients with asthma.

Anesthetic agents such as diethyl ether and cyclopropane liberate endogenous catecholamines. Elevation of peripheral resistance in the presence of myocardial depression can be detrimental to the left ventricle. On the other hand, judicious administration of halothane, narcotics, and methoxyflurane is used successfully for cardiac operations in patients taking propranolol.[91] Although enflurane is also used successfully in cardiac operations, hypotension during induction is common, which probably is not from myocardial depression per se.[92–94] Overall, enflurane is compatible with propranolol for coronary revascularization operations. It is difficult to be specific because data on the interaction of propranolol and general anesthetics are lacking.

Chlorpromazine and Lithium Carbonate. Twenty per cent of all prescriptions written in the United States are for medications intended to treat psychiatric disorders.[95] Chlorpromazine, the prototype of the phenothiazine derivatives, is still widely used. Chlorpromazine produces many pharmacologic actions including antihyperthermia, antihistamine, CNS sedation, antiemesis, and *alpha*-adrenergic inhibition.[96] The last is the result of the blockade of postsynaptic *alpha*-adrenergic receptors and reuptake of norepinephrine into adrenergic nerve terminals (Fig. 6–1). Orthostatic hypotension and reflex tachycardia are common in patients taking chlorpromazine. Discontinuance is probably unnecessary if the drug is required for maintaining psychiatric equilibrium in the patient. Since it also possesses a CNS-depressant action, the effect of preoperative sedatives may be potentiated. Intraoperative management is not a major problem, but the anesthesiologist should be aware of the potential hypotensive additive effects of general anesthetics and of narcotic analgesics in combination with chlorpromazine and other phenothiazines. Direct-acting *alpha*-adrenergic stimulants (methoxamine or phenylephrine) would be more effective than indirect-acting *alpha*-adrenergic stimulants in overcoming the phenothiazine-induced hypotension.

Lithium carbonate is becoming popular in the treatment of various psychiatric disorders.[97] Lithium inhibits acetylcholine synthesis and release from the cholinergic nerve terminal. It also replaces sodium during cellular depolarization and antagonizes the pressor response to norepinephrine in man.[98] Lithium carbonate has been shown to potentiate the neuromuscular blocking actions of pancuronium, succinylcholine, and decamethonium.[99,100] (See Chap. 13.)

General Guidelines. Reasons for uninterrupted antihypertensive therapy:

1. Temporary withdrawal of antihypertensive drugs may be helpful, but it does not insure a more stable anesthetic course.
2. Withdrawal of drugs in patients with severe hypertension may precipitate:
   a. Renal damage by diastolic pressures above 140 torr.
   b. Cardiac failure from left ventricular strain.
   c. Cerebral vascular accident.
   d. Decreased blood volume.
   e. Inconveniences of delay to the patient and the hospital.

When antihypertensive therapy is not interrupted, the following considerations are helpful:

1. Prophylactic intravascular replacement with crystalloids and plasma expanders.
2. Importance of assuring a smooth induction of anesthesia.
3. Avoidance of abrupt postural changes and excessive intra-abdominal manipulation.
4. Avoidance of abrupt increases in anesthetic concentration.
5. Avoidance of playing "catch-up" in blood loss.

Agents that increase sympathetic activity

Monoamine Oxidase (MAO) Inhibitors (Pargyline, Phenelzine, Tranylcypromine). The MAO inhibitors block oxidative deamination (Figs. 6–1 and 6–2) of naturally occurring monoamines. These inhibitors do not inhibit synthesis of biogenic amines, which accumulate in the adrenergic nerve terminal.[22] After the administration of a large dose of MAO inhibitor, norepinephrine, epinephrine, dopamine, and 5-hydroxytryptamine levels increase in the brain, heart, intestine, and blood.[101] Successful treatment of psychotic depressions may be related to their ability to elevate endogenous amines. Although MAO inhibitors may be present in the body for a short time only, they produce long-lasting, irreversible inhibition of the enzyme. Regeneration of MAO after the discontinuance of drug therapy may take weeks.

Acute overdosage may produce agitation, hallucinations, hyperpyrexia, convulsions, hypertension, or hypotension. Orthostatic hypotension is common in patients taking MAO inhibitors. The action of sympathomimetic amines is potentiated by MAO inhibitors; adrenergic drugs with partial or complete indirect actions (for example, ephedrine, amphetamine, tyramine) may produce exaggerated release of neuronal catecholamines.[101] The ingestion of cheese, wine, and pickled herring, which have a high tyramine content, can precipitate a hypertensive crisis.[21] Reflex sympathetic stimulation is similarly intensified. MAO inhibitors can also prolong and intensify the effects of CNS depressants including alcohol, barbiturates, anesthetics, and potent analgesics, although the mechanism of this potentiating effect of MAO inhibitors is unclear.[101] Adverse CNS interactions, such as convulsions, coma, and hyperthermia, have been reported with tricyclic antidepressants, especially imipramine and amitriptyline.[102] To change a patient from a MAO inhibitor to a tricyclic antidepressant requires a respite of two weeks. Hyperpyrexia is a serious reaction to the combined use of MAO inhibitors and meperidine.

The discontinuance of MAO inhibitors for at least two weeks is advisable prior to an elective operation. When a surgical procedure is performed on an emergency basis, conduction anesthesia without sympathomimetic drugs is preferable. If general anesthesia is required, an inhalation anesthetic with a low propensity to induce catecholamine-dependent dysrhythmias is advised (see the discussion on general anesthetics and catecholamines). Balanced anesthesia using large doses of morphine should be approached with care, since morphine in large quantities releases catecholamines from the adrenals.[16] If hypertensive episodes occur, agents that produce *alpha*-adrenergic blockade (chlorpromazine, phentolamine), ganglionic blockade (trimethaphan, pentolinium), or direct vasodilation (nitroprusside) may be used.

Other Antidepressants.

Tricyclic Antidepressants. Imipramine, desipramine, amitriptyline, and other closely related drugs have almost replaced MAO inhibitors in the treatment of psychotic depression because there are fewer side effects associated with the continued use of the tricyclic antidepressants.[103] The mechanism by which imipramine exerts its antidepressant action in psychotic depression is not clear. All tricyclic antidepressants block the reuptake of norepinephrine by adrenergic nerve terminals (Fig. 6–1). Synthesis and release of catecholamines are not affected. About two to five weeks must pass before the CNS-therapeutic effects of the drug are evident. With a reduction in catecholamine storage and a demonstrable anticholinergic effect of these drugs, orthostatic hypotension, tachycardia, and cardiac dysrhythmias are commonly observed.[103] The most frequent ECG change following imipramine therapy is inversion or flattening of the T wave. The combined use of imipramine and guanethidine may result in cardiac standstill.[104] The concurrent administration of MAO inhibitors and these drugs can produce convulsions, coma, and hyperpyrexia.[102] Other drug interactions include the potentiation of CNS depressants, the antagonism of the antihypertensive effects of guanethidine, and the potentiation of the pressor effects of sympathomimetic amines.[105] Similarly, imipramine is expected to augment intraoperatively induced sympathetic activity.[106] In spite of these unusual problems, the discontinuance of tricyclic antidepressants prior to an operation is probably unnecessary.

Amphetamine. Amphetamine is structurally similar to sympathomimetic amines except that it has a powerful CNS-stimulating action in addition to its peripheral *alpha*- and *beta*-adrenergic stimulatory effects. The acute toxic effects of amphetamine are an extension of its therapeutic effects and are usually the result of overdosage. The CNS effects commonly include restlessness, hyperreflexia, fever, and irritability. The cardiovascular effects may include hypertension, tachycardia, cardiac dysrhythmias, and circulatory collapse.

There is a lack of published data on the interaction of amphetamine and anesthetics on the CNS and cardiovascular systems. With normal anorexic and cerebral-stimulating doses, no serious anesthetic problems are likely. Chlorpromazine is helpful in controlling CNS symptoms and hypertension resulting from an acute amphetamine overdose. Amphetamine has been shown to increase anesthetic requirement in dogs by virtue of its CNS-stimulatory effects.[106a] The depletion of CNS catecholamines with repeated amphetamine intake may reduce the required anesthetic dose.[106a]

Cocaine. Cocaine is an alkaloid of *Erythroxylon coca.* It was introduced as a local anesthetic in clinical practice in 1884 by Koller.[107]

The structural similarities of cocaine, procaine, and atropine may account for some of the important pharmacologic actions of cocaine (Fig. 6–3), such as (a) local anesthesia, (b) CNS stimulation, (c) peripheral vascular constriction and tachycardia, (d) blockage of the uptake of catecholamines at adrenergic nerve endings (Fig. 6–1) and subsequent potentiation of the responses of sympathetic innervated organs to epinephrine and norepinephrine.

The significant vasoconstrictor property of cocaine is desirable for hemostasis in otolaryngologic surgery. The addition of epinephrine to cocaine for additional vasoconstriction is of questionable value, especially when one considers the hazards of hypertension and cardiac arrhythmias produced by the cocaine-epinephrine interaction.[108] Anderton and Nassar show that, in patients undergoing nasal operations and anesthetized with halothane-N_2O-O_2, the topical administration of cocaine, 20 mg, dissolved in 2 ml of saline without epinephrine produces adequate nasal decongestion without serious cardiovascular problems.[109]

The fatal dose of cocaine in man is estimated at 1.2 g, but the usual maximal dose in clinical practice is about 200 mg.[110] Toxic effects are reported from doses as low as 20 mg.[110] Habitual use of cocaine could enhance intrinsic sympathetic activity in man as well as potentiate the effects of sympathomimetic agents.

ANESTHETIC INFLUENCE ON SYMPATHOMIMETIC AGENTS

In 1895, Oliver and Schaefer first showed that adrenal extract produced ventricular fibrillation in a dog anesthetized with chloroform.[111] The pioneering work of Meek et al. used an arrhythmogenic dose of 10 μg/kg epinephrine diluted in 5 ml of normal saline solution, which was injected into dogs at the rate of 1 ml/10 sec.[112] Electrocardiographic changes were carefully monitored. More recently, other researchers have used the appearance of ventricular extrasystoles as the endpoint following incremental doses of epinephrine.[113–117] The study of exogenously administered epinephrine-induced cardiac dysrhythmias is a useful method of evaluating the arrhythmogenicity of anesthetics. Although there are other chemical or mechanical means of inducing cardiac dysrhythmias, the use of epinephrine has particular clinical relevance during anesthesia. Intraoperative cardiac dysrhythmias are frequently associated with the imbalance of the autonomic nervous system, usually a preponderance of sympathetic activity.

Epinephrine is commonly used to reduce

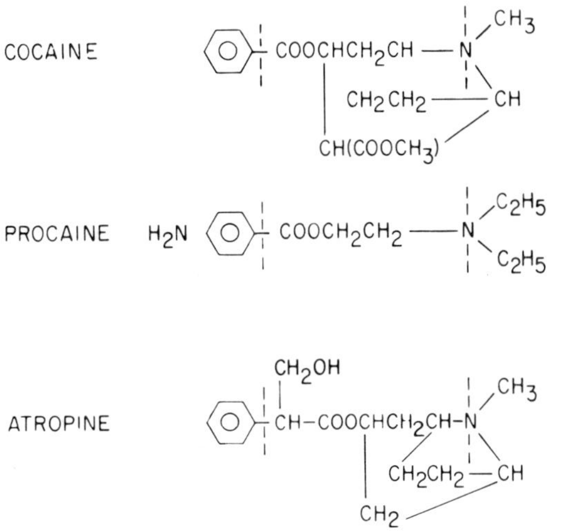

Fig. 6–3. Structural comparison of cocaine, procaine, and atropine.

surgical bleeding. The well-known publications of the Columbia group recommend that the epinephrine dose in adults for hemostasis during halothane-N_2O-O_2 anesthesia should not exceed 10 ml of 1:100,000 in any given 10-minute period nor 30 ml per hour.[10] Ten milliliters of 1:100,000 epinephrine is equal to 100 μg or to about 1.5 μg/kg/10 min (for a 70-kg person). This dosage guide may be safely used for other halogenated inhalation anesthetics, since the combination of halothane and epinephrine is more arrhythmogenic than the others. It is convenient to use a commercially prepared, dilute lidocaine-epinephrine solution, for example, Xylocaine 0.5% with epinephrine 1:100,000. Evidence suggests that the addition of Xylocaine may reduce the severity of potential dysrhythmias induced by epinephrine.[115] However, under conditions of increased endogenous sympathetic activity, hyperthyroidism or hypercapnia, for example, the arrhythmogenicity of epinephrine is enhanced.

Because of different experimental designs, it is difficult to compare the results from different studies. In spite of this, some conclusions are evident. Diethyl ether is still the least sensitizing drug, whereas cyclopropane is the most sensitizing to epinephrine-induced or intraoperative dysrhythmias (Table 6–2). The halogenated ethers are less sensitizing than halothane. The mechanism for this "sensitizing" effect on the myocardium is not understood; the elevation of arterial blood pressure, the slowing of the sinoatrial rate, and the increase of myocardial automaticity are components that contribute to catecholamine-induced dysrhythmias, as discussed. A rela-

Table 6–2

Dosage of epinephrine required to produce ventricular dysrhythmias in man and dog

Anesthetic	Species	Dosage (μg/kg)	Investigator
Diethyl ether	Dog	10*	Meek et al. (1937)[112]
	Man	10–20†	Wong et al. (1974 and unpublished data)[120]
Fluroxene	Dog	43–48	Joas & Stevens (1971)[116]
	Dog	10*	Wong et al. (1977)[185]
Isoflurane	Dog	22–37	Joas & Stevens (1971)[116]
	Man	6.72 ± 0.66	Johnston et al. (1976)[115]
Methoxyflurane	Dog	14.0 ± 4.7	Munson & Tucker (1975)[113]
	Dog	10–50	Bamforth (1961)[117]
	Man	1–2‡	Hudon (1961)[123]
Enflurane	Dog	17.1 ± 7.2	Munson & Tucker (1975)[113]
	Man	10.9 ± 8.9	Johnston et al. (1960)[115]
Halothane	Dog	4.6 ± 3.3	Munson & Tucker (1975)[113]
	Dog	5–8	Joas & Stevens (1971)[116]
	Man	2.11 ± 0.15	Johnston et al. (1976)[115]
	Man	1.7§	Katz et al. (1962)[10]
Cyclopropane	Dog	1–2	Dresel et al. (1960)[119]
	Man	up to 7 in 30 min**	Matteo et al. (1963)[122]
	Dog	10	Meek et al. (1937)[112]

* Occasional nodal rhythm.
† Occasional ventricular arrhythmias. Stable cardiac rhythm during induced hypothermia of infants requiring cardiac surgery.
‡ Occasional wandering pacemaker.
§ Recommended safe dose.
** Ventricular arrhythmias in 30% patients.

tive ranking of drug sensitivity to epinephrine-induced dysrhythmias is listed, as follows (1 = least sensitive, 5 = most sensitive):

Diethyl ether	1
Fluroxene (Fluoromar)	2
Isoflurane (Forane)	2
Methoxyflurane (Penthrane)	3
Enflurane (Ethrane)	3
Halothane (Fluothane)	4
Cyclopropane	5

The dog is more resistant than man to the arrhythmogenic effect of epinephrine (Table 6–2). However, there is a qualitative similarity between the two species in their response to the effects of anesthetic-epinephrine interaction. It is the general clinical impression that balanced anesthesia (that is, narcotic-N_2O-muscle relaxant) produces minimal disturbance of the cardiovascular system. Dogs anesthetized with a narcotic (morphine, fentanyl or meperidine), N_2O, and pancuronium demonstrated virtually no ventricular tachycardia from intravenous epinephrine; in contrast, dogs anesthetized with halothane or enflurane-N_2O-pancuronium were prone to develop ventricular tachycardia during the epinephrine challenge.[17a] Minimal anesthesia consisting of 70% N_2O and d-tubocurarine or gallamine also protected dogs from epinephrine-induced ventricular tachycardia or fibrillation.[118]

SYMPATHOMIMETIC ANESTHETICS

Phencyclidine (Ketamine)

Ketamine produces anesthesia by the stimulation of the medulla and limbic systems of the brain and by the simultaneous depression of the cortex.[124–126] The cardiovascular system is stimulated by anesthetic doses of ketamine, which causes a significant elevation in cerebrospinal fluid (CSF) pressure, heart rate, and mean arterial blood pressure. The work of Traber et al. suggests that this stimulation of the cardiovascular system may be of central origin

and thereby would require an intact sympathetic nervous system. Whether ketamine causes the depression of the baroreceptors is uncertain.[127–131]

Ketamine blocks the neuronal reuptake of catecholamines (Fig. 6–1) in a manner similar to that of cocaine.[132,133] Ketamine probably enhances the arrhythmogenicity of epinephrine in dogs anesthetized with halothane-N_2O-O_2.[134] In larger dogs, direct myocardial depression occurs.[130] We found that ketamine potentiates the cardiotonic effects of norepinephrine, epinephrine, and tyramine, whereas it antagonizes the cardiotonic effects of isoproterenol and dopamine.[135] A possible explanation for this difference is that there are two neuronal uptake processes for vasoactive amines. Uptake 1 (intraneuronal) has greater affinity for norepinephrine; Uptake 2 (extraneuronal) has greater affinity for isoproterenol. Cocaine and ketamine preferentially block the Uptake 1 process.

Ketamine should be used with caution in patients who have myocardial disease or who are taking drugs that further exaggerate sympathetic activities.

Dioxolanes (Dexoxadrol and Etoxadrol)

The dioxolanes possess pharmacologic properties similar to those of ketamine but are structurally quite dissimilar from ketamine. Etoxadrol (CL-1848C, Cutter Laboratories), 0.75 mg/kg, was administered intravenously to 11 adult male volunteers. The duration of unconsciousness induced by this single dose was from 50 to 85 minutes. Analgesia and amnesia usually surpassed the duration of unconsciousness. Cardiac output, heart rate, and arterial blood pressure were significantly elevated for 120 minutes following the drug injection with minimal undesirable psychologic side effects.[136] No subject experienced hallucination in the postarousal period. The clinical use of this longer-acting ketamine-like drug awaits further studies in man.

SYMPATHOMIMETIC AGENTS IN SHOCK

CASE REPORT

A 55-year-old man involved in an automobile accident arrived at the emergency room in shock. The only significant history was digoxin and furosemide intake for over five years for "heart trouble." He was complaining of severe pain in the left upper quadrant of the abdomen and rebound tenderness. Cuff arterial blood pressure, taken from the brachial artery, was 60/40 torr with a thready pulse of 160/min. His skin was pale, cold, and clammy to the touch. Laboratory tests showed a hematocrit of 24% and serum potassium concentration of 2.8 meq/L. No urine was obtainable for analysis. The ECG showed a depressed ST segment with first-degree AV block and occasional ventricular extrasystoles. Roentgenograms revealed fracture of ribs 7, 8, and 9 on the right side; the flat and upright films of the abdomen suggested increased opacity with demonstrable air under the diaphragm. Bloody fluid was aspirated by paracentesis. A presumptive diagnosis of ruptured spleen and bowel with hemorrhagic shock was made. Preoperative preparation of the patient was carried out in the surgical intensive care unit for a scheduled exploratory laparotomy and splenectomy.

However, before the patient was brought to the operating room, he developed episodes of ventricular fibrillation in the intensive care unit. Electrical countershock was effective in defibrillating the heart, but each time ventricular fibrillation recurred after a few minutes of regular cardiac rhythm. Assuming there was continued intra-abdominal bleeding perpetuating the labile cardiovascular state, the physicians rushed the patient to the operating room. Upon arrival, the following were noted: (1) the patient's trachea had been intubated (during the cardiopulmonary resuscitation) and the lungs mechanically ventilated; (2) one liter of 5% dextrose in water and a unit of albumin were running into a peripheral venous catheter; (3) one liter of dilute epinephrine (1 μg/ml) in 5% dextrose in water was being administered through a central venous pressure (CVP) catheter; (4) the bladder was catheterized, but there was no urine in the receptacle; (5) no auscultatory pressures were obtainable from a pressure cuff around the upper arm, but there was a palpable carotid pulse; (6) his temperature was 34.5°C; and (7) the patient was still conscious.

Diazepam 10 mg and pancuronium 7 mg were administered intravenously while another intravenous catheter was established. The patient was mechanically ventilated with 100% O_2 and the operation began. Intravenous replacement now consisted of albumin and 5% dextrose in lactated Ringer's solution with KCl 40 meq/L added. The patient continued to exhibit ventricular extrasystoles. When the radial pulse became palpable, a percutaneous catheter was placed in the radial artery for continuous pressure monitoring. An immediate arterial blood gas yielded P_{O_2}—120 torr, P_{CO_2}—24 torr, pH—7.2 and negative base excess—8.4 meq/L; serum [Na]—142 meq/L and serum [K]—2.7 meq/L. The metabolic acidosis was corrected following two injections of $NaHCO_3$ 50 meq, and the respiratory alkalosis was corrected by reduction of mechanical ventilation.

The epinephrine solution was replaced by dopamine (5 to 10 μg/kg/min). Following infusion of four units of warmed whole blood, two liters of crystalloid solution, and two units of albumin, there was evidence of urine formation and of increased need for anesthesia. Serum [K] had increased from 2.7 to 3.4 meq/L without additional intravenous KCl. The number of ventricular extrasystoles appearing on the ECG reduced to one to two per minute. Hemorrhage was controlled after the removal of the ruptured spleen and the operation was successful. The patient was discharged after 22 days of hospitalization.

What may be some of the contributing factors to the patient's repeated occurrences of ventricular fibrillation prior to the operation? These factors include hypotension, hypoxia, acidosis, hypothermia, hypocapnia, and hypokalemia. Adverse responses to epinephrine and other catecholamines are common under such circumstances. These factors will be discussed further.

The pathophysiology of low perfusion states will be reviewed before the discussion of the sympathomimetic drugs. Comments will then be directed toward the anesthetic management of the hypotensive patient.

Pathogenesis of shock

Shock is a state of inadequate tissue perfusion. The low-flow state in vital organs is the final common denominator in all forms of shock, which results from failure of one or more of the following separate but interrelated factors:[137] (1) the pump (heart), (2) the content and volume of the intravascular space (blood), (3) the arteriolar tone, and (4) the venous tone. Thus it is clinically useful to classify shock in terms of (1) primary pump failure—cardiogenic shock, (2) reduction of intravascular volume—hypovolemic shock, and (3) changes in arteriolar or venous tone—neurogenic and/or septic shock.

Microcirculation. The result of inadequate tissue perfusion is the lack of tissue-blood exchange of gases and metabolic substrates that occurs primarily at the terminal vascular bed, that is, in the arterioles, capillaries, and venules (Fig. 6–4). The arterioles are especially sensitive to sympathetic stimulation. Changes in the caliber of the arterioles provide for the maintenance of blood pressure and volume flow through the capillary beds. However, without adequate intra-arterial volume, arteriolar constriction would reduce capillary perfusion. The venous system normally contains about two-thirds of the total intravascular volume. Sympathetic stimulation also increases venous tone, thus delivering more blood to the arterial system. Humoral agents, pH, and acidic metabolites are important factors in the regulation of capillary blood flow through actions exerted on terminal arterioles, pre- and postcapillary sphincters, venules, and capillaries, where transcapillary exchange occurs.[138-142] Cardiac filling and regulation of active (arterial) blood volume are governed by the muscular venules and veins.

Vasomotion is a unique feature of the microcirculation that provides a cyclic opening and closing of the pre- and postcapillary sphincters to change the perfusion pattern of capillary beds. Vasomotion is probably the most important vasomotor determinant of capillary blood flow and transcapillary ex-

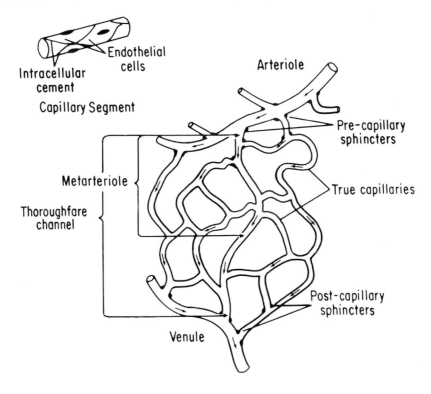

Fig. 6–4. Schematic drawing of the microcirculation. See details in text. (Adapted from Zauder, H. L.: *Pharmacology of Adjuvant Drugs.* (Clinical Anesthesia Series.) Philadelphia, F. A. Davis, 1973.)

change. It can be influenced by local tissue and humoral agents as well as by physical factors.[138–142]

The terminal-phase shock, then, represents a decompensation of the physiologic controls of microcirculation. Since this is a simplistic approach to a complex problem, the reader is referred to several excellent sources for more complete treatment of the subject.[137–144]

Classification of sympathomimetic agents

Alpha- *and* **Beta-***Adrenergic Receptors.* In 1948, Ahlquist postulated the existence of *alpha-* and *beta*-adrenergic receptors in the body.[78] The stimulation of *alpha*-adrenergic receptors leads to vasoconstriction and pupillary dilation, whereas the stimulation of *beta*-adrenergic receptors leads to positive inotropic and chronotropic effects on the heart, vasodilation, and bronchodilation. As described, *beta*-adrenergic receptors have been further differentiated more recently into the categories *beta* 1 (exerting cardiac stimulation) and *beta* 2 (exerting bronchial and peripheral vasodilation).[79,80]

The action of dopamine on adrenergic receptors is different from that of the other catecholamines. The renal vasodilatory effect of dopamine is not antagonized by *beta*-adrenergic blockers, atropine, or antihistamines. Thus the term "dopaminergic receptor" is used to describe its actions.

Direct Versus Indirect Action. Direct action implies a drug-receptor interaction without releasing endogenous catecholamines from the adrenergic nerve terminals for its pharmacologic action. Direct-acting sympathomimetic amines are the catecholamines—epinephrine, norepinephrine, isoproterenol, and dopamine; and the adrenergic amines—methoxamine and phenylephrine. Indirect action implies that the drug acts primarily at a catecholamine storage site and requires the presence of endogenous catecholamines. Indirect-acting sympathomimetics include tyramine (an endogenous amine), amphetamine, and the more clinically useful agents ephedrine, metaraminol, and mephentermine.

Sympathomimetic drug actions

The use of sympathomimetic amines as an adjunct during anesthesia is ideally to improve tissue perfusion. Rational choice of a drug can be made only following the diagnosis of the cause of the hypotension or shock. Is it pump failure, hypovolemia, increased vascular capacitance, or a combination of these? The choice should be further weighed against its efficacy in patients with a history of drug therapy that influences the normal adrenergic mechanism. The vasoactive drugs should also be compatible with the anesthetic regimen. The rationale for the use of sympathomimetic agents should focus on the temporary support of the circulatory system until the cause can be corrected.

Common causes of hypotension during anesthesia are excessive depth of anesthesia, hypoxia, intravascular fluid loss, and surgical manipulation. Less common causes include myocardial infarction, pulmonary embolism, and cerebral vascular accident. The pharmacologic actions and arrhythmogenicity of several sympathomimetic agents used to treat hypotensive states are summarized in Table 6–3. Those agents with similar actions are expected to have similar interactions with drugs as well as pathophysiologic conditions discussed in this chapter. Table 6–3 is intended to assist the reader with the appropriate selection of a vasoactive agent. The pharmacologic actions of vasoactive agents are discussed briefly.

Catecholamines. All catecholamines are direct-acting agents. All except isoproterenol are synthesized in the body (Fig. 6–1). They are called "catechol" because they all possess a dihydroxybenzene (catechol) moiety.

Epinephrine (Adrenalin). Epinephrine, predominantly *beta* at low concentrations,

Table 6–3

Adrenergic drugs used in hypotension or shock

Drugs	Action		Cardiovascular Effects			Cardiac Output	Intravenous Dose	Arrhythmogenicity
	Receptor	Type	VC	VD	CS			
Catecholamines								
Epinephrine	α & β	Direct	++++	+++	++++	Increased	0.1–0.25 mg	+++++
Norepinephrine	α & β	Direct	+++++	0	+++	Unchanged or decreased	2–8 μg/min	++++
Isoproterenol	β_1 & β_2	Direct	0	+++++	++++	Increased	2–4 μg/min	++++
Dopamine	α & β	Direct & some indirect	++	++*	++	Increased	50–200 μg/min	+++
Sympathomimetics								
Methoxamine	α	Direct	++++	0	0	Decreased	5–10 mg	+
Phenylephrine	α	Direct	++++	0	0	Decreased	0.1–0.5 mg	+
Ephedrine	α & β	Indirect & some direct	++	+	+++	Increased	10–25 mg	++
Metaraminol	α & β	Indirect & some direct	+++	++	+	Decreased	0.5–5.0 mg	++
Mephentermine	α & β	Indirect	+	+++	++	Increased	5–15 mg	+

VC = vasoconstriction; VD = vasodilation; CS = cardiac stimulation
* Renal and mesenteric vasodilation caused by stimulation of "dopaminergic receptors."

stimulates both the *alpha* and *beta* receptors. In higher doses through *alpha*-adrenergic stimulation it constricts arterioles, precapillary sphincters, veins, and large arteries. Epinephrine is useful for cardiopulmonary resuscitation because it takes advantage of its positive inotropic and chronotropic effects (*beta*-receptor stimulation) and of the increase in coronary blood flow.[145] However, acidosis antagonizes the cardiovascular-stimulant actions of epinephrine and must be corrected in order to maximize the effect of epinephrine and other sympathomimetic amines. Hypothermia, hypercapnia, hypoxia, and hypokalemia potentiate epinephrine-induced cardiac dysrhythmias. Ventricular fibrillation should be corrected by countershock before the administration of intravenous bolus epinephrine for resuscitation. The simultaneous administration of lidocaine, 1 to 3 mg/kg, helps to reduce cardiac excitability and automaticity.

Epinephrine should be reserved for the most difficult cases during anesthesia and is generally contraindicated in patients with severe coronary disease. Epinephrine is the most arrhythmogenic of the catecholamines and is frequently used for hemostasis during an operation. Its interaction with halothane is of great concern to the anesthesiologist, as discussed.

Norepinephrine (Levophed). By means of *alpha*-adrenergic stimulation, norepinephrine causes marked vasoconstriction.[145,146] By means of *beta*-adrenergic stimulation, it also causes a positive inotropic and chronotropic effect. Its *alpha*-stimulating effect is dominant, and causes hypertension by an increase in peripheral vascular resistance with compensatory vagal reflex bradycardia. Cardiac output may decrease or remain unchanged. Coronary blood flow is elevated, as with epinephrine. The circulating volume may be reduced following the prolonged use of norepinephrine, probably owing to an increase in postcapillary vasoconstriction and a loss of protein-free fluid caused by the increased capillary pressure.

Norepinephrine should only be administered intravenously in dilute concentrations (4 μg/ml). The infusion site should be checked frequently for possible extravasation into the tissues, since local necrosis and sloughing of the skin is a dreaded complication. Sometimes without obvious extravasation, blanching along the course of the infused vein is seen. Infusion of an *alpha*-adrenergic blocker (for example, phentolamine, 5 to 10 mg) in the norepinephrine-extravasated tissue may reduce the severity of tissue ischemia. Stellate ganglion block of the same side of the infiltrated arm may also improve circulation to the ischemic area.

Norepinephrine also has significant arrhythmogenic effects. Like epinephrine, intraoperative use of norepinephrine should be reserved for the most severe cases only. Norepinephrine has been used in patients who develop hypotension from loss of vasomotor tone as a consequence of spinal anesthesia or surgical sympathectomy, but other less hazardous vasopressor agents such as ephedrine and methoxamine are effective and should be used in preference to norepinephrine.[147]

Isoproterenol (Isuprel). Isoproterenol is almost a pure *beta*-adrenergic stimulant possessing both *beta* 1 and *beta* 2 stimulatory effects. Its bronchodilating effect makes it important as an aerosol mist in the treatment of asthma and other bronchoconstricting diseases.

The potent cardiac stimulatory action of isoproterenol is accompanied by peripheral vasodilation. Cardiac output is raised by an increase in the venous return to the heart, combined with the positive inotropic and chronotropic actions of the drug. The increase in cardiac output usually maintains systolic pressure, but mean arterial pressure may be reduced. Renal blood flow is elevated in patients in cardiogenic or septicemic shock, where intravascular volume is not reduced.[145,148] *Beta*-adrenergic stimulation increases AV conduction. Since isoproterenol is devoid of *alpha*-adrenergic stimulating activity, reflex bradycardia (more frequently observed with epinephrine and norepinephrine) does not occur. Thus isoproterenol is effective in treating atrioventricular heart block and for cardiac resuscitation, as well as in supporting the cardiovascular system during open heart operations.[145,149]

Isoproterenol is also helpful in treating cor pulmonale and pulmonary embolism.[150–152] The arrhythmogenicity of isoproterenol is less than that of epinephrine or norepinephrine.[145,153]

Dopamine (Intropin). Dopamine is the immediate precursor in the synthesis of norepinephrine in the body (see earlier discussion). Like the other catecholamines, it exerts a positive inotropic action. Cardiac output is increased but there is little change in arterial blood pressure or heart rate. Peripheral vascular resistance is usually decreased. Dopamine produces mesenteric and renal vasodilation. Renal blood flow, glomerular filtration rate, urine flow, and sodium excretion are enhanced.[145,148,154–156]

The drug is less likely than other catecholamines to cause cardiac dysrhythmia or tachycardia, but these are dose-related phenomena, since, for example, tachycardia is not uncommon during open heart operations when dopamine is used to support the circulation.[153] Tachycardia is less likely to develop if dopamine is infused at a rate of less than 5 μg/kg/min.[155]

The advantage of dopamine over the other catecholamines is its ability to maintain renal blood flow while providing a stimulatory effect on the myocardium. It is well known that renal perfusion is sacrificed during low-perfusion states in an attempt by the body to shunt more blood to the brain and the heart. Urinary output is thus an important monitor for assessing the adequacy of organ perfusion.

The experimental and clinical observations with dopamine suggest that it has good therapeutic potentials for the treatment of shock.[140–145,157–159]

Noncatecholamines.

Methoxamine (Vasoxyl) and Phenylephrine (Neo-Synephrine). Both sympathomimetic amines act directly on *alpha* receptors and are almost pure peripheral vasoconstrictor agents. They are devoid of cardiac stimulatory actions at the usual concentrations used to treat hypotension.[145,160,161] Reflex vagal bradycardia is common with both agents; therefore, these drugs are used clinically to relieve attacks of paroxysmal atrial tachycardia. Most vascular beds are constricted; renal, splanchnic, and cutaneous blood flows are reduced, but coronary blood flow may increase as the result of increased mean arterial pressure and increased coronary filling time (that is, reflex bradycardia). Cardiac dysrhythmias are infrequently observed during anesthesia. Large doses of phenylephrine given during halothane anesthesia produce ventricular arrhythmias in dogs.[162] These drugs are useful for the temporary treatment of acute hypotension resulting from the discrepancy between intravascular volume and peripheral vascular capacitance.

Methoxamine and phenylephrine are useful for such common clinical situations as hypotension associated with spinal anesthesia;[147] controlled hypotension, which does not reverse when the hypotensive agent (for example, nitroprusside or trimethaphan) has been removed; and low-perfusion pressure during cardiopulmonary bypass when there appears to be adequate intravascular volume.

Ephedrine. Ephedrine is an alkaloid occurring in various plants of the genus *Ephedra* and has been used in China for over 5,000 years. The Chinese herb containing ephedrine and called *Ma huang* (yellow astringent) was introduced into Western medicine by Chen and Schmidt in 1924.[163] These researchers reported the cardiovascular effects of the alkaloid and noted its similarities to epinephrine.

Ephedrine is a partially indirect-acting sympathomimetic amine that exerts its effects by the release of endogenous catecholamines from the adrenergic nerve terminals and the adrenal medulla. Some direct effect also exists.[145,164] Thus both *alpha-* and *beta*-adrenergic receptors are stimulated by ephedrine.

The cardiovascular stimulatory effects of

ephedrine diminish with rapidly repeated doses. The mechanism of this tachyphylaxis response is not clear, but the depletion of catecholamine stores is a factor. The drug usually elevates both systolic and diastolic pressures in man. Cardiac output is increased, provided there is adequate venous return to the heart.

Effects on renal circulation appear to be a dose-dependent phenomenon: at lower concentrations, *beta*-adrenergic effects are more prominent, with the result that renal blood flow is increased; whereas at high concentrations, *alpha*-adrenergic stimulation predominates and produces constriction of renal blood vessels.[145,165] Splanchnic circulation is reduced.

Placental blood flow is preserved by ephedrine in concentrations effective for supporting the maternal circulation, thus making this sympathomimetic drug the best choice in treating hypotension in the parturient patient.[166,167] One intravenous administration of ephedrine (10 to 25 mg) sustains an elevated blood pressure for seven to ten minutes, with little tendency to an exaggerated rise in systolic pressure.

The effects of ephedrine on cardiac electrophysiology are complex. Local effects of the drug include an increase in the excitability of ventricular muscle that is manifested by ventricular tachycardia and fibrillation, and an increase in idioventricular rhythm.[168,169] However, in the anesthetized dog ephedrine prevents the atrial fibrillation induced by epinephrine and the ventricular fibrillation induced by an electrical current applied to the ventricle. Cardiac dysrhythmias have been demonstrated in the dog with halothane and ephedrine,[11] but no apparent problem is associated with the administration of ephedrine during methoxyflurane anesthesia.[170]

Metaraminol (Aramine). Metaraminol has both direct and indirect actions and overall effects similar to those of norepinephrine.[145] Its pressor action is of longer duration than its cardiac stimulatory action; therefore, in man its *alpha*-adrenergic

stimulatory effect predominates.[171] Both systolic and diastolic pressures are elevated. Metaraminol increases venous tone and reduces cerebral blood flow. The effect of metaraminol on renal blood flow depends on the preexisting conditions of the patient; for instance, it reduces renal blood flow in hypotensive individuals.[172] Pulmonary vasoconstriction results in elevated pulmonary blood pressure even when cardiac output is reduced.

Metaraminol is a potent agent for depleting norepinephrine stores in adrenergic nerve terminals.[173] Consequently, the continuous infusion of metaraminol leads to reduced cardiovascular stimulation. Furthermore, metaraminol is taken up by the adrenergic nerve terminal and acts as a false transmitter, but it is much less potent than endogenous catecholamines. Hypotension may result from the prolonged use of metaraminol.[173,174] It may be useful to think of metaraminol as a "potent ephedrine."

Mephentermine (Wyamine). Mephentermine is pharmacologically similar to ephedrine and metaraminol in that it acts in part by releasing catecholamines. Hence it elicits cardiac stimulation, vasodilation, and vasoconstriction. The cardiac effects of mephentermine are more consistent than its vascular effects. Cardiac output is increased in normal subjects as well as in patients suffering from shock.[175,176] Systemic vascular resistance may increase, decrease, or show no change. Coronary blood flow is usually increased following intravenous mephentermine as the result of increased blood pressure and local vasodilation.[177,178]

The responses of the renal and splanchnic circulations to intravenous mephentermine are variable. Cardiac dysrhythmias induced by halothane in man may be prevented by mephentermine,[162] which is less likely to produce renal vasoconstriction and cardiac dysrhythmias than other sympathomimetic amines that stimulate *alpha* and *beta* receptors. It also abolishes cardiac dysrhythmias induced by digitalis and myocardial infarction.[159,179] Thus the use of mephentermine has advantages over metaraminol in the treatment of hemorrhagic or cardiogenic shock.[177]

Anesthetic management of hypotension or shock

Sympathomimetic agents should support the cardiovascular system until the cause of hypotension has been adequately treated. An accurate diagnosis of the cause of hypotension allows a more rational choice of drug therapy. It should be reemphasized that common causes of hypotension during anesthesia are excessive depth of anesthesia, hypoxia, intravascular loss, and surgical manipulation. The previous administration of drugs that interfere with endogenous catecholamine stores or metabolism of catecholamines can also affect the patient's tolerance to anesthetics and sympathomimetic amines. Careful monitoring and preparation are important to successful anesthetic management.

When a patient has hemorrhaged sufficiently to cause severe hypotension or shock, his defensive mechanisms shunt most of his remaining blood volume to the brain and heart; there is a concomitant increase in sympathetic tone with the release of norepinephrine, angiotensin, and vasopressin. To institute proper treatment, the anesthesiologist should monitor several physiologic parameters: direct arterial pressure, central venous pressure, urinary output, temperature, and ECG. The anesthesiologist should also make a repeated determination of hematocrit, blood gases, and osmolality of plasma and urine. Direct measurements of cardiac output with oxygen-transport calculations are becoming more common in this context. The use of a Swan-Ganz catheter in the pulmonary artery allows the sampling of mixed venous blood from which venous P_{O_2} or oxygen saturation can be determined.[180] A venous P_{O_2} of less than 30 torr (normal-40) or a venous oxygen saturation of less than 60% (normal-75%) indicate a severe decrease in cardiac output

and/or an increase in tissue extraction of oxygen.[181,182]

Mixed venous oxygen saturation is especially useful when acid-base disturbance is severe or when large quantities of stored bank blood with reduced 2, 3-DPG (diphosphoglycerate) are transfused, because both alkalosis and a reduction of 2, 3-DPG of red blood cells can decrease P-50 (that is, the P_{O_2} at which 50% of the hemoglobin is saturated).[181,183] Pulmonary shunt of 20 to 30% is not uncommon in the shocked patient. Frequent arterial blood-gas determinations, with an appropriate inspired concentration of oxygen to maintain the arterial P_{O_2} above 100 torr, are desirable. Positive end-expiratory pressure is often necessary to improve the ventilation-perfusion ratio of the lungs in order to reduce pulmonary shunting.

The central venous pressure is used as an estimate of adequate intravascular volume replacement and right atrial filling pressure; 15 cm H_2O may be used as the upper limit of venous pressure. Pulmonary wedge pressure measured with a Swan-Ganz catheter is helpful when a filling pressure of 15 cm H_2O does not improve cardiac output or arterial pressure. Pulmonary wedge pressure can help to differentiate circulatory overload from left ventricular failure.[180] The normal pulmonary wedge pressure is 8 to 12 torr.

Continuous urinary output monitoring from a catheter placed in the bladder is the most useful method of assessing organ perfusion.

The first and most important aspect of treating a patient in shock is replacing intravascular volume. Crystalloid solutions are helpful but should not be used alone, since redistribution of crystalloid solutions can produce excessive fluid in the interstitial space. Intravascular colloidal osmotic pressure should be maintained by the administration of albumin or plasma substitute to minimize pulmonary interstitial edema. Whole blood should be administered without exceeding a hematocrit of 40%. Body temperature may decrease, necessitating the use of warm intravascular replacements. Hypothermia can reduce peripheral perfusion, potentiate cardiac dysrhythmias, produce acidosis, and depress the nervous system. Hyperventilation leads to respiratory alkalosis (hypocapnia) and hypokalemia, which produce vasoconstriction (reduced perfusion) and irritable myocardium, respectively. Cardiac output can be increased with inotropic drugs. Dopamine, isoproterenol, and norepinephrine, chosen judiciously, may improve the efficiency and the distribution of perfusion. Large doses of glucocorticoids may be helpful.[184]

The ultimate choice of general anesthetic agents may not be important, since a patient in shock requires far less anesthetic than a healthy person. The compatibility of the anesthetic chosen with the sympathomimetic agent used to support circulation is important. Unfortunately, there is little relevant published data. In general, sympathomimetic agents with greater *beta*-adrenergic activity are more arrhythmogenic than agents with primarily *alpha*-adrenergic activity (Table 6–2); and the interaction of inhalation anesthetics that are ether derivatives is less arrhythmogenic than that of inhalation anesthetics that are not ether derivatives. The combined use of narcotic, N_2O-O_2 and nondepolarizing muscle relaxant ("balanced" anesthesia) appears to have clinically minimal cardiovascular-depressant effects. Data from our laboratory suggest that balanced anesthesia renders the canine heart more resistant to epinephrine-induced dysrhythmias than does either enflurane or halothane anesthesia.[17a] Potent sympathomimetic drugs should be administered in a dilute solution, with microdrip control to minimize overdosing as manifested by cardiac arrhythmias or excessive hypertension.

Finally, special care should be taken in the anesthetic management of the hypokalemic patient. There are no published data on the interaction between sympathomimetic agents and hypokalemia in man. In the dog, depletion of body potassium with serum hypokalemia is associated with a sudden onset of ventricular tachycardia or fibrillation during the intravenous infusion of epinephrine.

Serum potassium represents only about 1.5% of total body potassium. When there is a significant reduction of extracellular potassium, a comparable decrease is necessary intracellularly in order to maintain a proper transmembrane potassium gradient for cellular membrane stability. Chronic hypokalemia and potassium depletion resulting from digitalis and diuretic therapy cannot be replenished suddenly by intravenous potassium. Hypokalemic dogs pretreated with furosemide are more sensitive to the cardiac arrhythmic effects of intravenous potassium than are healthy, untreated dogs.[186] Serum alkalosis can produce hypokalemia from cellular H^+ exchange for extracellular K^+.[187] Respiratory alkalosis potentiates cardiac dysrhythmias in patients whose body potassium has been depleted by long-term digitalis and diuretic therapy.[188] Cardiac arrhythmias are corrected by eucapnia or by KCl infusion.[187,189] If possible, chronically hypokalemic patients should be allowed 48 hours for replenishment of potassium before elective surgery. However, in emergency situations, potassium chloride, 0.5 mg/kg/hr, in concentrations of 40 to 80 meq/L in the infusion fluid, may be administered under careful monitoring of ECG and urinary output. Insulin and glucose can facilitate the cellular uptake of potassium and minimize the acute toxicity of hyperkalemia.[190] One unit of regular insulin is used for each four grams of glucose.

Hyperkalemia can also potentiate the arrhythmogenic effects of catecholamines. A disproportionate increase in serum potassium concentration with respect to intracellular potassium can inhibit repolarization of the cardiac cell. This cardiac effect is reflected on the ECG as an elevation of the T wave, a depression of the ST segment, and a prolongation of the PR interval. Further increases in serum potassium can lead to complete heart block and cardiac arrest. Important in enhancing catecholamine-induced dysrhythmias is vagal (cholinergic) stimulation, which suppresses the spontaneous depolarization of the sinoatrial node and of AV conduction (see earlier discussion). Hyperkalemia, then, mimics excessive cholinergic stimulation to the heart, allowing ventricular dysrhythmias to develop more readily. Direct-acting *alpha*-adrenergic stimulants are more desirable for managing the hyperkalemic, hypotensive patient (Table 6–2). Common causes of hyperkalemia in the operating room are (1) inappropriate exogenous intravenous replacement, (2) the administration of old blood that has increased potassium concentration,[191,192] and (3) the use of succinylcholine in patients with severe burns, trauma, or spinal cord injury.[193–195]

The rational use of sympathomimetic agents for circulatory support is based on a proper appreciation of the pharmacology and pathophysiology of the sympathetic nervous system. Drugs that influence the normal adrenergic mechanisms must be considered in relation to possible interactions with certain general anesthetics. I took a simplified approach to the complex subject of low-flow state or shock and pointed out common problems that lead to circulatory failure. Optimal anesthetic management of the patient in shock requires recognition and treatment of the cause; temporary circulatory support can be provided by a properly chosen sympathomimetic agent in conjunction with a compatible anesthetic regimen.

REFERENCES

1. Hauswirth, O., and Schaer, H.: Effects of halothane on the sinoatrial node. J. Pharmacol. Exp. Ther., *158*:36, 1967.
2. Atlee, J. L. III, and Rusy, B. F.: Halothane depression of A–V conduction studied by electrograms of the bundle of His in dogs. Anesthesiology, *36*:112, 1972.
3. Biscoe, T. J., and Millar, R. A.: The effect of halothane on carotid sinus baroreceptor activity. J. Physiol. (Lond.), *173*:24, 1964.
4. Price, H. L., Linde, H. W., and Morse, H. T.: Central nervous actions of halothane affecting the systemic circulation. Anesthesiology, *24*:770, 1963.
5. Galindo, A., Wyte, S. R., and Wetherhold, J. W.: Junctional rhythm induced by halothane anesthesia—Treatment with succinylcholine. Anesthesiology, *37*:261, 1972.
6. Reynolds, A. K., Chia, J. F., and Pasquet, A. F.: Halothane and methoxyflurane—A comparison of their effects on cardiac pacemaker fibers. Anesthesiology, *33*:602, 1970.
7. Pick, A., and Langendorf, R.: Recent advances in the differential diagnosis of V–A junctional arrhythmias. Am. Heart J., *76*:553, 1968.
8. Hamlin, R. L., and Smith, R.: Effects of vagal stimulation on S–A and A–V nodes. Am. J. Physiol., *215*:560, 1968.
9. Russell, R., and Warner, H.R.: Effect of combined sympathetic and vagal stimulation on heart rate. Physiologist, *10*:295, 1967.
10. Katz, R. L., Matteo, R. S., and Papper, E. M.: The injection of epinephrine during general anesthesia with halogenated hydrocarbons and cyclopropane in man. 2. Halothane. Anesthesiology, *23*:597, 1962.
11. Takaori, M., and Loehning, R. W.: Ventricular arrhythmias during halothane anesthesia: Effect of isoproterenol, aminophylline and ephedrine. Can. Anaesth. Soc. J., *12*:275, 1965.
12. Katz, R. L., and Bigger, T.: Cardiac arrhythmias during anesthesia and operation. Anesthesiology, *33*:193, 1973.
13. Eisele, J. H., and Smith, N. T.: Cardiovascular effects of 40 percent nitrous oxide in man. Anesth. Analg. (Cleve.), *51*:956, 1972.
14. Smith, N. T., et al.: The cardiovascular and sympathomimetic response to the addition of nitrous oxide to halothane in man. Anesthesiology, *32*:410, 1970.
15. Smith, N. T., et al.: The cardiovascular responses to the addition of nitrous oxide to diethyl ether in man. Can. Anaesth. Soc. J., *19*:42, 1972.
16. Wong, K. C., et al.: The cardiovascular effects of morphine sulfate with oxygen and with nitrous oxide in man. Anesthesiology, *38*:542, 1973.
17. Smith, N. T., et al.: The cardiovascular responses to the addition of nitrous oxide to fluroxene in man. Br. J. Anaesth., *44*:142, 1972.
17a. Puerto, B. A., Wong, K. C., et al.: Epinephrine-induced dysrhythmias: comparison during anaesthesia with narcotics and with halogenated inhalation agents in dogs. Can. Anaesth. Soc. J., *26*:263, 1979.
18. Axelrod, J.: The formation, metabolism, uptake and release of noradrenaline and adrenaline. *In* The Clinical Chemistry of Monoamines. Edited by H. Varley and A. H. Gawenlock. Amsterdam, Elsevier Publishing Co., 1963.
19. Blaschko, H., and Muscholl, E. (Eds.): Catecholamines. Vol. 33, Handbook of Experimental Pharmocology. Berlin, Springer-Verlag, 1972.
20. Axelrod, J.: Methylation reactions in the formation and metabolism of catecholamines and other biogenic amines: The enzyme conversion of norepinephrine (NE) to epinephrine (E). Pharmacol. Rev., *18*:95, 1966.
21. Marley, E., and Blackwell, B.: Interactions of

monoamine oxidase inhibitors, amines and foodstuff. Adv. Pharmacol. Chemother., *8*:185, 1970.

22. Perks, E. R.: Monoamine oxidase inhibitors. Anaesthesia, *19*:376, 1964.

23. Rosen, M. R., Hoffman, B. F., and Andrew, L.W.: Electrophysiology and pharmacology of cardiac arrhythmias. V. Cardiac antiarrhythmic effects of lidocaine. Am. Heart J., *89*:526, 1975.

24. Collinsworth, K. A., Kalman, S. M., and Harrison, D. C.: The clinical pharmacology of lidocaine as an antiarrhythmic drug. Circulation, *50*:1217, 1974.

25. Shand, D. G.: Propranolol. N. Engl. J. Med., *293*:280, 1975.

26. Nies, A. S., and Shand, D. G.: Clinical pharmacology of propranolol. Circulation, *52*:6, 1975.

27. Price, H. L.: Effect of carbon dioxide on the cardiovascular system. Anesthesiology, *21*:652, 1960.

28. Tenney, S. M., and Lamb, T. W.: Physiologic consequences of hypoventilation and hyperventilation. *In* Handbook of Physiology. Section 3, Respiration. Washington, D.C., American Physiology Society, 1965, Vol. II.

29. Gross, B. A., and Silver, I. A.: Central activation of the sympathetico-adrenal system by hypoxia and hypercapnia. J. Endocrinol., *24*:91, 1962.

30. Brunjes, S., Johns, V. J., and Crane, M. G.: Pheochromocytoma. N. Engl. J. Med., *262*:393, 1960.

31. Goldfien, A.: Pheochromocytoma: Diagnosis and anesthetic and surgical management. Anesthesiology, *24*:462, 1963.

32. Brewster, W. R., et al.: The hemodynamics and metabolic inter-relationships in the activity of epinephrine, norepinephrine and the thyroid hormones. Circulation, *13*:1, 1956.

33. Parsons, V., and Ramsey, I.: Thyroid and adrenal relationships. Postgrad. Med. J., *44*:377, 1969.

34. Murray, J. F., and Kelly, J. J.: The relation of thyroidal hormone level to epinephrine response: A diagnostic test for hyperthyroidism. Ann. Intern. Med., *51*:309, 1959.

35. Chidsey, C. A., Braunwald, E., and Morrow, A. G.: Catecholamine excretion and cardiac stores of norepinephrine in congestive heart failure. Am. J. Med., *39*:442, 1965.

36. Chidsey, C. A., et al.: Myocardial norepinephrine concentration in man. Effects of reserpine and of congestive heart failure. N. Engl. J. Med., *269*:653, 1963.

37. Braunwald, E.: The sympathetic nervous system in heart failure. Hosp. Pract., *5*:31, 1970.

38. Chidsey, C. A., and Braunwald, E.: Sympathetic activity and neurotransmitter depletion in congestive heart failure. Pharmacol. Rev., *18*:685, 1966.

39. Trendelenburg, U.: Supersensitivity and subsensitivity to sympathomimetic amines. Pharmacol. Rev., *15*:225, 1963.

40. Johnson, B., et al.: Autonomic hyperreflexia: A review. Milit. Med., *140*:345, 1975.

41. Morgan, R., and Cagan, E. J.: Acute alcoholic intoxication reaction and methyl alcohol intoxication. *In* The Biology of Alcoholism. Vol. 3, Clinical Pathology. Edited by B. Kissin and H. Begleiter. New York, Plenum Press, 1974.

42. Goldstein, M., et al.: Inhibition of dopamine *beta*-hydroxylase by disulfiram. Life Sci., *3*:763, 1964.

43. Goldstein, M., and Nakajima, K.: The effects of disulfiram on the repletion of brain catecholamine stores. Life Sci., *5*:1133, 1966.

44. Sellers, A. M., Itskovitz, H. D., and Linduer, M. A.: Systemic arterial hypertension. *In* Cardiac and Vascular Diseases. Edited by H. L. Conn, Jr., and O. Horwitz. Philadelphia, Lea & Febiger, 1971. Vol. II.

45. Tyce, G. M., Sheps, S. G., and Frock, E. V.: Determination of urinary metabolites of catecholamines after the administration of methyldopa. Mayo Clin. Proc., *38*:571, 1963.

46. Onesti, G., et al.: Pharmacodynamics and clinical use of *alpha*-methyldopa in the treatment of essential hypertension. Am. J. Cardiol., *9*:863, 1962.

47. Onesti, G., et al.: Pharmacodynamic effects of *alpha*-methyldopa in hypertensive patients. Am. Heart J., *67*:32, 1964.

48. Dollery, C. T.: Methyldopa in the treatment of hypertension. Prog. Cardiovasc. Dis., *8*:278, 1965.

49. Weil, M. H., Barbour, B. H., and Chesne, R. B.: *Alpha*-methyldopa for the treatment of hypertension: Clinical and pharmacodynamic studies. Circulation, *28*:165, 1963.

50. Kalsner, S., and Nickerson, M.: Effects of reserpine on the disposition of sympathomimetic amines in vascular tissue. Br. J. Pharmacol., *35*:394, 1969.

51. Alper, M. H., Flacke, W., and Krayer, O.: Pharmacology of reserpine and its implications for anesthesia. Anesthesiology, *24*:524, 1963.

52. Sannerstedt, R., and Conway, J.: Hemodynamic and vascular responses to antihypertensive treatment with adrenergic blocking agents. A review. Am. Heart J., *79*:122, 1970.

53. Gaffney, T. E., Chidsey, C. A., and Braunwald, E.: Study of the relationship between the neurotransmitter store and adrenergic nerve block induced by reserpine and guanethidine. Circ. Res., *12*:264, 1963.

54. Ziegler, C. H., and Lovette, J. B.: Operative complications after therapy with reserpine and reserpine compounds. J.A.M.A., *176*:916, 1961.

55. Coakley, C. S., Alpert, S., and Boling, J. S.: Circulatory responses during anesthesia of patients on rauwolfia therapy. J.A.M.A., *161*:1143, 1956.

56. Naylor, W. G.: A direct effect of reserpine on ventricular contractility. J. Pharmacol. Exp. Ther., *139*:222, 1962.

57. Freedman, D. X., and Benton, A. J.: Persisting effects of reserpine in man. N. Engl. J. Med., *264*:529, 1961.

58. Dingle, H. R.: Antihypertensive drugs and anesthesia. Anaesthesia, *21*:151, 1966.

59. Munson, W. M., and Jenicek, J. A.: Effect of anesthetic agents on patients receiving reserpine therapy. Anesthesiology, *23*:741, 1962.

60. Katz, R. L., Weintraub, H. D., and Papper, E. M.: Anesthesia, surgery and rauwolfia. Anesthesiology, 25:142, 1964.
61. Rocklin, D. B., Shohl, T., and Blakemore, W. S.: Blood volume changes associated with essential hypertension. Surg. Gynecol. Obstet., 111:569, 1960.
62. Finnerty, F. A., Bucholz, J. H., and Guillauden, R. L.: Blood volumes and plasma protein during levarterenol-induced hypertension. J. Clin. Invest., 37:425, 1958.
63. Papper, E. M.: Selection and management of anaesthesia in those suffering from diseases and disorders of the heart. Can. Anaesth. Soc. J., 12:245, 1965.
64. Ominsky, A. J., and Wollman, H.: Hazards of general anesthesia in the reserpinized patient. Anesthesiology, 30:443, 1969.
65. Aviado, D. M.: Sympathomimetic drugs. Springfield, Ill., Charles C Thomas, 1970.
66. Zaimis, E.: Vasopressor drugs and catecholamines. Anesthesiology, 29:732, 1968.
67. Rosenblum, R.: Physiologic basis for the therapeutic use of catecholamines. Am. Heart J., 87:527, 1974.
68. Eger, E. I., and Hamilton, W. K.: The effect of reserpine on the action of various vasopressors. Anesthesiology, 20:641, 1959.
69. Fries, E.D.: Guanethidine. Prog. Cardiovasc. Dis., 8:183, 1965.
70. Page, I. H., Hurley, R. E., and Dustan, H. P.: The prolonged treatment of hypertension with guanethidine. J.A.M.A., 175:543, 1961.
71. Fielden, R., and Green, A. L.: A comparative study of the noradrenaline-depleting and sympathetic-blocking action of guanethidine and (−)-B-hydroxy-phenethylquanidine. Br. J. Pharmacol. Chemother., 30:155, 1967.
72. Mitchell, J. R., et al.: Guanethidine and related agents. III. Antagonism by drugs which inhibit the norepinephrine pump in man. J. Clin. Invest., 49:1596, 1970.
73. Goodman, L. S., and Gilman, A.: The Pharmacological Basis of Therapeutics. 5th Edition. New York, Macmillan, 1975, p. 710.
74. Van Zwieten, P. A.: The central action of antihypertensive drugs medicated via central *alpha*-receptors. J. Pharm. Pharmacol., 25:89, 1973.
75. Werner, U., Starke, K., and Schumann, H. J.: Actions of clonidine and 2-(2-methyl-6-ethyl-cyclohexylamino)-2-oxazoline on postganglionic autonomic nerves. Arch. Int. Pharmacodyn. Ther., 195:282, 1972.
76. Hansson, L., et al.: Blood pressure crisis following withdrawal of clonidine (Catapres, Catapresan) with special reference to arterial and urinary catecholamine levels and suggestions for acute management. Am. Heart J., 85:605, 1973.
77. Brodsky, J. D., and Bravo, J. J.: Acute postoperative clonidine withdrawal syndrome. Anesthesiology, 44:519, 1976.
78. Ahlquist, R. P.: A study of adrenotropic receptors. Am. J. Physiol., 153:586, 1948.
79. Lands, A. M., Luduena, F. P., and Buzzo, H. J.: Differentiation of receptors responsive to isoproterenol. Life Sci., 6:2241, 1967.
80. Levy, B., and Wilkenfield, B. E.: Selective interactions with *beta*-adrenergic receptors. Fed. Proc., 29:1362, 1970.
81. Epstein, S. E., and Braunwald, E.: *Beta*-adrenergic receptors blocking drugs. Mechanism of action and clinical application. N. Engl. J. Med., 275:1106, 1175, 1975.
82. Nies, A. S., Evans, G. H., and Shand, D. G.: Regional hemodynamic effects of *beta*-adrenergic blockade with propranolol in the unanesthetized primate. Am. Heart J., 85:97, 1973.
83. Malcolm, J.: Adrenergic *beta*-receptor inhibition and hyperthyroidism. Acta Cardiol. (Brux.), 15:320, 1972.
84. Shand, D. G., Nuckolls, E. M., and Oates, J. A.: Plasma propranolol levels in adults with observations in four children. Clin. Pharmacol. Ther., 11:112, 1970.
85. Faulkner, S. L., et al.: Time required for complete recovery from chronic propranolol therapy. N. Engl. J. Med., 293:280, 1975.
86. Nellen, M.: Withdrawal of propranolol and myocardial infarction. Lancet, 1:558, 1973.
87. Diaz, R. G., et al.: Myocardial infarction after propranolol withdrawal. Am. Heart J., 88:257, 1974.
88. Alderman, E. L., et al.: Coronary artery syndrome after sudden propranolol withdrawal. Ann. Intern. Med., 81:625, 1974.
89. Kaplan, J. A., et al.: Propranolol and cardiac surgery: A problem for the anesthesiologist? Anesth. Analg. (Cleve.), 54:571, 1975.
90. Eckenhoff, J. E., and Oech, S. R.: The effects of narcotics and antagonists upon respiration and circulation in man. Clin. Pharmacol. Ther., 1:483, 1960.
91. Viljoen, J. F., Estafanous, F. G., and Kellner, G. A.: Propranolol and cardiac surgery. J. Thorac. Cardiovasc. Surg., 64:826, 1972.
92. Graves, C. L., and Downs, N. H.: Cardiovascular and renal effects of enflurane in surgical patients. Anesth. Analg. (Cleve.), 53:898, 1974.
93. Dobkin, A. B., et al.: Ethrane (compound 347) anesthesia: A clinical and laboratory review of 700 cases. Anesth. Analg., (Cleve.), 48:477, 1969.
94. Shimosato, S., and Etsten, B. E.: Effect of anesthetic drugs on the heart: A critical review of myocardial contractility and its relationship to hemodynamics. Clin. Anesth., 3:17, 1969.
95. Goodman, L. S., and Gilman, A.: The Pharmacological Basis of Therapeutics. 5th edition. New York, Macmillan, 1975, p. 152.
96. Webster, R. A.: The antiadrenaline activity of some phenothiazine derivatives. Br. J. Pharmacol. Chemother., 25:566, 1965.
97. Schou, M.: Lithium in psychiatric therapy and prophylaxis. J. Psychiatr. Res., 6:67, 1968.
98. Goodman, L. S., and Gilman, A.: The Pharmacological Basis of Therapeutics. 5th Edition. New York, Macmillan, 1975, p. 791.
99. Borden, H., Clarke, M., and Katz, H.: The use of

pancuronium bromides in patients receiving lithium carbonate. Can. Anaesth. Soc. J., *21*:79, 1974.

100. Hill, G. E., Wong, K. C., and Hodges, M. R.: Lithium carbonate and neuromuscular blocking agents. Anesthesiology, *46*:122, 1977.

101. Goodman, L. S., and Gilman, A.: The Pharmacological Basis of Therapeutics. 5th Edition. New York, Macmillan, 1975, p. 180.

102. Goodman, L. S., and Gilman, A.: The Pharmacological Basis of Therapeutics. 5th Edition. New York, Macmillan, 1975, p. 174.

103. Klerman, G. L., and Cole, J. O.: Clinical pharmacology of imipramine and related antidepressant compounds. Pharmacol. Rev., *17*:101, 1965.

104. Williams, R. B., and Sherter, C.: Cardiac complications of tricyclic antidepressant therapy. Ann. Intern. Med., *74*:395, 1971.

105. Jenkins, L. C., and Graves, H. B.: Potential hazards of psychoactive drugs in association with anesthesia. Can. Anaesth. Soc. J., *12*:121, 1965.

106. Boaker, A. J., et al.: Interactions between sympathomimetic anines and antidepressant agents in man. Br. Med. J., *10*:311, 1973.

106a. Johnston, R. R., Way, W. L., and Miller, R. D.: The effect of CNS catecholamine-depleting drugs on dextroamphetamine-induced elevation of halothane MAC. Anesthesiology, *41*:57, 1974.

107. Koller, K.: Uebec die Verivendurg des Concein zur Anasthesirung. Auge. Wien. Med. Bul., *7*:1352, 1884.

108. Adriani, J.: Appraisal of Current Concepts in Anesthesiology. St. Louis, C. V. Mosby Co., 1968, Vol. 4.

109. Anderton, J. M., and Nassar, W. Y.: Topical cocaine and general anaesthesia: An investigation of the efficacy and side effects of cocaine on the nasal mucosae. Anaesthesia, *30*:809, 1975.

110. Goodman, L. S., and Gilman, A.: The Pharmacological Basis of Therapeutics. 5th Edition. New York, Macmillan, 1975, p. 386.

111. Oliver, G., and Schaefer, E. A.: The physiological effects of extracts of the suprarenal capsules. J. Physiol. (Lond.), *18*:230, 1895.

112. Meek, W. J., Hathaway, H. R., and Orth, O. S.: The effects of ether, chloroform and cyclopropane on cardiac automaticity. J. Pharmacol. Exp. Ther., *61*:240, 1937.

113. Munson, E. S., and Tucker, W. K.: Doses of epinephrine causing arrhythmia during enflurane, methoxyflurane and halothane anesthesia in dogs. Can. Anaesth. Soc. J., *22*:495, 1975.

114. Tucker, W. K., Rackstein, A. D., and Munson, E. S.: Comparison of arrhythmic doses of adrenaline, metaraminol, epinephrine and phenylephrine during isoflurane and halothane anaesthesia in dogs. Br. J. Anaesth., *46*:392, 1974.

115. Johnston, R. R., Eger, E. I. II, and Wilson, C.: A comparative interaction of epinephrine with enflurane, isoflurane and halothane in man. Anesth. Analg. (Cleve.), *55*:709, 1976.

116. Joas, T. A., and Stevens, W.: Comparison of the arrhythmic doses of epinephrine during Forane, halothane and fluroxene anesthesia in dogs. Anesthesiology, *35*:48, 1971.

117. Bamforth, B. J., et al.: Effect of epinephrine on the dog heart during methoxyflurane anesthesia. Anesthesiology, *22*:169, 1961.

118. Wong, K. C., et al.: Antiarrhythmic effects of skeletal muscle relaxants. Anesthesiology, *34*:458, 1971.

119. Dresel, P. E., MacCannell, K. L., and Nickerson, M.: Cardiac arrhythmias induced by minimal doses of epinephrine in cyclopropane-anesthetized dogs. Circ. Res., *8*:948, 1960.

120. Wong, K. C., et al.: Deep hypothermia and ether anesthesia for open-heart surgery in infants—A clinical report of eight years' experience. Anesth. Analg. (Cleve.), *53*:765, 1974.

121. This reference has been deleted.

122. Matteo, R. S., Katz, R. L., and Papper, E. M.: The injection of epinephrine during general anesthesia with halogenated hydrocarbons and cyclopropane in man. 3. Cyclopropane. Anesthesiology, *24*:327, 1963.

123. Hudon, F.: Methoxyflurane. Can. Anaesth. Soc. J., *8*:544, 1961.

124. Donino, E., Chodoff, P., and Corssen, G.: Pharmacologic effects of CI-581: A new dissociative anesthetic in man. J. Clin. Pharmacol. Ther., *6*:279, 1965.

125. Corssen, G., and Domino, E. F.: Dissociative anesthesia. Anesth. Analg. (Cleve.), *45*:29, 1966.

126. Wilson, R. D., et al.: Evaluation of CL-1848C: A new dissociative anesthetic in normal human volunteers. Anesth. Analg. (Cleve.), *49*:236, 1970.

127. Traber, D. L., Wilson, R. D., and Priano, L. L.: Differentiation of the cardiovascular effects of CI-581. Anesth. Analg. (Cleve.), *47*:769, 1968.

128. Traber, D. L., and Wilson, R. D.: Involvement of the sympathetic nervous system in the pressor response to ketamine. Anesth. Analg. (Cleve.), *48*:248, 1969.

129. Traber, D. L., Wilson, R. D., and Priano, L. L.: Blockade of the hypertensive response to ketamine. Anesth. Analg. (Cleve.), *49*:420, 1970.

130. Dowdy, E. G., and Kaya, K.: Studies of mechanism of cardiovascular response to CI-581. Anesthesiology, *29*:931, 1968.

131. Slogoff, S., and Allen, G. W.: The role of baroreceptors in the cardiovascular response to ketamine. Anesth. Analg. (Cleve.), *53*:704, 1974.

132. Nedergaard, O.: Cocaine-like effect of ketamine on vascular adrenergic neurons. Eur. J. Pharmacol., *23*:152, 1973.

133. Miletick, D. J., et al.: The effect of ketamine on catecholamine metabolism in the isolated perfused rat heart. Anesthesiology, *39*:271, 1973.

134. Kolhntop, D. E., Liao, J-C, and Van Bergen, F. H.: Effects on pharmacologic alterations of adrenergic mechanisms by cocaine, tropolone, aminophylline and ketamine on epinephrine-induced arrhythmias during halothane-nitrous oxide anesthesia. Anesthesiology, *46*:83, 1977.

135. Hill, G. E., et al.: Interaction of ketamine with vasoactive amines at normothermia and hypothermia in the isolated rabbit heart. Anesthesiology, *48*:315, 1978.

136. Chen, G.: Sympathomimetic anaesthetics. Can. Anaesth. Soc. J., *20*:180, 1973.

137. Shires, G. T.: Principles in the management of shock. *In* Care of the Trauma Patient. New York, McGraw-Hill, 1966.

138. Altura, B. M.: Chemical and humoral regulation of blood flow through the precapillary sphincter. Microvasc. Res., *3*:361, 1971.

139. Zweifach, B. W.: Functional Behavior of the Microcirculation. Springfield, Ill., Charles C Thomas, 1961.

140. Shepro, D., and Fulton, G. P. (Eds.): Microcirculation As Related to Shock (Symposium). New York, Academic Press, 1966.

141. Shoemaker, W. C.: Shock: Chemistry, Physiology and Therapy. Springfield, Ill., Charles C Thomas, 1967.

142. Hershey, S. G., and Altura, B. M.: Vasopressors and low-flow states. *In* Clinical Anesthesia. Edited by J. F. Artusio, Jr. Vol 10, Pharmacology of Adjuvant Drugs. Philadelphia, F. A. Davis, 1973.

143. Hardaway, R. M., III: Clinical Management of Shock: Surgical and Medical. Springfield, Ill. Charles C Thomas, 1968.

144. Nickerson, M.: Drug therapy of shock. *In* Shock: Pathogenesis and Therapy (Ciba Foundation Symposium). Edited by K. D. Bock. Berlin, Springer-Verlag, 1962.

145. Aviado, D. M.: Sympathomimetic Drugs. Springfield, Ill., Charles C Thomas, 1970.

146. Dundee, J. W.: L-noradrenaline as vasoconstrictor. Br. Med. J., *1*:547, 1952.

147. Bromage, P. R.: Vasopressors. Can. Anaesth. Soc. J., 7:310, 1960.

148. McNay, J. L., and Goldberg, L. I.: Comparison of the effects of dopanine, isoproterenol, norepinephrine and bradykinin on canine renal and femoral blood flow. J. Pharmacol. Exp. Ther., *151*:23, 1966.

149. Redding, J. S., and Pearson, J. W.: Resuscitation from asphyxia. J.A.M.A., *182*:283, 1962.

150. Halmagyi, D. F. J., et al.: Effect of isoproterenol in "severe" experimental lung embolism with and without post-embolic collapse. Am. Heart J., 65:208, 1963.

151. Halmagyi, D. F. J., Horner, F. J., and Starzecki, B.: Acute cor pulmonale and shock. Med. J. Aust., 2:143, 1965.

152. McDonald, I. G., et al.: Isoproterenol in massive pulmonary embolism: Haemodynamic and clinical effects. Med. J. Aust., 2:201, 1968.

153. Gilbert, J. L., et al.: Effects of vasoconstrictor agents on cardiac irritability. J. Pharmacol. Exp. Ther., *123*:9, 1958.

154. Goldberg, L. I.: Dopamine—Clinical uses of an endogenous catecholamine. N. Engl. J. Med., *291*:707, 1974.

155. Goldberg, L. I.: Cardiovascular and renal actions of dopamine: Potential clinical applications. Pharmacol. Rev., *24*:1, 1974.

156. Allwood, M. J., Cobbold, A. F., and Gensburg, J.: Peripheral vascular effects of noradrenaline, isoproprylnoradrenaline and dopamine. Br. Med. Bull., *19*:132, 1963.

157. Kuhn, L. A.: Shock in myocardial infarction—Medical treatment. Am. J. Cardiol., *26*:578, 1970.

158. Bernstein, A., et al.: The treatment of shock accompanying myocardial infarction. Angiology, *14*:559, 1963.

159. Bernstein, A., et al.: Treatment of shock in myocardial infarction. Am. J. Cardiol., *9*:74, 1962.

160. Eckstein, J. W., and Abboud, F. M.: Circulatory effects of sympathomimetic amines. Am. Heart J., *63*:119, 1962.

161. Schmid, P. G., Eckstein, J. W., and Abboud, F. M.: Comparison of the effects of several sympathomimetic amines on resistance and capacitance vessels in the forearm of man. Circulation (Suppl. 3), *34*:3, 1966.

162. Catehacci, A. J., et al.: Serious arrhythmias with vasopressors during halothane anesthesia in man. J.A.M.A., *183*:662, 1963.

163. Chen, K. K., and Schmidt, C. F.: The action of ephedrine, the active principle of the Chinese drug, Ma huang. J. Pharmacol. Exp. Ther., 24:339, 1924.

164. Zaimis, E.: Vasopressor drugs and catecholamines. Anesthesiology, 29:732, 1968.

165. Moyer, J. H., Morris, G., and Beazley, L.: Renal hemodynamic response to vasopressor agents in treatment of shock. Circulation, *12*:96, 1955.

166. James, F. M., III, et al.: An evaluation of vasopressor therapy for maternal hypotension during spinal anesthesia. Anesthesiology, *33*:25, 1970.

167. Eng, M., et al.: The effects of methoxamine and ephedrine in normotensive pregnant primates. Anesthesiology, *35*:354, 1971.

168. Seevers, M. H., and Meek, W. J.: The cardiac irregularities produced by ephedrine after digitalis. J. Pharmacol. Exp. Ther., *53*:295, 1935.

169. Meek, W. J., and Seevers, M. H.: The cardiac irregularities produced by ephedrine and a protective action of sodium barbital. J. Pharmacol. Exp. Ther., *51*:287, 1934.

170. Sphire, R. D.: Hypotension and other problems associated with methoxyflurane administration. Anesth. Analg. (Cleve.), *45*:737, 1966.

171. Livesay, W. R., Moyer, J. H., and Chapman, D. W.: The cardiovascular and renal hemodynamic effects of aramine. Am. Heart J., *47*:745, 1954.

172. Moyer, J. H., Morris, G., and Snyder, H.: A comparison of cerebral hemodynamics response to aramine and norepinephrine in the normotensive and hypotensive subjects. Circulation, *10*:265, 1954.

173. Shore, P. A.: The mechanism of norepinephrine depletion by reserpine, metaraminol and related agents. The role of monoamine oxidase. Pharmacol. Rev., *18*:561, 1966.

174. Crout, J. R., et al.: The antihypertensive action of metaraminol in man. Clin. Res., *13*:204, 1965.

175. Udhoji, V. N., and Weil, M. H.: Vasodilator action of a pressor amine mephentermine in circulatory shock. Am. J. Cardiol., *16*:841, 1965.

176. Andersen, T. W., and Gravenstein, J. S.: Mephentermine and ephedrine in man. A comparison study on cardiovascular effects. Clin. Pharmacol. Ther., *5*:281, 1964.

177. Brofman, B. L., Hellerstein, H. K., and Caskey,

W. H.: Mephentermine—An effective pressor amine. Am. Heart J., *44*:396, 1952.

178. Welch, G. H., et al.: The effect of mephentermine sulfate on myocardial oxygen consumption, myocardial efficiency and peripheral vascular resistance. Am. J. Med., *24*:871, 1958.

179. Regan, T. J., et al.: Sympathomimetics as antagonists of strophanthidin's ionic and arrhythmic effects. Circ. Res., *11*:17, 1962.

180. Swan, H. J. C., and Ganz, W.: Use of balloon flotation catheters in critically ill patients. Surg. Clin. North Am., *55*:501, 1975.

181. Martin, W. E., et al.: Continuous monitoring of mixed venous oxygen saturation in man. Anesth. Analg. (Cleve.), *52*:784, 1973.

182. Stanley, T. H., and Isern-Amaral, J.: Periodic analysis of mixed venous oxygen tension to monitor the adequacy of perfusion during and after cardiopulmonary bypass. Can. Anaesth. Soc. J., *21*:454, 1974.

183. Scheinman, M. M., Brown, M. A., and Rappaport, E.: Critical assessment of use of central venous oxygen saturation as a mirror of mixed venous oxygen in severely ill cardiac patients. Circulation, *40*:165, 1969.

184. Antonaccio, M. J.: Cardiovascular pharmacology. New York, Raven Press, 1977.

185. This reference has been deleted.

186. Wong, K. C., et al.: Acute intravenous administration of potassium chloride to furosemide pretreated dogs. Can. Anaesth. Soc. J., *24*:203, 1977.

187. Schribner, B. H., and Burnell, J. M.: Interpretation of the serum potassium concentration. Metabolism, *5*:468, 1956.

188. Wright, B. D., and DiGiovanni, A. J.: Respiratory alkalosis, hypokalemia and repeated ventricular fibrillation associated with mechanical ventilation. Anesth. Analg. (Cleve.), *48*:467, 1969.

189. Surawicz, B., and Gettes, L. S.: Effect of electrolyte abnormalities on the heart and circulation. *In* Cardiac and Vascular Diseases. Edited by H. L. Conn, Jr., and O. Horwitz. Philadelphia, Lea & Febiger, 1971.

190. Zierler, K. L.: Insulin, ions and membrane potentials. *In* Endocrinology. Vol. 1. Handbook of Physiology, Section 7. Edited by D. F. Steiner and N. Freinkel. Washington, D. C., American Physiological Society, 1972.

191. Miller, R. D.: Complications of massive blood transfusions. Anesthesiology, *39*:82, 1973.

192. Bunker, J. P.: Metabolic effects of blood transfusion. Anesthesiology, *27*:446, 1966.

193. Tolmic, J. D., Joyce, T. H., and Mitchell, G. D.: Succinylcholine danger in the burned patient. Anesthesiology, *39*:29, 1967.

194. Mazze, R. I., Escue, H. M., and Houston, J. B.: Hyperkalemia and cardiovascular collapse following administration of succinylcholine to traumatized patient. Anesthesiology, *31*:540, 1969.

195. Tobey, R. E.: Paraplegia, succinylcholine and cardiac arrest. Anesthesiology, *32*:359, 1970.

I express deep appreciation for the technical aid of Mrs. Vicky Larsen and Mr. Richard Blatnick in preparing this manuscript.

Chapter 7

Beta-Adrenergic Blockers

EDWARD LOWENSTEIN

Drugs that antagonize the *beta* functions of the sympathetic nervous system (*beta*-adrenergic blockers) are widely used in medicine. Their introduction caused major concern to the anesthesiologist, who approached the *beta*-blocked patient with trepidation. Indeed, the initial experience confirmed the anesthesiologist's worst fears.[1,2] However, the opposite view now prevails, namely, that the discontinuance of *beta*-adrenergic blocking agents may be inadvisable, and that their prophylactic administration may be beneficial.[3,5] In this chapter I examine the reasons for this dramatic reversal of opinion.

THE SYMPATHETIC NEUROEFFECTOR JUNCTION

The adrenergic neuroeffector junction consists of a postganglionic nerve terminal, a synaptic gap, and an adjacent effector cell. The last contains the adrenergic receptors, which are specific cellular structures capable of the selective binding of agonists and antagonists (Fig. 7–1).[6] The mediator, bound to the neuron, is released into the synaptic gap when a nerve action potential traverses the nerve terminal. As more of the mediator is released, more becomes bound to the receptor by the law of mass action. When a sufficient number of receptors is occupied by the mediator, the effect caused by that receptor occurs by the "all or none" principle. The effect is often mediated by the adenyl cyclase system acting as the "second-messenger." The binding is reversible, since the mediator may be metabolized in the junction, diffused into the capillaries, or become rebound to the nerve terminals.

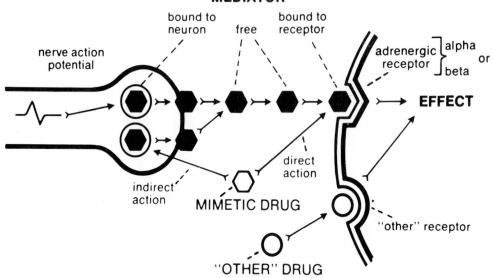

Fig. 7–1. A schematic representation of the sympathetic neuroeffector junction. See text for details. (From Moran, N. C.: The role of *alpha-* and *beta*-adrenergic receptors in the control of the circulation and in the actions of drugs on the cardiovascular system. *In* Cardiovascular Therapy. Edited by H. I. Russek and B. L. Zohman. Baltimore, Williams & Wilkins, 1971.)

When a mimetic drug is administered, it may work either directly or indirectly (Fig. 7–1).

Recent research has identified the *beta*-adrenergic receptor.[7] In man, the mediator of the *beta*-adrenergic nervous system is norepinephrine.

Antagonists of this system act by competitive inhibition. This term implies that agonists and antagonists compete for the same binding sites, and that their success in securing these locations depends on the specific affinity of the drug for the site and the number of molecules available for binding. Furthermore, it implies that the binding is reversible, that the antagonist may be overcome by sufficient quantities of agonist (and is therefore never "complete"), and that the slope of the dose-response curve is unchanged by the antagonist.

The binding process is further complicated because the prolonged occupation of the receptor by a *beta* agonist (isoproterenol) leads in a few hours to "inactiva-

tion," or a functional reduction in the number of *beta*-adrenergic receptors (similar to epinephrine resistance in asthma). Furthermore, there is evidence that the chronic occupation of *beta* receptors by *beta* antagonists can *increase* the number of *beta* receptors (Fig. 7–2).[8] This means that the prolonged administration of a *beta* blocker could induce catecholamine hypersensitivity, which could cause problems on withdrawal of the *beta* blocker. Hypersensitivity has been convincingly demonstrated, and may indeed be due to this mechanism.[8]

CLASSIFICATION OF ADRENERGIC RECEPTORS

The adrenergic receptors were initially divided into *alpha* and *beta* categories by Ahlquist.[9] In 1967 Lands further subdivided the *beta*-adrenergic system into *beta* 1 and *beta* 2 receptors.[10] The primary actions of

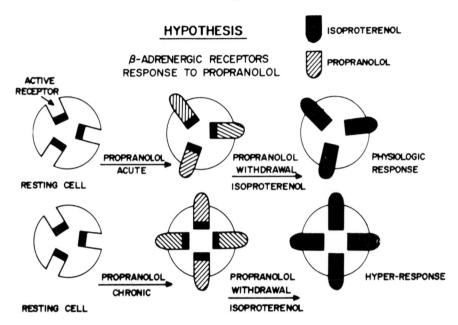

Fig. 7–2. Diagram of the mechanism for hypersensitivity of the *beta*-adrenergic nervous system following cessation of chronic propranolol therapy, as hypothesized by Boudoulas, H., et al.: Hypersensitivity to adrenergic stimulation after propranolol withdrawal in normal subjects. Ann. Intern. Med., 87:433, 1977. Top: When propranolol is administered on a short-term basis, active receptors are occupied by the antagonist. Following cessation, receptors are no longer occupied, and isoproterenol is associated with a response of normal magnitude. Repeated propranolol therapy (bottom) is associated with an increase in the number of receptors. Cessation of administration leaves an increased number of active, unbound receptors, so that isoproterenol administration causes an exaggerated response.

beta 1 receptor stimulation are exerted on the heart, whereas the primary actions of *beta* 2 receptor stimulation are arteriolar vasodilation, bronchodilation, and metabolic effects.

The specific effects of *beta* stimulation on the heart are on myocardial and electrophysiologic functions (Fig. 7–3). The former include increased ventricular ejection rate, decreased ejection time, and decreased ventricular volume, whereas the latter include increased automaticity, increased conduction velocity, and decreased atrioventricular node refractoriness. The myocardial effects are therefore associated with increased inotropy, and the electrophysiologic effects with increased heart rate and ventricular irritability.

Whether there is a direct effect of *beta*-adrenergic stimulation on the coronary arteries is undecided. Coronary dilation does occur, but it is considered by many to be due to autoregulation caused by local metabolic factors that are secondary to the increased contractile state and heart rate associated with *beta*-adrenergic stimulation.

Recent investigations indicate that further subdivision of the *beta* 1 receptors may be warranted. This is suggested by the manufacture of relatively chronotropic-selective stimulating drugs,[11] as well as by the longer persistence of chronotropic over inotropic blockade after the discontinuance of propranolol.[12]

Most sympathetically active compounds, whether endogenous or exogenous, have both *alpha*- and *beta*-stimulating capabilities. For example, although norepinephrine is frequently considered to have only vasoconstrictor *(alpha*-adrenergic) properties, its potent *beta*-adrenergic activity is apparent when the *alpha*-adrenergic system is

CARDIAC EFFECTS BETA STIMULATION

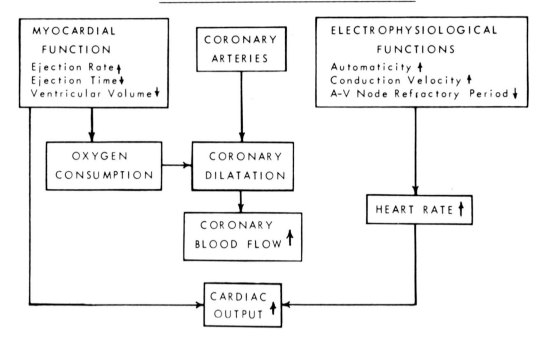

Fig. 7–3. Cardiac effects of *beta*-adrenergic stimulation. See text for details.

blocked. Isoproterenol is a pure *beta*-adrenergic stimulating compound and methoxamine appears to be a pure *alpha*-adrenergic compound. These drugs represent the exception rather than the rule.

PROPERTIES OF *BETA*-ADRENERGIC BLOCKING DRUGS

As a group, *beta*-adrenergic blockers have four principal actions on the cardiovascular system. These include actions mediated by the *beta*-adrenergic nervous system, plus other actions:

1. Antagonism of *beta* 1 receptors.
2. Antagonism of *beta* 2 receptors.
3. Membrane-stabilizing or "quinidine-like" activity.
4. Sympathomimetic activity.

One must consider the relative actions of each specific drug in order to predict its effect. For example, it is theoretically possible to synthesize either cardioselective (*beta* 1) or cardiac-sparing (*beta* 2) *beta*-adrenergic

blocking drugs. Practolol is an example of the former, whereas butoxamine is an example of the latter. However, the terms "cardiac-sparing" and "cardioselective" are relative because when sufficiently high doses are administered, both *beta* 1 and *beta* 2 systems are affected.

At present, only one *beta*-adrenergic blocking drug, propranolol, is available for clinical use in the United States. In contrast, 12 are available in the Netherlands. Propranolol acts almost equally on the *beta* 1 and *beta* 2 receptors. It is devoid of sympathomimetic activities, but it does have an important membrane-stabilization effect, particularly in large doses. The latter property is primarily responsible for the myocardial depression that may be observed when large doses of propranolol are administered. This membrane-stabilization activity also accounts for the effectiveness of propranolol in the therapy of digitalis intoxication. In addition, propranolol has an antirenin effect that has recently come under increasing scrutiny, and that appears to have an important relation to the role of this drug in the therapy of essential hypertension.[13] Finally, it appears that the antihypertensive effect may also have a central nervous system component.[14]

METABOLISM OF PROPRANOLOL

The metabolism of propranolol is imperfectly understood. When ingested orally, the drug is absorbed completely, but up to 70% of the administered dose undergoes first pass metabolism in the liver. Thus an oral dose of propranolol is less effective than an intravenous dose of the drug. The effect of a single intravenous dose two hours after injection is less than the effect of an oral dose two hours later, even though the same propranolol concentration has been achieved in the blood. This disparity in effect between similar blood concentrations disappears by six hours and is thought to be due to an active short-lived metabolite (4 hydroxypropranolol) that is formed in the liver after oral administration.[15] After repeated oral administration neither drug dosage nor plasma level is reliably related to the degree of *beta* blockade.[16] This may be due to the factors discussed or it may be connected to the previously mentioned potential increase in the number of receptor sites.

The plasma half-life of propranolol has been studied in man after both intravenous and oral administration. The half-life after oral administration varies from 3½ to six hours.[17] Assuming a six-hour half-life, a 24-hour period of discontinuance means a plasma level of approximately 5%. Propranolol is no longer detectable in the plasma five minutes after the intravenous injection of 1 mg[18] (Fig. 7–4). In addition, a comparison of the decline of propranolol levels in the heart and the plasma of animals reveals that the decline in myocardial levels parallels the decline in plasma and indicates that there is no reservoir of propranolol in the heart after the discontinuance of the drug.[17] However, it is documented that the negative chrono-

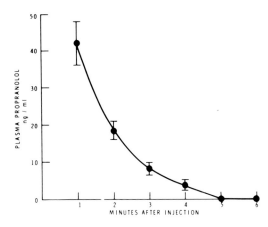

Fig. 7–4. Plasma propranolol concentration following administration of 1 mg intravenously in man. Although the drug is no longer detectable after five minutes, the duration of action appears to be between 15 and 30 minutes. (From Romagnoli, A., and Keats, A. S.: Plasma and atrial propranolol after preoperative withdrawal. Circulation, 52:1123, 1975.)

tropic effect of propranolol persists after the drug is no longer detectable in serum.[12]

CLINICAL APPLICATIONS

Nonsurgical indications for use of *beta*-adrenergic blockers

As is often the case with newly popular drugs, propranolol has been advised for many conditions, with or without justification. For example, on the basis of a double-blind crossover trial in which *beta* blockade appeared to improve the musical performance of solo string musicians, it was recommended that such drugs be considered when "career prospects or livelihood" were at stake.[19] More conventional indications include hypertrophic ventricular outflow tract obstruction of both the left ventricle (idiopathic hypertrophic subaortic stenosis, asymmetrical septal hypertrophy, disproportionate upper septal thickening,) and the right ventricle,[20] digitalis toxicity, essential hypertension (in combination with other drugs or by itself),[13,14,21] thyrotoxicosis, myocardial infarction, angina pectoris, hyperdynamic septic shock,[22] migraine headache, and opiate addiction.

It is beyond the scope of this chapter to discuss each indication in detail. However, it is not *beta* blockade itself that affects digitalis toxicity, but rather the membrane-stabilizing properties of propranolol. In addition, *beta*-adrenergic blockade does not affect the underlying increase in cardiac contractility present in thyrotoxicosis.[23]

The sensitivity of essential hypertension to propranolol depends on the nature of the disease.[13] High- and normal-renin-associated hypertension responds to modest (160 mg/day) doses of propranolol. Low-renin hypertension responds only to higher doses (320 mg/day and greater). Patients with low-renin hypertension may receive up to 3 g/day of propranolol to the time of an operation.[13]

Ischemic heart disease (angina pectoris, postmyocardial-infarction arrhythmias,

acute myocardial infarction) constitutes the best documented and most common indication for the administration of *beta*-adrenergic blockers. *Beta*-blockers clearly prolong the lifespan, enhance exercise tolerance in angina pectoris, help salvage ischemic myocardium in the presence of acute myocardial infarction, and effectively treat life-threatening arrhythmias, particularly atrial tachyarrhythmias.[24] The consequence of these many indications is the large number of surgical patients with a history of recent propranolol intake.

ANESTHETICS AND *BETA* BLOCKERS. A RATIONALE FOR CAUTION

Figure 7–5 schematically illustrates the function of the normal heart and the *beta*-adrenergically blocked heart. The normal heart easily handles its ordinary work load and has a large reserve besides. *Beta*-adrenergic blockade, by inhibiting the re-

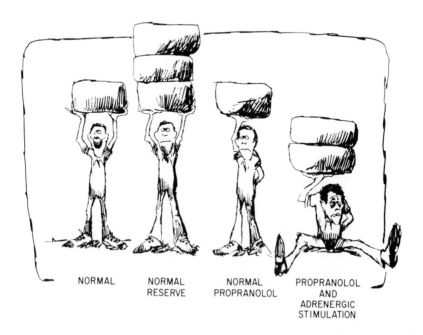

| NORMAL | NORMAL RESERVE | NORMAL PROPRANOLOL | PROPRANOLOL AND ADRENERGIC STIMULATION |

Fig. 7–5. Schematic illustration of the action of propranolol upon the normal heart. The heart is represented by the man, and the load (work) performed by the boulders he is lifting. Propranolol "ties one hand behind the heart's back." This allows the heart to accomplish a normal amount of work, but causes it to collapse when required to perform more, as in the presence of a catecholamine with *alpha*-agonist properties. See text for details.

sponse of the heart to endogenous (or exogenous) neurohumoral influences, limits the ability of the heart to respond to an increased load. In addition, *beta* 2-mediated vasodilation is prevented, whereas *alpha*-mediated vasoconstriction is not affected. Thus, although the heart may be able to tolerate a normal work load, it may not be able to fulfill the demands of the additional flow or pressure associated with stress. The combination of an insufficient inotropic and chronotropic response to catecholamines and unopposed vasoconstriction may lead to heart failure and cardiovascular collapse.

There are many perioperative interventions and situations that may provoke sympathoadrenal discharge. Although some anesthetic agents may induce the liberation of catecholamines, surgical or nonsurgical stimulation (for example, preoperative apprehension, surgical incision, retraction, blood loss, tracheal intubation, postoperative pain) may present the heart with *alpha* and *beta* stimulation. Since the *beta* receptors are already occupied by the blocking agent, the heart's ability to increase its contractile state or heart rate is impaired. Since the *alpha* receptors are not occupied, the peripheral arterial circulation may constrict, increasing the work demand of the heart. Thus the "handicapped" heart, with one hand symbolically tied behind its back (Fig. 7–5), may collapse.

Initial clinical experiences confirmed the fear of anesthetizing patients who were *beta* blocked. For example, 5 mg propranolol was associated with bradycardia and hypotension when administered intravenously in the presence of diethyl ether, an anesthetic known to rely on the liberation of endogenous catecholamines to maintain circulatory stability.[1] Cardiogenic shock refractory to maximal therapy was reported at the conclusion of cardiopulmonary bypass in a series of patients who had received large doses of propranolol until shortly before their operations.[2]

The fears of anesthetists regarding *beta*-blocked patients involve (1) the latent im-

balance of the sympathetic system during *beta* blockade, (2) the clinical inability to reverse *beta* blockade, and (3) the side effect of direct myocardial depression due to the membrane-stabilizing effect.

Mechanisms of *beta* adrenergic agents in the presence of ischemic heart disease

Beta-adrenergic blockers appear to benefit ischemic or potentially ischemic myocardium by correcting, minimizing, or preventing an imbalance between myocardial oxygen demand and myocardial oxygen supply. The principal determinants of myocardial oxygen demand include myocardial wall tension, which is proportional to the ventricular systolic pressure and the ventricular volume, the contractile state of the heart, and the heart rate.[25] (Under most circumstances, the left ventricle, which performs "pressure work," is responsible for the major portion of myocardial oxygen demand. When severe right ventricular hypertension or hypertrophy is present, that ventricle may have similar requirements.) Thus propranolol may decrease or prevent increases in left ventricular systolic pressure and heart rate, and may reduce the contractile state, all of which decrease myocardial oxygen demand (Table 7–1). On the other hand, the drug may dilate the ventricles and increase systolic ejection

Table 7–1

Effects of propranolol in relation to myocardial oxygen consumption ($M\dot{V}_{O_2}$)

		$M\dot{V}_{O_2}$
1.	Decrease (prevent increase) left ventricular systolic pressure	↓
2.	Decrease (prevent increase) heart rate	↓
3.	Decrease (prevent increase) contractile state	↓
4.	Increase systolic ejection period	↑
5.	Cause left ventricular dilation	↑

Propranolol may also affect myocardial oxygen supply by two mechanisms. See text for details.

time, both of which increase myocardial oxygen demand. The balance between the beneficial and detrimental effects on the net myocardial oxygen balance is the primary determinant of whether the response is beneficial or detrimental.[26]

In addition, *beta*-adrenergic blockers may promote the intramyocardial redistribution of blood flow to those areas most ischemic, a type of "Robin Hood" effect (Fig. 7–6). This concept was originally postulated by McGregor.[27] Although decreased coronary artery blood flow and increased coronary vascular resistance are documented after propranolol, this is thought to occur only in normal, nonischemic situations. Local metabolic regulation supervenes in the presence of ischemia.

CONDUCTANCE
VESSELS
(α receptors)   RESISTANCE
VESSELS
(β receptors)

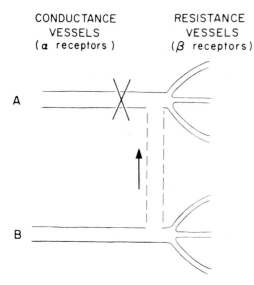

Fig. 7–6.   Schematic diagram of the mechanism by which *beta*-adrenergic blockers may redistribute blood flow from normal to ischemic areas of myocardium. Occlusion in vascular bed A renders tissues ischemic, and thus reduces local resistance by producing maximal vasodilation. Collaterals (dashed lines) are the only source of blood for the ischemic area. *Beta* blockade enhances vascular resistance in nonischemic bed B, which results in favoring blood flow through the collaterals from B to A. Experimental confirmation of this hypothesis has been presented by Pitt. (From *Cardiovascular Beta Adrenergic Responses.* Edited by A. A. Kattus, G. Ross, and V. Hall. (UCLA Forum in Medical Sciences, No. 13.) Los Angeles, University of California Press, 1970.)

CORONARY ARTERY DISEASE

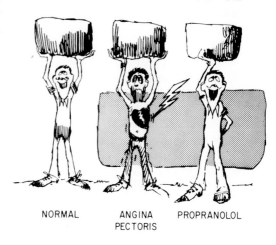

NORMAL   ANGINA   PROPRANOLOL
PECTORIS

Fig. 7–7.   Schematic representation of the situation pertaining in the presence of coronary artery disease. Angina pectoris occurs when the heart is performing a normal amount of work; propranolol allows the same amount of work to be accomplished without evidence of myocardial ischemia.

Thus *beta* blockade relieves myocardial ischemia and angina pectoris by reestablishing a balance between myocardial oxygen demand and myocardial oxygen supply, which is limited in the patient with ischemic heart disease (Fig. 7–7).

Intraoperative administration of *beta*-adrenergic blocking agents

Intraoperative situations occur in which it is theoretically desirable to administer a *beta*-adrenergic blocker. Experience proves that in this instance theory and practice coincide. These situations include sinus tachycardia, such as associated with the administration of atropine, gallamine, and pancuronium; the prevention of tachycardia, hypertension, ventricular arrhythmias, and myocardial ischemia during laryngoscopy and tracheal intubation of patients with hypertensive heart disease[5] (Fig. 7–8); a tachycardia in patients with evidence of acute myocardial ischemia (Fig. 7–9); an increase in heart rate and ventricular irritabil-

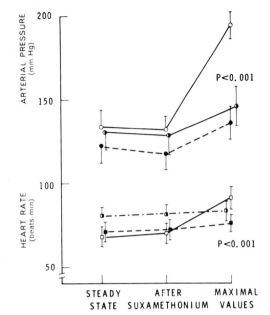

Fig. 7–8. Response of arterial blood pressure and heart rate to suxamethonium (succinylcholine) administration followed by laryngoscopy and tracheal intubation ("maximal values") during a standard anesthetic in three groups of patients with essential hypertension. Patients designated by the solid and half-filled squares and circles had received a *beta*-blocking drug, whereas those designated by the open circles and squares had not. The heart rate and blood pressure increases normally associated with laryngoscopy were attenuated by *beta* blockade. Incidence of ischemic ECG changes was reduced from 38 to 4%. (From Prys-Roberts, C., et al.: Studies of anesthesia in relation to hypertension. V. Adrenergic *beta*-receptor blockade. Br. J. Anaesth., *45*:671, 1973.)

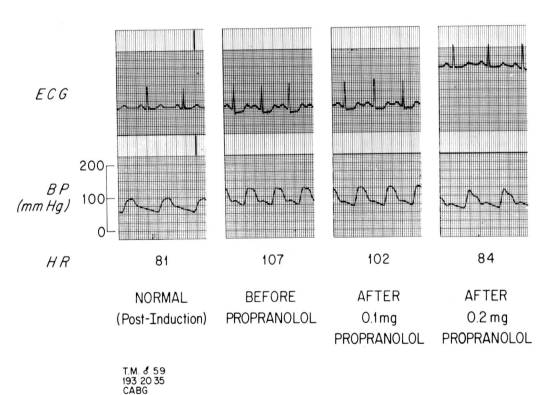

Fig. 7–9. Relief of electrocardiographic evidence of myocardial ischemia by propranolol administration. A modest rise in heart rate (81 to 107) and blood pressure (100/55 to 125/75), consequent to surgical stimulation was associated with a 2 mm depression of ST segment. Two 0.1 mg increments of propranolol were associated with return of blood pressure and heart rate to pre-ischemic levels, and restoration of ST segment to normal.

ity consequent to catecholamine release secondary to the manipulation of a pheochromocytoma (only in the presence of *alpha*-adrenergic receptor blockade); and hyperthyroid crisis.

The administration of propranolol prior to cardiopulmonary bypass in patients with ventricular hypertrophy, particularly in patients with severe aortic valve disease, is associated with a decrease in the incidence of ischemic contracture of the ventricle ("stone heart").[28] The dose recommended in adults is 1 to 2 mg. The acute hemodynamic effects of such a dose are minor under these circumstances. In some centers the success of this regimen has led to its routine use prior to aortic cross-clamping and cardiopulmonary bypass in patients without hypertrophic ventricles. Objective evidence that this practice is beneficial awaits confirmation.

The administration of propranolol for the relief of life-threatening ventricular or atrial tachyarrhythmias is also a success (Fig. 7–10). In some centers propranolol is used initially for the relief of ventricular irritability, although lidocaine is still generally preferred. Atrial tachyarrhythmias are particularly devastating in patients with cardiac diseases (coronary artery disease, aortic stenosis). Propranolol is effective in these situations.

The suggested dose-rates at which propranolol is administered intravenously vary greatly. Prys-Roberts recommends a 5 mg bolus in adults, and the earlier Swedish studies with ether and halothane anesthesia also used this regimen.[1,30] In most hospitals, increments of 0.25 to 1 mg to a total dose of .075 to 0.15 mg/kg maximum in adults are used. In children, the increments are smaller but the maximum total dose range is similar.

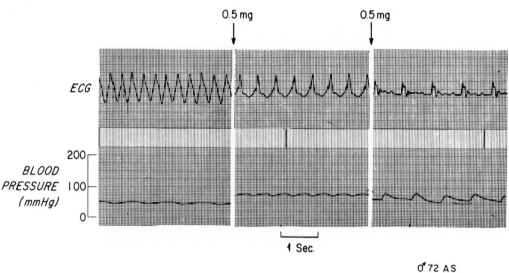

Fig. 7–10. Resolution by propranolol of chaotic ventricular rhythm prior to termination of cardiopulmonary bypass. Left panel: Chaotic rhythm persisted despite multiple attempts at electrical defibrillation and drug therapy including lidocaine, procaine amide, phenytoin, and bretyllium tolsylate at termination of cardiopulmonary bypass. Center panel: Propranolol (0.5 mg) produced an organized ventricular rhythm. Right panel: A further 0.5 mg propranolol was associated with sinus rhythm with AV and intraventricular block, increased ventricular ejection as indicated on the blood pressure tracing, and effective heart action. The patient's further course was uneventful.

Contraindications to *beta*-adrenergic blockade

The primary contraindications to *beta*-adrenergic blockade are congestive heart failure, second- or third-degree heart block, and asthma. It is important to differentiate congestive heart failure, in which the heart is dependent on a catacholamine drive to maintain an adequate cardiac output, from acute elevations in left ventricular filling pressure associated with tachyarrhythmias. In the former, a *beta* blocker may be disastrous; in the latter it may be lifesaving (Fig. 7–11). A *beta* blocker should not be administered in the presence of second- or third-degree heart block unless pacing capabilities are immediately available. At present, no cardioselective *beta* blocker for use in patients with asthma is available in the United States for therapy in patients with asthma. However, bronchoconstriction has been described in asthmatic patients even when a cardioselective drug has been employed,[29] emphasizing that cardioselectivity is a relative term.

Reversal of propranolol-associated circulatory depression (Table 7–2)

In most instances, circulatory depression associated with *beta*-adrenergic blockade consists of the combination of bradycardia and hypotension, which is usually relieved by atropine.[1,30] If readily available, as in cardiac surgical situations, cardiac pacing (preferably atrial) is equally effective. If bradycardia is not present, calcium chloride, up to 7 mg/kg by intravenous

Table 7–2
Therapy of propranolol-associated circulatory depression

1. Bradycardia
   Atropine
   Cardiac pacing
2. Pharmacologic antagonist
   Isoproterenol
3. Action beyond the block
   Digitalis
   Calcium chloride
4. Empiric
   Epinephrine in low doses

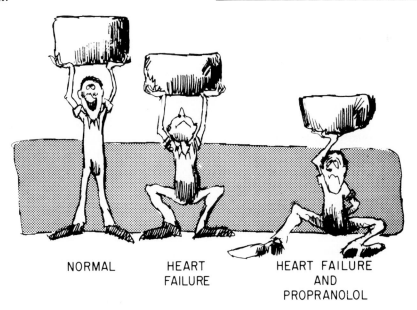

NORMAL   HEART   HEART FAILURE
                FAILURE   AND
                              PROPRANOLOL

Fig. 7–11. Schematic diagram of the effect of propranolol administration in heart failure. Chronic heart failure is associated with progressive dependence on catecholamines for maintenance of circulatory integrity. Propranolol induces acute interruption of this support, and collapse may occur without increasing the burden of the heart. Compare situation here to that depicted in the normal heart (Fig. 7–5) and the heart with coronary artery disease (Fig. 7–7).

bolus, usually reverses hypotension. Whether this response is due to enhanced myocardial contractility or to increased systemic vascular resistance is not known. Whereas the specific pharmacologic *beta* agonist isoproterenol may be able to antagonize both the negative chronotropic and inotropic effects of propranolol, one must employ enormous doses. For example, in the presence of normal doses of propranolol (80 to 240 mg/day), the standard dose of isoproterenol must be increased 25 to 50 times[17] (see Table 7–3). The inotropic response may be less affected, but still required eight and 13 times the preblockade dose of isoproterenol in two patients receiving 160 and 240 mg/day.[17] On a long-term basis, digitalis is sometimes used to prevent the circulatory depression caused by large doses of propranolol, although this has little relevance to anesthesia. In spite of its theoretical contraindication, low doses of epinephrine (< 2 μg/min) are sometimes used to reverse hypotension. The effect on cardiac output and systemic vascular resistance under these circumstances is not adequately defined.

Interactions between anesthesia and *beta*-adrenergic blockade

The study of the interaction between anesthesia and *beta*-adrenergic blockade raises two questions: First, is there an additive and/or synergistic interaction between the circulatory-depressant action of the *beta*-adrenergic blocking agents and that of the anesthetic agents? Second, should *beta* blockers be withheld or withdrawn prior to cardiac or noncardiac operations? These questions have been investigated in animals, and much information has been accumulated by experience in man.

Anesthetic agents can be divided into those that depend on the release of endogenous catecholamines to counteract their depressant effects (and therefore to maintain circulatory stability), and those that do not. There is certainly some overlap between these categories. Ether and cyclopropane typify anesthetic agents that depend on endogenous catecholamine liberation to support the circulation. Although narcotic anesthesia is believed to be associated with catecholamine liberation during operations, circulatory competence does not appear to be dependent on this release. Whether other anesthetic agents, specifically isoflurane, are associated with catecholamine release is still undecided.[31,32] With the recent development of more sensitive techniques of measuring the blood levels of catecholamines, however, this association should soon be understood, not only for isoflurane, but for all anesthetic drugs.

For the reasons cited previously, it appears prudent to avoid *beta*-adrenergic blockade during ether and cyclopropane, since they depend on catecholamine release for the maintenance of circulatory integrity. In healthy volunteers, a 5 mg bolus of propranolol injected intravenously during ether anesthesia induced decreased heart rate, stroke volume, cardiac output, and increased systemic vascular resistance. The single episode of severe circulatory depression (hypotension, bradycardia) observed was reversed by atropine. Although data on intravenous induction agents are presently insufficient, ketamine appears to be similar to ether anesthesia in its dependence on endogenous catecholamines for circulatory integrity. Thus it may be wise to avoid the combination of *beta*-adrenergic blockers and this drug.

Those anesthetic agents that do not depend on catecholamine release for circulatory stability include halothane,[33] narcotics, methoxyflurane, trichloroethylene, enflurane, and isoflurane. Clinical and experimental data indicate that the combination of *beta* blockers with either narcotics or halothane is safe. For instance, the circulatory response to halothane in the normovolemic or hypovolemic animal is similar at several levels of halothane anesthesia, whether or not the animal has received a *beta*-adrenergic blocker.[34] Kopriva et al. re-

Table 7–3

Effect of beta blockade on subsequent response to isoproterenol in man

Dose Propranolol (mg/day)	Chronotropic		Inotropic	
	Multiple	Absolute	Multiple	Absolute
80	× 50	(40 μg)	—	—
160	× 23	(42 μg)	× 13	(17 μg)
240	× 38	(34 μg)	× 8	(6 μg)

Effect of *beta*-blockade with oral propranolol (80 to 240 mg/day) on the subsequent response to intravenous isoproterenol in three subjects with coronary artery disease. Note the enormous increase in the dose of isoproterenol (23 to 50 times the original dose) required to increase heart rate by the same increment as before blockade. The dose required to increase contractility is also greatly elevated, but the increase is less than that required to elevate heart rate. (Data from Faulkner, S. L., et al.: Time required for complete recovery from chronic propranolol therapy. N. Engl. J. Med., *289:*607, 1973.)

ported the response of two groups of patients with ischemic heart disease to an anesthetic regimen consisting of thiopental, succinylcholine, nitrous oxide, halothane, and pancuronium.[35] One group received an average of 140 mg propranolol per day until a few hours before general anesthesia, whereas the other group did not receive the drug. The only difference between the groups was the lower heart rate in the group treated with propranolol. No differences in mean arterial pressure, cardiac output, stroke volume, or systemic vascular resistance were present in response to anesthesia or endotracheal intubation. Ventricular filling pressures were not measured in this study. Slogoff et al.[36] compared the response to isoproteronol *beta*-adrenergic stimulation of propranolol-blocked dogs receiving either halothane or morphine anesthesia. The researchers demonstrated that propranolol is associated with dose-related decreases in heart rate, cardiac index, stroke volume index, and left ventricular contractility, as well as increases in mean aortic pressure, systemic vascular resistance, and pulmonary capillary wedge pressure. However, no increased sensitivity to any measured effect of propranolol, expressed as the slope of the log dose-response curve, was observed. The researchers concluded that there was no potentiation by morphine or halothane of the effects of propranolol.

Studies with enflurane, trilene, and methoxyflurane, however, cause concern. For instance, enflurane is associated with marginally greater impairment of left ventricular function than halothane anesthesia in the normovolemic *beta*-adrenergically blocked dog. However, withdrawal of 20% of estimated blood volume is tolerated poorly by the circulation during enflurane anesthesia.[37] The degree of circulatory depression produced under these circumstances would be clinically unacceptable. The relevance of these particular animal studies to the clinical situation is still in question, however. Enflurane is widely used to anesthetize patients receiving propranolol for cardiac operations, and there is little evidence that unacceptable circulatory depression is induced. The resolution of the disparity between the implications of animal studies and the apparently benign clinical experience awaits investigation.

Trichloroethylene anesthesia in the normovolemic *beta*-blocked dog, pretreated for three weeks with 20 mg/kg/day of propranolol orally, did not inhibit adequate cardiovascular function.[38] However, the response to graded hemorrhage was associated with a decrease in cardiac output that precluded recovery in some animals. The cause of the circulatory collapse appeared to be direct myocardial depression, since normal left ventricular filling pressures were associated with inadequate stroke volumes.

The most alarming observations have been made with the combination of methoxyflurane 0.4% and practolol.[39] Three of ten dogs receiving practolol under these circumstances died within 15 minutes. These are the only deaths encountered by the investigators at Oxford when using this model. In the seven survivors, cardiac output and left ventricular dP/dt decreased, and left ventricular end diastolic pressure increased in the presence of normal heart rate, blood pressure, and systemic vascular resistance. The clinical applicability of these studies is indicated by the report of a series of cardiac surgical patients who demonstrated irreversible circulatory depression at the termination of cardiopulmonary bypass after having received methoxyflurane.[2]

In contrast, experimental evidence suggests that isoflurane might be the ideal anesthetic agent to employ in the presence of *beta*-adrenergic blockade. Philbin and Lowenstein found no difference in cardiac output, arterial blood pressure, systemic vascular resistance, heart rate, or left ventricular filling pressure in dogs anesthetized with one and two MAC (minimum alveolar concentrations) isoflurane before and after administration of 0.5 mg/kg propranolol[31,40] (Fig. 7–12). These investigators were therefore unable to confirm any *beta*-adrenergic receptor effects of isoflurane.

Sensitive indices of ventricular performance are now found to be minimally depressed when 0.3 mg/kg propranolol is administered to dogs receiving isoflurane.[32] Thus isoflurane may be associated with a *beta*-adrenergic receptor-stimulating effect, although the effect may be small, and its clinical importance remains uncertain. However, although the dose of propranolol used in these studies is reputed not to cause myocardial depression, an ordinarily undetectable depression by propranolol in addition to a similar degree of depression by isoflurane might be responsible for these findings.

The studies performed to date in both man and animals thus indicate that myocardial depression from anesthetic agents and *beta*-adrenergic blockers is additive, and that a spectrum of tolerance to the combination of different anesthetic agents and a *beta* blocker exists (see Fig. 7–13). The clinical

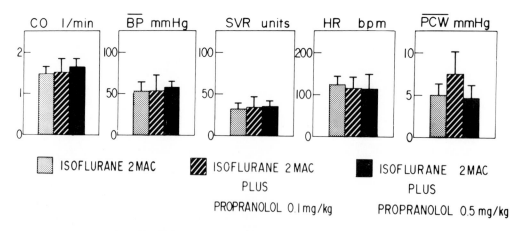

Fig. 7–12. Hemodynamic effect of propranolol during 2MAC isoflurane anesthesia in the dog. There was no detectable difference in cardiac output, arterial blood pressure, systemic vascular resistance, heart rate, and pulmonary capillary wedge pressure among three groups of dogs receiving isoflurane anesthesia, despite the absence of propranolol in one group, a modest dose (0.1 mg/kg) in a second group, and a large dose (0.5 mg/kg) in the third. The data suggest that isoflurane administration is associated with little if any *beta*-adrenergic agonism. (From Philbin, D. M., and Lowenstein, E.: Lack of *beta*-adrenergic activity of isoflurane in the dog: A comparison of circulatory effects of halothane and isoflurane after propranolol administration. Br. J. Anaesth., *48*:1165, 1976.)

MOF
ETHER
CYCLO
TRILENE
ENFLURANE
HALOTHANE
NARCOTICS
ISOFLURANE

Fig. 7–13. Pyramid denoting the spectrum of compatibility of the combination of various anesthetic agents and *beta* blockade. See text for detail.

implications of the data are that an absolute indication for the use of methoxyflurane, diethyl ether, trichloroethylene, or cyclopropane must exist before these drugs should be used in combination with *beta*-adrenergic blockers. The status of the combination of *beta* blockers and enflurane is undecided.

DISCONTINUANCE PRIOR TO ANESTHESIA AND OPERATION

Whether to discontinue *beta*-adrenergic blockade prior to the administration of general anesthesia is a controversial question. The proponents of discontinuance believe that circulatory depression from the anesthetic-*beta* blocker combination is possibly fatal. Those opposed to discontinuance feel strongly about the hazards of the former course of action. They base their arguments on the following factors: (1) if a patient needs *beta* blockade for relief of angina pectoris and myocardial insufficiency, withdrawal of a drug essential to the patient is irrational and hazardous, particularly in view of the formidable stress of the perioperative period;[4,41,42] and (2) the discontinuance of a *beta*-adrenergic blockade may lead to a situ-

ation analogous to denervation supersensitivity.[8]

Obviously, *beta* blockade could be safely discontinued in patients who did not initially present a valid indication for it. Only anecdotal clinical data exist to support the contention that *beta*-adrenergic blockers should be withheld or decreased in dose. Since some of these recommendations come from respected anesthesiologists in highly regarded clinical centers, it seems unwarranted to dismiss them. However, evidence exists that favors the continuance of *beta*-adrenergic blockers until anesthesia and operation. In fact, this evidence argues for the prophylactic administration of *beta* blockers prior to anesthesia in some instances, as well as their continuance throughout the postoperative period. The most compelling argument is the evidence that the discontinuance of *beta*-adrenergic blocking agents in patients who require these drugs for the control of severe angina is associated with an unacceptably high incidence of acute life-threatening, or even fatal, complications (Fig. 7–14).

In one carefully controlled study[4] (see Table 7–4), such complications, including two deaths, were observed in six of 20 pa-

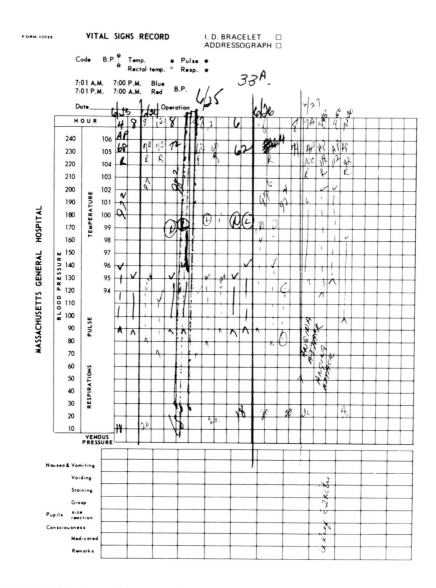

Fig. 7–14. Vital signs record demonstrating the hazard of preoperative discontinuance of propranolol in a patient with severe coronary artery disease. The last dose of propranolol was administered at 10 P.M. 6/25. Less than 36 hours later, the blood pressure had risen from a steady value of 130/90 to 200/130, and the heart rate from the low 60's to a maximum of 118 beats/min. These changes were associated with angina pectoris and severe (up to 6 mm) depression of the ST segment in the precordial leads.

tients. Increased severity of angina pectoris was observed in an additional four. Those patients who had the most severe angina pectoris were the ones who experienced the

Table 7–4
Complications associated with acute cessation of propranolol in 20 patients receiving it for symptoms of coronary artery disease

Fatalities	2
(Sudden death . . . . 1)	
(Fatal myocardial infarction . . . . 1)	
Acute life-threatening events	4
(Unstable angina pectoris . . . . 3)	
(Ventricular tachycardia . . . . 1)	
Increased severity of angina pectoris	4

(Data from Miller, R. R., et al.: Propranolol-withdrawal rebound phenomenon. N. Engl. J. Med., 293:416, 1975.)

greatest difficulty. Other studies confirm these data.[42,43]

An additional factor may be the enhanced sensitivity to catecholamines subsequent to withdrawal of *beta* blockers, a phenomenon now confirmed in man.[8] Finally, systematic prospective studies have failed to demonstrate an increased incidence of untoward circulatory complications during anesthesia in the presence of *beta*-adrenergic blockade[3,43] (Fig. 7–15). We still must determine whether there is a decreased incidence of perioperative myocardial infarctions in patients with ischemic heart disease who are subjected to cardiac or noncardiac operations and who are either given prophylactic propranolol or who continue to take it. Overall, I believe that *beta* blockade should not be discontinued prior to anesthesia and operation, since there appears to be consid-

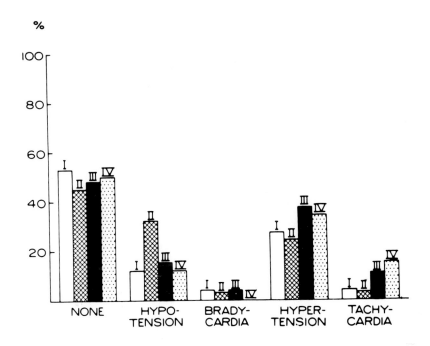

Fig. 7–15. Intra-anesthetic, precardiopulmonary bypass cardiovascular complications as a function of propranolol therapy in patients with coronary artery disease. Group I, propranolol discontinued less than 24 hours prior to surgery; Group II, 24 to 48 hours; Group III, greater than 48 hours; Group IV, no previous propranolol. No statistical differences existed between any of the groups. However, there is a suggestion that hypertension and tachycardia were more common in Group III and IV as compared to Group I and II. (From Jones, E. L., et al.: Propranolol therapy in patients undergoing myocardial revascularization. Am. J. Cardiol., *38*:697, 1976.)

erable benefit and little risk to its continuance.

REFERENCES

1. Jorfeldt, L., et al.: Propranolol in ether anesthesia. Acta Anaesthesiol. Scand., *11*:159, 1967.
2. Viljoen, J. F., Estafanous, F. G., and Kellner, G. A.: Propranolol and cardiac surgery. J. Thorac. Cardiovasc. Surg., *64*:826, 1972.
3. Kaplan, J. A., et al.: Propranolol and cardiac surgery: A problem for the anesthesiologist? Anesth. Analg. (Cleve.), *54*:571, 1975.
4. Miller, R. R., et al.: Propranolol-withdrawal rebound phenomenon. N. Engl. J. Med., *293*:416, 1975.
5. Prys-Roberts, C., et al.: Studies of anaesthesia in relation to hypertension. V: Adrenergic *beta*-receptor blockade. Br. J. Anaesth., *45*:671, 1973.
6. Moran, N.C.: The role of *alpha*- and *beta*-adrenergic receptors in the control of the circulation and in the actions of drugs. *In* Cardiovascular Therapy. Edited by H. R. Russek and B. L. Zoliman. Baltimore, Williams & Wilkins, 1971.
7. Lefkowitz, R. J.: *Beta*-adrenergic receptors: recognition and regulation. N. Engl. J. Med., *295*:323, 1976.
8. Boudoulas, H., et al.: Hypersensitivity to adrenergic stimulation after propranolol withdrawal in normal subjects. Ann. Intern. Med., *87*:433, 1977.
9. Ahlquist, R. P.: A study of the adrenotropic receptors. Am. J. Physiol., *153*:586, 1948.
10. Lands, A. M., et al.: Differentiation of receptor systems activated by sympathomimetic amines. Nature, *214*:597, 1967.
11. Dreyer, A. C., and Offermeier, J.: Indications for the existence of two types of cardiac *beta*-adrenergic receptors. Pharmacol. Res. Commun., *7*:151, 1975.
12. Boudoulas, H., et al.: Differential time course of inotropic and chronotropic blockade after oral propranolol. Cardiovasc. Med., *2*:511, 1977.
13. Hollifield, J. W., et al.: Proposed mechanisms of propranolol's antihypertensive effect in essential hypertension. N. Engl. J. Med., *295*:68, 1976.
14. Holland, O. B., and Kaplan, N. M.: Propranolol in the treatment of hypertension. N. Engl. J. Med., *294*:930, 1976.
15. Nies, A. S., and Shand, D. G.: Clinical pharmacology of propranolol. Circulation, *52*:6, 1975.
16. Coltart, D. J., and Shand, D. G.: Plasma propranolol levels in the quantitative assessment of *beta*-adrenergic blockade in man. Br. Med. J., *3*:731, 1970.
17. Faulkner, S. L., et al.: Time required for complete recovery from chronic propranolol therapy. N. Engl. J. Med., *289*:607, 1973.
18. Romagnoli, A., and Keats, A. S.: Plasma and atrial propranolol after preoperative withdrawal. Circulation, *52*:1123, 1975.
19. James, I. M., et al.: Effect of oxprenolol on stage-fright in musicians. Lancet, *2*:952, 1977.
20. Stenson, R. E., et al.: Hypertrophic subaortic stenosis: Clinical and hemodynamic effects of long-term propranolol therapy. Am. J. Cardiol., *31*:763, 1973.
21. Zacest, R., Gilmore, E., and Koch-Weser, J.: Treatment of essential hypertension with combined vasodilation and *beta*-adrenergic blockade. N. Engl. J. Med., *286*:617, 1972.
22. Berk, J. L., et al.: The treatment of shock with *beta*-adrenergic blockade. Arch. Surg., *104*:46, 1972.
23. Grossman, W., et al.: The enhanced myocardial contractility of thyrotoxicosis. Ann. Intern. Med., *74*:869, 1971.
24. Pitt, B., and Ross, R. S.: *Beta* adrenergic blockade in cardiovascular therapy. Mod. Concepts Cardiovasc. Dis., *38*:47, 1969.
25. Braunwald, E.: The determinants of myocardial oxygen consumption. Physiologist, *12*:65, 1969.
26. Aronow, W. S.: The medical treatment of angina pectoris. VI. Propranolol as an antianginal drug. Am. Heart. J., *84*:706, 1972.
27. McGregor, M.: Drugs for the treatment of angina. *In* International Encyclopedia of Pharmacology and Therapeutics. Edited by L. Lasagna. Oxford, Pergamon, 1966, Vol. II, Section 6.
28. Reul, G., et al.: Protective effect of propranolol on the hypertrophied heart during cardiopulmonary bypass. J. Thorac. Cardiovasc. Surg., *68*:283, 1974.
29. Bernecker, C., and Roetscher, I.: The *beta*-blocking effect of practolol in asthmatics. Lancet, *2*:662, 1970.
30. Jorfeldt, L., et al.: Cardiovascular effects of *beta*-receptor blocking drugs during halothane anaesthesia in man. Acta Anesthesiol. Scand., *14*:35, 1970.
31. Philbin, D. M., and Lowenstein, E.: Lack of *beta*-adrenergic activity of isoflurane in the dog: A comparison of circulatory effects of halothane and isoflurane after propranolol administration. Br. J. Anaesth., *48*:1165, 1976.
32. Horan, B. F., et al.: Haemodynamic responses to isoflurane anaesthesia and hypovolaemia in the dog, and their modification by propranolol. Br. J. Anaesth., *49*:1179, 1977.
33. Merin, R. G., and Tonnesen, A. S.: The effect of *beta*-adrenergic blockade on myocardial haemodynamics and metabolism during light halothane anaesthesia. Can. Anaesth. Soc. J., *16*:336, 1969.
34. Roberts, J. G., et al.: Haemodynamic interactions of high-dose propranolol pretreatment and anaesthesia in the dog. I: Halothane dose-response studies. Br. J. Anaesth., *48*:315, 1976.
35. Kopriva, C. J., Brown, A. C. D., and Pappas, G.: Hemodynamics during general anesthesia in patients receiving propranolol. Anesthesiology, *48*:28, 1978.
36. Slogoff, S., et al.: Failure of general anesthesia to potentiate propranolol activity. Anesthesiology, *47*:504, 1977.
37. Horan, B. F., et al.: Haemodynamic responses to enflurane anaesthesia and hypovolaemia in the dog, and their modification by propranolol. Br. J. Anaesth., *49*:1189, 1977.

38. Roberts, J. G., et al.: Haemodynamic interactions of high-dose propranolol pretreatment and anaesthesia in the dog. III: the effects of haemorrhage during halothane and trichloroethylene anaesthesia. Br. J. Anaesth., *48*:411, 1976.

39. Saner, C. A., et al.: Methoxyflurane and practolol: a dangerous combination? Br. J. Anaesth., *47*:1025, 1975.

40. Philbin, D. M., and Lowenstein, E.: Lack of *beta* adrenergic activity of isoflurane in the dog: A comparison of circulatory effects of halothane and isoflurane after propranolol administration. Br. J. Anaesth., *48*:1165, 1976.

41. Slome, R.: Withdrawal of propranolol and myocardial infarction. Lancet, *1*:156, 1973.

42. Mizgala, H. F., and Counsell, J.: Acute coronary syndromes following abrupt cessation of oral propranolol therapy. Can. Med. Assoc. J., *114*:1123, 1976.

43. Jones, E. L., et al.: Propranolol therapy in patients undergoing myocardial revascularization. Am. J. Cardiol., *38*:697, 1976.

Supported in part by United States Public Health Service grants GM15904–11 and HL17665–4.

Chapter **8**

Antihypertensives and *Alpha* Blockers

ROBERT K. STOELTING

An estimated 20 to 25 million Americans have essential hypertension. Two recent Veterans Administration cooperative studies confirm that pharmacologic treatment of hypertension decreases both the morbidity and the mortality associated with the disease.[1,2] These data and other studies that demonstrate the dangers of hypertension will likely increase the incidence of anesthesia and operation in patients receiving antihypertensive therapy.[3,4]

Drugs that selectively impair sympathetic nervous system (SNS) function are frequently selected as antihypertensive agents for the treatment of ambulatory essential hypertension. Antihypertensive drugs (Table 8–1) may act on the central nervous system, autonomic ganglia, adrenergic nerve endings (alter synthesis, storage, release, uptake, or metabolism of the neurotransmitter), adrenoceptive receptors (*alpha-* and *beta*-adrenergic blockers), or directly on the vascular smooth muscle. As with all potent drugs, the rational use of antihypertensives requires an understanding of their basic pharmacology. A knowledge of the anatomy and physiology of the peripheral autonomic nervous system (ANS) is needed for the safe anesthetic management of patients receiving antihypertensive drugs.

CASE REPORT

A 65-year-old, 85-kg man was admitted to the hospital with the diagnosis of an abdominal aortic aneurysm. The patient's current medications included a thiazide diuretic, methyldopa 1,000 mg/day, and hydralazine 80 mg/day for the treatment of essential hypertension. An

103

Table 8–1

Antihypertensive drugs used for the treatment of ambulatory essential hypertension

Drug	Trade Name	Oral Dose for Maintenance (70-kg patient)
reserpine	Serpasil	0.1 – 0.5 mg/day
alpha-methyldopa (methyldopa)	Aldomet	500 – 2,000 mg/day
guanethidine	Ismelin	10 – 200 mg/day
hydralazine	Apresoline	40– 300 mg/day
clonidine	Catapres	0.2– 0.8 mg/day
pargyline	Eutonyl	10 – 150 mg/day

unknown drug prescribed for the treatment of "depression" had not been taken for the past four weeks.

Preoperative laboratory measurements were:

Hemoglobin 15 gms %
Sodium 145 meq/L
Potassium 3.9 meq/L
Creatinine 0.8 mg %
Serum glutamic-oxaloacetic
transaminase—slightly elevated
Total bilirubin 0.8 mg %
Prothrombin time 100%
Plasma thromboplastin time—normal

The patient's supine blood pressure was 140/85 torr, and his heart rate was 56 beats/min. The electrocardiogram showed sinus bradycardia and left ventricular hypertrophy.

During the preoperative visit the patient complained of back pain, tiredness, and a "dizzy feeling" on arising in the morning. Pending a satisfactory type and crossmatch for ten units of whole blood, the operation was scheduled for the next morning.

Among the problems that this patient presented to the anesthesiologist were hypertension and the therapy for this condition.

ANATOMY AND PHYSIOLOGY OF THE PERIPHERAL AUTONOMIC NERVOUS SYSTEM

The peripheral ANS consists of sympathetic and parasympathetic divisions (Fig. 8–1). Preganglionic fibers from both divisions synapse in autonomic ganglia. Adrenergic postganglionic fibers release norepinephrine (NE) as the neurotransmit-

ter at adrenoceptive (*alpha, beta* 1, and *beta* 2) receptors. Preganglionic and postganglionic fibers that release acetylcholine as the neurotransmitter are termed cholinergic and the corresponding receptor sites are cholinoceptive. These receptors are further divided into nicotinic (autonomic ganglia and neuromuscular junction) and muscarinic (heart, airways, gastrointestinal tract, and genitourinary system). The SNS is most important with respect to the mechanism of antihypertensive drug action.

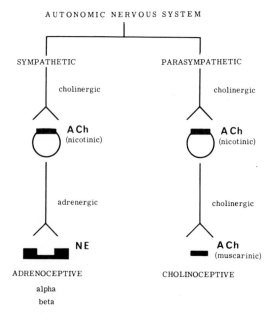

Fig. 8–1. A schematic diagram of the autonomic nervous system and its transmitters.

The postganglionic sympathetic nerve consists of a cell body, long axon, and a highly branched nerve terminal.[5] Varicosities of the nerve terminals are close to adrenoceptive sites. The varicosities contain vesicles or granules in which the neurotransmitter is both synthesized and stored. NE is synthesized from the amino acid tyrosine by a series of enzyme-controlled steps. Tyrosine is actively transported from the circulation into the varicosity of the nerve ending. The enzyme, tyrosine hydroxylase, converts tyrosine to dihydroxyphenylalanine (DOPA). The compound DOPA is decarboxylated to dopamine, which is then transported from the cytoplasm of the nerve ending into the storage vesicle where dopamine is converted to NE by dopamine *beta*-oxidase. An action potential causes NE to be extruded into the synaptic cleft so that a neurotransmitter-receptor interaction may occur.

Termination of NE activity at the adrenoceptive site is due primarily to uptake ("reuptake") of released NE back into the nerve terminal. The uptake process is not specific for NE. Structurally similar drugs, such as guanethidine, may enter the nerve ending and storage vesicle by the same process and ultimately deplete NE. In contrast, drugs such as ephedrine and cocaine may block this uptake process, making more NE available to adrenoceptive sites, which explains the exaggerated circulatory responses when sympathomimetics are administered. A small amount of NE is inactivated in the cytoplasm by monoamine oxidase (MAO) but most is delivered into the storage vesicle for reuse. The uptake and biosynthesis provide a large NE reserve and emphasize the difficulty in effecting a significant neurotransmitter depletion with antihypertensive drugs.

A small amount of NE escapes uptake and enters the circulation where it is metabolized by both MAO and catechol-O-methyl transferase (COMT). The final breakdown product is vanillylmandelic acid. Less than 5% of released NE escapes breakdown to appear unchanged in the urine. This factor emphasizes the difficulty in judging SNS activity at the receptor by measuring serum or urine NE concentrations.

INTERACTIONS OF ANTIHYPERTENSIVE DRUGS WITH ANESTHETICS

A properly functioning ANS permits adaptation to sudden environmental changes. Since antihypertensive drugs interfere with normal ANS function, the question whether to discontinue them preoperatively has been posed. Studies in patients receiving these drugs (usually reserpine) draw conflicting conclusions. Hypotension that occurs during anesthetic induction or maintenance and that responds poorly to sympathomimetic drugs is attributed to antihypertensive therapy and is the basis for the recommendation that such therapy be discontinued preoperatively.[6,7] In contrast, a controlled study demonstrated a greater incidence of blood pressure decrease in untreated hypertensive patients than in those treated with reserpine.[8] Furthermore, ephedrine (15 to 50 mg) was uniformly effective in increasing blood pressure in all patients requiring antihypertensive therapy. This suggests that sympathetic blockade after reserpine is incomplete and that it allows ephedrine to remain effective. Prys-Roberts et al. reported that treated or untreated hypertensive patients often developed hypotension accompanied by electrocardiographic evidence of myocardial ischemia during anesthetic induction, maintenance, or recovery.[9] In the same study, hypertensive patients who were rendered normotensive with drugs were indistinguishable from untreated normotensive patients. Furthermore, cardiac output fell to the same extent in all groups so that large decreases in blood pressure occurred in patients with a high resting peripheral vascular resistance.

Hypertensive patients, with or without antihypertensive therapy, are more likely to have marked fluctuations in blood pressure during anesthesia. *To discontinue anti-hypertensive drugs is undesirable if these drugs are necessary to keep the blood pressure in a normal range.* Better than the discontinuance of antihypertensive therapy is the understanding of the pharmacology of each drug and its possible interactions with anesthetics. Therefore, if problems occur, the anesthesiologist is prepared with proper pharmacologic or physiologic information.

Specific concerns during anesthesia for the patient receiving antihypertensive drugs have been reviewed by Dingle.[10] Some are the following.

Attenuated SNS activity

The impairment of circulatory homeostasis during anesthesia is related to the suppression of the SNS by antihypertensive drugs as manifested in the heart and peripheral vasculature. Orthostatic hypotension is an inevitable accompaniment to SNS inhibition. Sudden hypotension may reflect attenuated vasoconstriction during hemorrhage, positive pressure ventilation, sudden position change, or a response to vasodilation produced by anesthetics. In the presence of impaired SNS activity, the blood pressure varies with blood volume. Even minor blood loss may be followed by disproportionate decreases in blood pressure that reflect decreased venous return in the absence of adequate vasoconstrictor reflexes. Similarly, peripheral vasoconstriction is necessary to insure adequate venous return during positive pressure ventilation. Reduced cardiac sympathetic activity could decrease heart contractile force, and with vigorous volume expansion pulmonary edema might be more likely.

Preoperative evaluation of SNS function would be particularly valuable in patients taking antihypertensive drugs.[11]Unfortunately, no test reliably identifies that patient with neurovascular instability sufficient to pose an anesthetic risk. Orthostatic hypotension is the most commonly recog-nized abnormality of SNS dysfunction. Positive intrathoracic pressure (Valsalva maneuver) provides the most useful index of ANS function. However, it is not a practical clinical test, since the continuous recording of intra-arterial blood pressure is necessary for interpretation. A normal Valsalva response requires intact baroreceptors, vasomotor center, sympathetic and parasympathetic activity, and responsive end-organs. With an intact ANS a baroreceptor-mediated vasoconstriction and heart rate increase occur during the decrease in blood pressure produced by positive intrathoracic pressure. Following the release of the positive pressure, the heart rate slows in response to the blood pressure overshoot produced by the increased venous return. SNS impairment is evidenced by an unchanged heart rate during positive pressure and absence of a blood pressure overshoot when positive pressure is released.

Modification of response to sympathomimetic (vasopressor) drugs

The response to a sympathomimetic drug in the presence of antihypertensive therapy depends on the mechanism of action of both classes of drugs. To evoke a response, the sympathomimetic drug must excite the *alpha*-adrenergic effector site directly (direct-acting drug) or stimulate NE release, which then activates the *alpha*-effector site (indirect-acting drug). Many sympathomimetics exert a combination of direct and indirect effects, but one usually predominates. Antihypertensive drugs that deplete NE or that act on peripheral vascular smooth muscle decrease sensitivity to predominately indirect-acting sympathomimetics such as ephedrine (Table 8–2). In contrast, SNS block, which deprives the *alpha*-adrenergic receptors of tonic impulses, results in increased sensitivity to NE and direct-acting sympathomimetics.

Table 8–2

Effects of antihypertensive drugs on canine halothane anesthetic requirements (MAC) and response to intravenous ephedrine (0.5 mg/kg)[12]

	MAC decrease (%)	Systolic blood pressure increase (torr) in response to ephedrine	
		control	after drug
reserpine (0.2 mg/kg/day)	14 ± 5t	74 ± 20	33 ± 5
methyldopa (50 mg/kg/day)	16 ± 5	86 ± 14	30 ± 10
guanethidine (15 mg/kg/day)	1 ± 0.9	78 ± 21	19 ± 7

t = standard deviation; 5 animals in each group

Parasympathetic predominance

The selective impairment of SNS activity permits a predominance of parasympathetic tone as reflected by nasal stuffiness, bradycardia, increased gastric hydrogen ion secretion, and diarrhea. Bradycardia may limit the cardiac contribution to circulatory homeostasis and obscure signs of anesthetic depth, hypovolemia, or hypoventilation. Severe bradycardia could occur in combination with drugs administered during anesthesia that normally increase vagal activity.

Sedation

Drugs that deplete central catecholamine stores have been shown in animal studies to reduce halothane anesthetic requirements (Table 8–2).[12] More recent information suggests that the magnitude of reduction in anesthetic requirements depends on the SNS activity induced by the anesthetic drug.[13] For example, reserpine, 2 mg/kg, decreased halothane MAC (minimum alveolar concentration) 20% and cyclopropane 40%. Conceivably, an overdose of potent inhalation anesthetic drugs would be more likely if these anesthetics were administered in the usual manner. However, the doses of antihypertensive drugs employed in animals to reduce MAC far exceed the usual doses administered to patients (Tables 8–1 and 8–2). Nevertheless, clinical observations that preceded these animal studies suggest that patients receiving certain antihypertensives need smaller amounts of both inhalation or injectable anesthetic drugs.[12]

PHARMACOLOGY OF ANTIHYPERTENSIVE DRUGS

This section draws from the work of Melmon and of Gottlieb and Chidsey.[14,15]

Sympatholytic drugs

Reserpine. There is no generally accepted view as to the predominant mechanism of the hypotensive effects produced by reserpine, although actions on the central nervous system and peripheral SNS are felt to be essential. Peripherally, reserpine prevents NE accumulation in the storage vesicle but not in the nerve ending so that the neurotransmitter is vulnerable to oxidation by the enzyme monoamine oxidase. The net effect is gradual neurotransmitter depletion as the storage granules deplete their contents spontaneously or in response to nerve stimulation. This results in a dose-dependent impairment of SNS function. However, complete neurotransmitter depletion seems unlikely in man, as the drug's toxicity limits the total adult reserpine dose to about 0.5 mg/day.

The pharmacologic denervation produced by reserpine results in altered responses to sympathomimetic drugs. There may be increased sensitivity of the heart and smooth muscle to sympathomimetic stimulation as produced by direct-acting vasopressors. In contrast, drugs that act by releasing NE are less effective, since neurotransmitter stores are depleted. Ephedrine, which depends on both indirect and direct mechanisms for its pressor response, is less effective in animals treated with reserpine.[16] However, the reserpine doses administered in these animal studies (0.2 to 2.0 mg/kg) exceed the likely maximum dose used in man. Indeed, ephedrine is effective in increasing the blood pressure in reserpine-treated patients, which presumably reflects incomplete catecholamine depletion.[8]

In addition to the problems presented in the choice of a vasopressor during anesthesia, the reserpine-treated patient is theoretically susceptible to neurovascular instability from anesthetic drugs with resulting hypotension, position change, or blood loss. Nevertheless, the circulatory response to anesthetic drugs is not altered by prior reserpine.[17] Orthostatic hypotension is rare, suggesting that the reflex constrictor responses of capacitance vessels are not completely inhibited. Parenteral reserpine may result in sharp catecholamine release and thus should be avoided in patients anesthetized with halothane or cyclopropane. Sedation and tranquilization, mental depression, decreased anesthetic requirements, and occasional Parkinsonian-like rigidity reflect central nervous system depletion of NE or dopamine by reserpine. Parasympathetic predominance in reserpine-treated patients may be evidenced by bradycardia.

Alpha-methyldopa (methyldopa, Aldomet). Like that of reserpine, the mechanism of methyldopa action is not understood. One

theory is that methyldopa acts as a false transmitter. It is speculated that the drug is first converted to *alpha*-methyldopamine by DOPA decarboxylase. *Alpha* methyldopamine enters the storage vesicle and is converted by dopamine *beta*-oxidase to *alpha*-methylnorepinephrine, which has a weaker sympathomimetic effect than NE. The release of *alpha*-methylnorepinephrine in response to nerve stimulation results in a reduced peripheral vascular resistance and a lowered blood pressure. A more likely mechanism is the accumulation of *alpha*-methylated amines in the central nervous system, resulting in reduced central sympathetic outflow. Regardless of the mechanism, methyldopa results in a reduced blood pressure primarily by lowering peripheral vascular resistance with minimal changes in cardiac output.[18]

Parasympathetic predominance may be manifested as bradycardia. Orthostatic hypotension is rarely a problem. Sedation, although usually milder than that observed with reserpine, occurs with repeated therapy and is consistent with the reduced anesthetic requirements documented in treated animals (Table 8–2).[12] Reduced responses to ephedrine are recorded in animals, but the significance, if any, in patients is not established. Methyldopa is a logical choice in patients with renal disease, since the drug maintains or increases renal blood flow. About 20% of patients treated show a positive Coombs' test result, which indicates the possibility of an incompatible minor crossmatch. Methyldopa is chemically related to catecholamines. Therefore, false positive tests for pheochromocytoma may result when urinary catecholamines, but not vanillylmandelic acid, are measured. A rare but important side effect is methyldopa hepatitis.

Patients who are given methyldopa may manifest a hypertensive response on receiving propranolol.[19] It is speculated that propranolol blocks the usual vasodilating effects of *alpha*-methylnorepinephrine so that only the potent *alpha*-stimulating effects of this methyldopa metabolite are apparent. As such, the response now resembles that seen with NE. The anesthesiologist should consider this hazard when contemplating the intraoperative administration of propranolol to a patient receiving methyldopa.

Another consideration is dementia, reported in patients treated first with methyldopa and subsequently with the butyrophenone, haloperidol.[20] This dementia may be caused by the ability of both drugs to prevent dopamine from reaching the central nervous system receptor. Logic suggests caution in the use of Innovar, since this drug combination contains another butyrophenone, droperidol.

Guanethidine (Ismelin). Guanethidine acts solely on the peripheral SNS to depress postganglionic sympathetic nerve function. This selective action occurs because guanethidine uses the same uptake mechanism that transports NE into the nerve ending. Once in the storage vesicle, guanethidine causes NE release by a direct action and also inhibits the depolarization produced by nerve stimulation. Decreased SNS responses at *alpha-* and *beta*-effector sites result in decreased venous return and cardiac output and in guanethidine's characteristic blood-pressure-lowering effects.

Peripheral sympathetic block is also responsible for this drug's side effects. Orthostatic hypotension is the most frequent adverse effect of guanethidine therapy. It reflects a decreased responsiveness of resistance and capacitance vessels. Like reserpine and methyldopa, this drug sensitizes effector cells to catecholamines and direct-acting sympathomimetics. Therefore, the use of guanethidine in a patient with a pheochromocytoma is not appropriate. In contrast, the patient's response to indirect-acting drugs is impaired. Parasympathetic predominance is often manifested by bradycardia. Unlike reserpine and methyldopa, guanethidine does not enter the central nervous system. This means that psychic depression, sedation, and reduction of anesthetic requirements do not occur (Table 8–2).[12] Muscle weakness, presumably due to decreased neuromuscular transmission, occasionally results, but sensitivity to neuromuscular blockers has not been reported.

The control of blood pressure by guanethidine may be lost in patients receiving drugs that block the mechanism for NE uptake, since this mechanism is the same one used by guanethidine for entrance into the adrenergic nerve ending. Indeed, hypertension previously controlled with guanethidine has been reported following the initiation of tricyclic antidepressant therapy.[21] Since tricyclic antidepressants block the uptake of NE, it is assumed that guanethidine access to the nerve ending is also prevented. Other blockers include ephedrine (present in over-the-counter cold remedies), ketamine, cocaine, *alpha*-adrenergic blockers, and possibly pancuronium.

Autonomic ganglion blockers

Pentolinium (Ansolysen) and Trimethaphan (Arfonad). These drugs compete with acetylcholine at autonomic ganglia. They lower the blood pressure by reducing peripheral vascular resistance. Some intolerable side effects are related to both sympathetic and parasympathetic autonomic ganglion blockade. With the advent of selective SNS inhibitors, ganglionic blockers are seldom employed for the control of blood pressure in ambulatory patients.

Alpha-adrenergic blocking drugs

Phenoxybenzamine (Dibenzyline) and Phentolamine (Regitine). These drugs have no clinical value in treating ambulatory essential hypertension. Both phenoxybenzamine and phentolamine act as competitive blockers by occupying the *alpha*-receptor and by preventing the usual neurotransmitter-receptor interaction. The major disadvantage of *alpha*-adrenergic blockers is impairment of compensatory vasoconstriction and subsequent orthostatic hypertension. Marked decreases in blood pressure may occur with blood loss and conceivably in response to sudden position changes or positive intrathoracic pressure. Furthermore, increased myocardial oxygen requirements may result from lack of *beta*-receptor blockade, subsequent reflex tachycardia, and increased myocardial contractility. *Beta*-adrenergic effects, such as when local anesthetics are combined with epinephrine, may appear in the presence of preexisting *alpha*-adrenergic blockade. Prevention or treatment of hypertensive responses to endogenous (pheochromocytoma) or exogenous catecholamines is the most frequent indication for *alpha*-adrenergic blockade.

Vascular smooth muscle vasodilators

Hydralazine (Apresoline). Hydralazine probably interferes with calcium transport at the arterial vascular smooth muscle and lowers blood pressure by vasodilation. Since baroreceptors remain intact, increased sympathetic outflow to the myocardium and peripheral vasculature in response to lowered blood pressure may offset the desired antihypertensive effect. This reflex stimulation is prevented by combining this drug with other antihypertensives, such as guanethidine or propranolol. In contrast, orthostatic hypotension is not a problem since cardiovascular reflexes and SNS function are not altered. Because it either maintains or increases renal blood flow, hydralazine is a logical choice for patients with renal disease. In the anesthetized patient, exaggerated hypotension could reflect additive effects with other vasodilating anesthetic drugs.

Prazosin (Minipress). This drug is chemically unrelated to any other currently used antihypertensive.[22] Prazosin lowers blood pressure by decreasing peripheral vascular resistance through direct vascular smooth muscle vasodilation and *alpha*-adrenergic blockade. Compared with hydralazine, prazosin causes less tachycardia but may produce orthostatic hypotension and occasional first-dose syncopal reactions. This drug is indicated primarily in patients who cannot tolerate hydralazine.

Central nervous system acting drugs

Clonidine (Catapres). This drug is thought to stimulate *alpha*-adrenergic inhibitory receptors in the midbrain, which results in decreased sympathetic outflow and subsequent decreased peripheral vascular resistance and cardiac output.[23] Orthostatic hypotension is rare. This suggests that centrally acting drugs (reserpine and methyldopa as well) do not abolish sympathetic outflow. Sedation occurs. Decreased anesthetic requirements, although not documented, seem possible. The sudden discontinuance of clonidine is associated with rebound hypertension. We emphasize the need to withdraw this drug gradually if therapy is to be stopped.[24]

Monoamine oxidase inhibitors (MAOI, also known as MAO inhibitors)

Adverse drug interactions as well as the availability of more effective antihypertensives are the basis for the recommendation that these drugs not be the first choice in the control of blood pressure in ambulatory patients. Undesirable drug interactions may be caused because tyramine is no longer inactivated by MAO enzyme in the gastrointestinal tract. Hypertensive crises may occur with the ingestion of tyramine-containing foods (for example, cheese, beer, wine, chicken liver). Slowed or altered biotransformation may be responsible for atypical responses to meperidine (hyperthermia and excessive ventilatory depression) and barbiturates (prolonged sedation).

The speculated mechanism of MAOI action is the production of a false transmitter, octopamine, that produces less *alpha*-adrenergic stimulation than NE. Since MAOI prevent the oxidative determination of NE, the blood pressure response to indirect-acting sympathomimetic drugs (even to ephedrine in cold remedies) may be exaggerated. This response reflects the increased availability of neurotransmitter, since NE is no longer inactivated, whereas the production of NE continues normally. Direct-acting drugs should be less influenced, but exaggerated responses may still occur.

Pargyline (Eutonyl) is the only MAOI available for the control of blood pressure. It should be discontinued at least two weeks prior to any elective anesthetic and operation. The substitution of other antihypertensive drugs must be done carefully. For example, guanethidine and reserpine may stimulate NE release and cause hypertensive crises in the presence of a residual pargyline effect.

Veratrum alkaloids

These drugs lower blood pressure by setting the baroreceptors in the carotid sinus and aortic arch at lower levels, which results in increased parasympathetic and decreased sympathetic activity. *Veratrum* alkaloids are rarely used to control essential hypertension because of the high incidence of adverse side effects, such as nausea and vomiting. Interactions with anesthetic drugs are unlikely because of the small doses used to treat essential hypertension. However, as with any patient who takes antihypertensive drugs, the implications of an attenuated SNS must be appreciated. Similarly, increased vagal activity results in excessive bradycardia, especially if drugs that stimulate the vagus or act at cholinergic receptors are used during anesthesia.

HYPERTENSIVE CRISES

The most frequently chosen drugs for the management of intraoperative or postoperative hypertension are sodium nitroprusside (Nipride), trimethaphan (Arfonad) or diazoxide (Hyperstat).

Nitroprusside provides rapid control of blood pressure, but its extreme potency requires careful dose titration, preferably with an infusion pump. During anesthesia, an infusion rate of 0.5 to 5.0 μg/kg/min is usually adequate, with the lowest doses required in the presence of potent inhalation anesthetics. Since nitroprusside has no effect on the myocardium or the ANS, the cardiac output is usually unchanged or even increased when the blood pressure is lowered. Cyanide toxicity should be suspected in any patient who is resistant (who requires greater than 10 μg/kg/min) or who develops tachyphylaxis or metabolic acidosis. Nitroprusside should be immediately discontinued in such patients and appropriate cyanide antagonists should be employed if hypotension or metabolic acidosis persists.

Trimethaphan is a ganglionic blocking drug that acts rapidly but so briefly that it must be given by continuous intravenous infusion. As with nitroprusside, constant blood pressure monitoring is necessary. Because trimethaphan relaxes capacitance vessels and blocks sympathetic reflexes, it lowers blood pressure both by arteriolar vasodilation and by decreasing cardiac output. Accompanying tachycardia may offset reductions in blood pressure and may contribute to occasional resistance to the blood-pressure-lowering effects of this drug. Histamine release secondary to trimethaphan administration makes this drug inappropriate in the treatment of the patient with a pheochromocytoma. Large doses of trimethaphan may potentiate nondepolarizing neuromuscular blockers by an unknown mechanism.[25]

Diazoxide is a nondiuretic thiazide derivative that has been used for the management of postoperative hypertension.[26] This drug reduces systolic and diastolic blood pressure by a direct relaxant action on arteriolar smooth muscle. It has no significant effect on sympathetic reflexes, so that the decrease in peripheral vascular resistance is accompanied by a reflex increase in heart rate and cardiac output. A single intravenous injection of diazoxide of 2.5 to 5.0

mg/kg over 10 to 20 seconds rapidly lowers blood pressure to an acceptable level in two to five minutes without the need for constant monitoring. Since at least 90% of the drug is bound to protein, slow injection may not permit sufficient free drug to reduce blood pressure appropriately. Blood pressure gradually returns to control levels over the next 12 hours. The absence of a sedative effect allows the physician to evaluate the patient's mental status. Although excessive hypotension is unlikely, a disadvantage compared with nitroprusside is the inability to adjust the dose of diazoxide in accordance with the patient's response. It must be remembered that the response to diazoxide is accentuated in patients who are given drugs such as propranolol or guanethidine, since the reflex-sympathetic responses to decreased blood pressure are blocked. When used in patients with eclampsia, diazoxide acts as a powerful uterine relaxant, but contractions may be reestablished with oxytocin. Diazoxide inhibits the release of insulin from the pancreas, but hypoglycemia is not a factor with the administration of a single dose. Stimulation of catecholamine release contraindicates using this drug in patients with a pheochromocytoma.

REFERENCES

1. Veteran's Administration Cooperative Study Group on Antihypertensive Agents: Effects of treatment on morbidity and hypertension. J.A.M.A., *202*:1028, 1967.
2. Veteran's Administration Cooperative Study Group on Antihypertensive Agents: Effects of treatment on morbidity and hypertension. J.A.M.A., *213*:1143, 1971.
3. McKee, P. A., et al.: The natural history of congestive heart failure: The Framingham study. N. Engl. J. Med., *285*:1441, 1971.
4. Breckenridge, A., Dollery, C. T., and Parry, E. H. O.: Prognosis of treated hypertension: changes in life expectancy and causes of death between 1952 and 1967. Q. J. Med., *39*:411, 1970.
5. Axelrod, J., and Weinshilbaum, R.: Catecholamines. N. Engl. J. Med., *287*:237, 1972.
6. Coakley, C. A., Alpert, S., and Boling, J. S.: Circulatory responses during anesthesia of patients on rauwolfia therapy. J.A.M.A., *161*:1143, 1956.
7. Crandell, D. L.: The anesthetic hazards in patients on antihypertensive therapy. J.A.M.A., *179*:495, 1962.
8. Katz, R. L., Weintraub, H. D., and Papper, E. M.: Anesthesia, surgery and rauwolfia. Anesthesiology, *25*:142, 1964.
9. Prys-Roberts, C., Meloche, R., and Foex, P.: Studies of anesthesia in relation to hypertension I: Cardiovascular responses to treated and untreated patients. Br. J. Anaesth., *43*:122, 1971.
10. Dingle, H. R.: Antihypertensive drugs and anaesthesia. Anaesthesia, *21*:151, 1966.
11. Thomson, P. D., and Melmon, K. L.: Clinical assessment of autonomic function. Anesthesiology, *29*:724, 1968.
12. Miller, R. D., Way, W. L., and Eger, E. I., II: The effects of *alpha*-methyldopa, reserpine, guanethidine and iproniazid on minimum alveolar anesthetic requirement (MAC). Anesthesiology, *29*:1153, 1969.
13. Mueller, R. A., et al.: Central monaminergic neuronal effects on minimum alveolar concentrations (MAC) of halothane and cyclopropane in rats. Anesthesiology, *42*:143, 1975.
14. Melmon, K. L.: The clinical pharmacology of commonly used antihypertensive drugs. *In* Cardiovascular Drug Therapy. Edited by K. L. Melmon. Philadelphia, F. A. Davis Co., 1974.
15. Gottlieb, T. R., and Chidsey, C. A.: The clinician's guide to pharmacology of antihypertensive agents. Geriatrics, *31*:99, 1976.
16. Eger, E. I., II, and Hamilton, W. K.: The effect of reserpine on the action of various vasopressors. Anesthesiology, *20*:641, 1959.
17. Bagwell, E. E., and Woods, E. F.: Influence of reserpine on the cardiovascular responses to cyclopropane anesthesia. Fed. Proc.,*22*:186, 1963.
18. Dollery, C. T., Harrington, M., and Hodge, J. V.: Haemodynamic studies with methyldopa: Effect on cardiac output and response to pressor amines. Br. Heart J., *25*:670, 1963.
19. Nies, A. S., and Shand, D. G.: Hypertensive response to propranolol in a patient treated with methyldopa—a proposed mechanism. Clin. Pharmacol. Ther., *14*:823, 1973.
20. Thornton, W. E.: Dementia induced by methyldopa with haloperidol. N. Engl. J. Med.,*294*:1122, 1976.
21. Mitchell, J. R., and Oates, J. A.: Guanethidine and related agents I. Mechanism of the selective blockade of adrenergic neurons and its antagonism by drugs. J. Pharmacol. Exp. Ther., *172*:100, 1970.
22. Kosman, M. E.: Evaluation of a new antihypertensive agent. Prazosin hydrochloride (Minipress). J.A.M.A., *238*:157, 1977.
23. VanZwieten, P.A.: The central action of antihypertensive drugs mediated via central *alpha* receptors. J. Pharm. Pharmacol., *25*:89, 1973.
24. Brodsky, J. B., and Bravo, J. J.: Acute postoperative clonidine withdrawal syndrome. Anesthesiology, *44*:519, 1976.
25. Wilson, S. L., et al.: Prolonged neuromuscular blockade associated with trimethaphan: A case report. Anesth. Analg. (Cleve.), *55*:353, 1976.
26. Weser, J. K.: Diazoxide. N. Engl. J. Med., *294*:1271, 1976.

Chapter **9**

Cholinergic and Anticholinergic Agents

WERNER E. FLACKE
and
JOAN W. FLACKE

CASE REPORT

A 38-year-old, 60-kg nurse, underwent a cholecystectomy. Except for gallbladder disease, her past history was essentially negative. The only item of note was a history of severe bronchial asthma as a child. The frequency of attacks had decreased with age, and the last asthmatic episode had been more than ten years earlier. The patient had had general anesthesia at age 15 for an appendectomy, apparently without incident, but no anesthetics since that time.

Anesthesia was induced with intravenous thiopental and maintained uneventfully with nitrous oxide, 60% in oxygen, intravenous meperidine, and pancuronium for muscle relaxation. Near the conclusion of the operation, the patient was given atropine, 1 mg intravenously, followed by neostigmine, 2.5 mg intravenously. Good reversal of neuromuscular block (as ascertained by nerve stimulation and by respiratory efforts) was obtained. The patient's chest was clear, and there was no bradycardia. The patient was allowed to breathe spontaneously, and an additional dose of thiopental (50 mg) was given to keep her asleep for the placement of skin sutures. Approximately ten minutes after the neostigmine had been given, nitrous oxide was discontinued. The patient awoke and promptly developed severe bronchospasm with a prolonged expiratory phase and little air entry bilaterally. Her heart rate fell from 85 to less than 60 per minute. The endotracheal tube was removed immediately, which resulted in sufficient improvement that it was possible to ventilate her with oxygen by mask. Neither intravenous aminophylline (300 mg) nor another dose of atropine (2 mg) relieved the bronchospasm, although they did abolish the bradycardia. The patient was taken to the recovery room, treated with manually assisted ventilation by mask with oxygen, 100%, and with Vaponefrin mist inhalation. She gradually improved over the next hour.

Comment. The crux of this case is the abnormal sensitivity of the patient's airway musculature to bronchoconstrictor agents (acetylcholine) and the endogenous vagal nervous activity depending on the state of consciousness. The dose of atropine given prior to neostigmine was sufficient to prevent early vagal effects on the heart and bronchial smooth musculature. When atropine was given, the patient was still anesthetized and apparently had a low vagal tone. However, the buildup with time of acetylcholine (ACh) at the cholinergic receptors and the sudden increase in vagal activity and ACh release associated with awaking overcame the antagonistic effect of the previously effective dose of atropine and resulted in bradycardia and bronchospasm. The additional 2 mg of atropine might have been sufficient to alleviate this, but by now other bronchospastic humoral agents may have been maintaining the bronchoconstriction. Airway smooth muscle in sensitive patients is much more responsive not only to acetylcholine but also to other bronchospastic agonists, such as histamine and slow-reacting substance.

This chapter discusses the interactions of cholinergic and anticholinergic agents, with emphasis on their pharmacology and their use in anesthesia.

MORPHOLOGY, BIOCHEMISTRY, AND PHYSIOLOGY

Acetylcholine was the first chemical identified as a neurohumoral transmitter by the classic experiments of Otto Loewi, who demonstrated that the effects of vagal nerve stimulation on the frog heart could be transferred to a second heart by the bathing fluid of the first heart taken during the stimulation.[1]

Loewi's demonstration was in a postganglionic parasympathetic system, but Sir Henry Dale had recognized earlier the similarity between the effects of ACh and the responses to stimulation of different peripheral nerves.[2] Within 15 years of Loewi's ex-

periment, the transmitter role of ACh was firmly established at all preganglionic autonomic nerve endings, parasympathetic postganglionic nerve endings, and the terminals of motor nerves (neuromuscular junction). Somewhat later, convincing evidence was added that ACh is a transmitter also in the central nervous system.[3] It is further known that ACh can stimulate sensory nerve endings, but this effect probably has no physiologic significance. Moreover, not all tissues that possess receptors for and therefore respond to ACh have cholinergic innervation (for example, vascular smooth muscle).

Sir Henry Dale also posited that different effects of ACh could be mimicked or blocked by different drugs: *muscarine* and atropine at postganglionic parasympathetic effector sites, *nicotine* at autonomic ganglia and at the neuromuscular junction. These observations have led to the classification of "muscarinic" and "nicotinic" cholinergic systems. Nicotinic effects can be further subdivided because *hexamethonium* and related agents block ganglionic effects relatively selectively, whereas *curare*-type drugs do the same at the neuromuscular junction.

Synthesis of ACh in all cholinergic nerve endings is catalyzed by choline acetylase in the presence of coenzyme A. ACh is then stored in the nerve terminals and is inactive until released into the extracellular space or synaptic junction during nerve activity. (Reid Hunt of Harvard Medical School early recognized the high potency of ACh, which he had synthetized from choline extracted from the adrenal medulla, but he rejected the idea of a biological role of ACh because it was "much too toxic" to exist in the body. This shows how difficult it was to conceive of storage of a chemical in the body in such a way that it was inactive or "nontoxic" but so that it could be released as a free or active compound.) Free ACh is rapidly hydrolyzed by cholinesterases, which are among the most widely distributed enzymes in the body and occur both in solution and bound to tissue components. Thus free ACh, that is ACh in a nonstorage condition, has a brief lifetime and is present only during nerve activity near the terminals of cholinergic nerves.

For the physiologic functions of ACh, or of any transmitter, morphologic as well as biochemical factors are important. The synaptic gap, the distance from the site of release to the site of the receptors on postsynaptic or effector cell membranes, differs greatly. At the neuromuscular junction the gap is about 400 to 500 Å wide; in autonomic ganglia and in the central nervous system (CNS) gaps of only 50 to 150 Å occur; at postganglionic parasympathetic junctions (for example, in the heart, in smooth muscle tissues in the airways, or in the intestine) the distance from the site of release to the receptor sites may be 10,000 Å or more. The transmitter must diffuse to the receptor sites, and the time required is determined by the distance. The time varies from one millisecond or less at the neuromuscular junction or in autonomic ganglia to several hundred milliseconds or more in the case of postganglionic junctions.

The size of the synaptic (or junctional) gap also determines the importance of the hydrolyzing enzymes for terminating the lifetime of the transmitter. When the gap is small, little ACh needs to be released to produce an effective concentration in the vicinity of the receptors, and this localized amount may be diminished rapidly by diffusion alone. When the gap is large, much more transmitter must be released to produce the same concentration at the distant receptor sites, and enzymatic hydrolysis is essential for rapid termination of free ACh. The total process is (1) transmitter release, (2) diffusion to the receptor, and (3) destruction of free transmitter. This process determines the speed of the cycle or the speed with which the postsynaptic effect can be turned on and off. The speed is of the order of milliseconds in neuromuscular transmission or in ganglionic transmission but of seconds in the case of parasympathetic end-organ function, such

as cardiac effects or smooth muscle contraction-relaxation. Inhibition of cholinesterase has little effect on impulse transmission in the autonomic ganglia, more effect at the neuromuscular junction, and much more effect at the parasympathetic postganglionic junctions.

The functional role of cholinergic systems is clear at the neuromuscular junction, where it transmits the nerve signal to the muscle fiber one-to-one with a high margin of safety. At autonomic ganglia the functions broaden. The preganglionic-postganglionic ratio may vary widely, and there is increasing evidence of mechanisms that permit modulation of signal transmission in ganglia. We know little about the physiologic and pathophysiologic role of these mechanisms.[4]

There are still questions regarding the functioning of the parasympathetic postganglionic system. Transmission is not "all or nothing" as it is at the neuromuscular junction, but rather it is graded, and there seems to be no "margin of safety." The magnitude of the end-organ response is a function of the number of active nerve units and their frequency of firing. A decrease in transmitter release causes a proportionate decrease of end-organ response and vice versa. One might say that the parasympathetic is an integrating system rather than a system concerned with single-unit transmission.

The overall role of the parasympathetic nervous system has been described as serving recuperation, in contrast to the role of the sympathetic/adrenergic system, which subserves activity: fight or flight.[5] However, these concepts are too broad to be of much practical value. More specifically, many important autonomic functions are mediated by the parasympathetic nervous system, and both hypo- and hyperactivity may be detrimental. Salivary secretions are necessary, but either excessive or insufficient secretions may hinder function. This is even more obvious in the airways. A proper amount of secretions protects the integrity of the mucosa and permits effective clearing by the ciliary system. Insufficient secretions may lead to inspissation of mucus with a resulting breakdown of ciliary function. The importance of maintaining heart rate, impulse conduction, and automaticity within reasonable limits is obvious, and here both the sympathetic and the parasympathetic system are involved in keeping cardiac functions within these limits. Recently, the role of the vagus nerve in the parasympathetic control of the heart has become the target of renewed interest by anatomists, physiologists, pharmacologists, and clinicians.[6]

Vagal stimulation and infusion of methacholine reduce the vulnerability of the heart to ventricular fibrillation.[7-10] This effect is minor under normal conditions, but becomes marked during sympathetic nerve stimulation or infusion of norepinephrine.[11] This is a specific example of the old concept of sympathetic/parasympathetic balance. Observations in human beings have been in agreement: parasympathetic stimulation, evoked by carotid sinus stimulation or by administration of vagotonic agents, decreases the frequency of premature ventricular beats and abolishes ventricular tachycardia.[12-17] It has been observed that the frequency and severity of ventricular arrhythmias are lower during sleep, that is, a condition in which the sympathetic/parasympathetic balance is shifted in the direction of the latter.[18]

These observations may have their basis partially in the recently observed peripheral interaction between sympathetic and parasympathetic nerves in organs with dual, antagonistic innervation. Muscarinic agents and vagal nerve stimulation reduce the release of the sympathetic transmitter norepinephrine.[19-20] In the heart there is a definite morphologic basis for such interaction. Sympathetic and parasympathetic nerve terminals are found in such close approximation that transmitter from one can easily reach the other terminal and affect transmitter release there.[21-22] Thus the ef-

fect of vagal activation is possibly mediated by a modulation of release of sympathetic transmitter. Vagal activity may reduce oxygen requirements of the myocardium not only by a direct negative chronotropic and inotropic effect on effector cells, but also by its inhibition of transmitter release from sympathetic nerve endings. Both factors may be involved in stabilizing the myocardium and in antagonizing the arrhythmogenic effect of catecholamines and sympathetic nerve activity.

PHARMACOLOGY OF CHOLINERGIC MECHANISMS

The classification of drugs that affect cholinergic functions follows logically from their physiology and morphology:

1. Cholinomimetic agents
   a. Nicotinic
      (neuromuscular transmission)
      autonomic ganglionic transmission
   b. Muscarinic
      direct-acting
      indirect-acting
2. Cholinolytic agents
   a. Nicotinic
      (neuromuscular transmission)
      autonomic ganglionic transmission
   b. Muscarinic

(mimetic = agonistic or stimulant, lytic = antagonistic or blocking)

Neuromuscular transmission, which has been discussed in detail elsewhere in this book, is not covered here except to mention that it can be blocked either by nicotinic agonists such as succinylcholine or decamethonium (so-called depolarizing block) or by antagonists such as curare and pancuronium (nondepolarizing block).

Cholinomimetic agents

Nicotinic. Ganglionic nicotinic cholinomimetic or stimulant effects are not used in therapy. Ganglionic stimulation may be seen as a side or toxic effect of the depolarizing neuromuscular blocking agents. Ganglionic stimulation by succinylcholine has been observed in animals, and may cause some of the undesirable effects that have been reported with this drug. Nicotine itself, although it is not administered therapeutically, is widely used in the form of tobacco. Occasionally, ganglionic stimulation may be seen in acute nicotine overdose, manifested by bradycardia, possibly leading to hypotension, diarrhea (parasympathetic stimulation), nausea, and vomiting, perhaps followed by tachycardia and hypertension (sympathetic stimulation).

Nicotinic cholinomimetic agents are capable also of stimulating sensory nerve endings, especially the carotid body chemoreceptors. This is a possible alternate mechanism for the tachycardia and hypertension occasionally seen with succinylcholine. In Russia, the effect of dicholine esters on chemoreceptors is used clinically to stimulate respiration.[23]

Muscarinic. Of the direct-acting muscarinic cholinomimetic agents, acetylcholine itself is not used clinically. Methacholine, carbachol, and bethanechol are less rapidly hydrolyzed, and therefore their effects are longer lasting. Although they can be given subcutaneously or even by mouth, their importance and their use is limited.

Pilocarpine is a plant-derived alkaloid with muscarinic activity, and is used widely in the treatment of glaucoma. Although systemic effects can occur with overdosage or with special sensitivity, the ophthalmic use of pilocarpine is one of the few examples of successful localized drug application, and toxicity is not common.

A common characteristic of the systemic effects of the muscarinic cholinomimetic agents is that they affect homeostatically controlled systems, such as heart rate and blood pressure, less than they affect functions that lack such compensatory mechanisms, for example bronchial constriction and airway secretions, salivation, sweating, and cardiac impulse conduction. All the last effects are antagonized easily by small doses of any anticholinergic drug.

Of much greater importance than the foregoing directly produced muscarinic cholinomimetic effects are those produced indirectly as a result of the inhibition of cholinesterases. Anticholinesterase drugs are used routinely in anesthesia to reverse nondepolarizing neuromuscular block. They are also used in the treatment of myasthenia gravis[24] and glaucoma. Furthermore, since organophosphate anticholinesterase agents are widely encountered in the environment as household and agricultural pesticides, exposure to such agents is common.

Among anticholinesterase drugs one must distinguish between those that do and those that do not enter the CNS. The anticholinesterase drugs used for their effects on neuromuscular transmission are carbamic acid esters and quaternary ammonium compounds. They do not pass the blood-brain barrier to any significant extent. The compounds used as pesticides must have high lipid solubility, and all of these agents do have CNS effects. Most of the pesticide anticholinesterase agents are organophosphates. In contrast to the carbamates, these agents are not competitive, surmountable inhibitors of cholinesterase; rather they are nonsurmountable and, for practical purposes, irreversible enzyme inhibitors. Thus their effect is much longer lasting and is cumulative. Fortunately, the only members of this group in medicinal use are the eyedrops echothiophate and isoflurophate. Theoretically the functional consequences of cholinesterase inhibition should parallel the degree of inhibition, and measurement of plasma cholinesterase or, even better, of red cell cholinesterase, should be an important diagnostic and predictive tool. However, this has not proven to be the case, as the symptomatology caused by anticholinesterase inhibitors does not seem to correlate well with the degree of enzyme inhibition.[25]

One factor that may explain this discrepancy in part is that the consequence of the inhibition of cholinesterase depends not only on the dose of the inhibitor and the magnitude of the biochemical effect, but especially on the degree of the nerve activity, that is, on the amount of ACh being released at the time of enzyme inhibition. For example, there may be no parasympathomimetic effects resulting from an anticholinesterase drug when parasympathetic nerve activity is low or absent. For a given dose in a given system, the effect of an anticholinesterase drug is proportional to the magnitude of parasympathetic nerve activity.

The organophosphate eyedrops can be important clinically. Patients may be careless about the amount of eyedrops that they use. Absorption is variable, but usually considerable. They only safe way to avoid an interaction is to elicit from the patient a history of taking these drugs. Since the inhibition is long-term, agents such as succinylcholine that require cholinesterase to terminate their action should be avoided for two to three weeks after the cessation of eyedrop therapy.

Cholinolytic agents

Nicotinic. This group of drugs, which acts on autonomic ganglia, produces a nondepolarizing ganglionic block. Hexamethonium, pentolinium, trimethaphan, and chlorisondamine are examples of such drugs. These agents were the first to be used in the treatment of hypertension, but they produce block of impulse transmission in all ganglia, sympathetic and parasympathetic, with little selectivity. Hence their side effects are global and severe: fully effective doses produce almost complete pharmacologic autonomic denervation. For this reason, they have been replaced by more selective agents for the treatment of chronic hypertension. In anesthesia, they have a limited application for deliberate, controlled, short-lasting hypotension. Ganglion blocking drugs have been advocated also for the acute treatment of congestive heart failure, since they lower arterial pressure and thus reduce the load on the failing heart.

The overriding characteristic of ganglion blocking drugs is their lack of selectivity. Ganglion block implies the interruption of sympathetic and parasympathetic efferent pathways, with the consequent paralysis of autonomic functions, from tear production to cessation of intestinal motility. Such a condition requires special care on the part of the anesthetist to substitute for the missing "protective" effect of the autonomic system. Fortunately, however, complete ganglionic block is unnecessary for the foregoing uses of ganglionic blocking drugs in anesthesia.

It is not surprising that ganglion blocking activity is a side effect of some of the nondepolarizing neuromuscular blocking drugs in view of the close pharmacologic relationship between the two classes of agents. Among the neuromuscular blocking drugs presently in use, d-tubocurarine is the most potent ganglionic blocker. Several inhalation anesthetic agents also inhibit nicotinic ganglionic transmission to some degree in commonly used concentrations.[26] The clinical significance of this phenomenon has not been determined. In addition, it has been established that impulse transmission through some autonomic ganglia is not fully blocked by nicotinic blocking drugs, and that the remaining transmission is sensitive to small doses of atropine-type agents; that is, it is muscarinic in nature.[27,28] Again, the clinical relevance of these findings has not been established.

Muscarinic. The pharmacology of the cholinolytic, antimuscarinic drugs, often somewhat inaccurately called "anticholinergic" or "atropine-like," is too well known to be repeated here except for some special points.[29-32] Several, if not all, of these agents are not "pure" antagonists. Atropine and scopolamine in small doses produce bradycardia and, perhaps, slowing of impulse conduction. These effects were earlier attributed to a central vagal stimulating effect at a time when the concentration in the periphery was too small to produce vagal blockage.[33,34] Homatropine, which combines a weak peripheral blocking effect with a potent central stimulation, causes the most pronounced dose-related bradycardia.[35] However, methylatropine, the quaternary congener of atropine, does not enter the CNS easily, yet still produces bradycardia.[36] Bradycardia from these drugs has been seen even after bilateral vagotomy. Thus, although a central component cannot be excluded, these cholinolytics must have a peripheral site of action. This is further supported by the observation that both salivation and pupillary accommodation are initially stimulated before being paralyzed.[32] These phenomena may be due to a partial agonist effect of the antagonists.

A distinction must be made between the antagonistic effect of these drugs against circulating cholinomimetic agents (including ACh, if it should "spill over" during massive anticholinesterase poisoning) and the usual effect of blocking parasympathetic nerve activity. The former situation is relatively simple, involves more or less equilibrated agonist (generally of low concentrations), and is sensitive to small doses of antimuscarinic drugs. However, when the agonist is released from nerve endings, a situation more commonly encountered in the operating room, it may be much more concentrated in time and in space. Whereas block of low-magnitude nerve activity, associated with small and transient concentrations of transmitter, can be achieved with relatively small doses of antagonist, the same doses may not block a massive burst of nerve activity, which results in high and more prolonged transmitter concentrations. The situation is aggravated by the inhibition of cholinesterase and by the consequent potentiation of parasympathetic nerve activity. These conditions can be demonstrated in the experimental animal, and there is reason to believe that analogous clinical situations do occur.

The recent observations of the interaction of sympathetic and parasympathetic nerve activity in the periphery may give a new dimension to the understanding of the effects of anticholinergic agents. These observations imply that such effects involve not only the antagonism of parasympathetic activity directly on effector systems, but also an indirect effect resulting from a block of the inhibition or attenuation of release of the sympathetic transmitter, norepinephrine, in organs or systems with dual, antagonistic innervation. This effect of atropine on the release of norepinephrine during simultaneous stimulation of sympathetic and vagal nerves has indeed been observed in the heart,[19,20] and this phenomenon may shed a new light on clinical observations of a "sympathomimetic" effect of atropine. However, more work is required in order to clarify the situation both in animals and in man.

There are variations in sensitivity of different effector systems to anticholinergic drugs and differences among different agents in relative potency.[30,32] The effects on salivary secretion and, probably, airway secretion—which have, however, not been measured—and on sweating are the most sensitive. These occur in man with drug doses that have little or no cardiac vagolytic action.[30,31] Atropine is a more potent agent in blocking cardiac vagal effects than scopolamine, whereas scopolamine is more potent as an antisialogogue.[32] Both these alkaloids have more marked central and ocular effects than do the quaternary ammonium antimuscarinic agents, as expected. The central effects are discussed separately in this chapter.

CLINICAL USE OF CHOLINERGIC DRUGS IN ANESTHESIA

Two main types of drugs that affect the parasympathetic nervous system are used in anesthesia:
1. antimuscarinic anticholinergic agents (atropine-like)
   a. for premedication
   b. as protection against the mus-

carinic consequences of cholinesterase inhibition
2. anticholinesterase agents to improve transmission after nondepolarizing neuromuscular blocking drugs

We shall first consider the use of atropine-like drugs for premedication, which is the most controversial question.

Antimuscarinic anticholinergic agents

Historically, atropine was introduced to protect the heart from vagal influences during chloroform anesthesia, and to prevent excessive secretions during diethyl ether anesthesia. Since these agents are now used infrequently in this country, the question has been asked whether the routine use of anticholinergic drugs prior to anesthesia is justified.[37-39]

Eger[30] concluded over 15 years ago that belladonna drugs should "not be given by rote" and Gravenstein and Anton have written:[40] "Anticholinergic drugs often can be omitted from premedication. A healthy young woman coming for a minor operative procedure, such as dilatation and curettage, does not require premedication with an anticholinergic drug if thiopental and nitrous oxide are used as exclusive anesthetics." This is a cautious statement from researchers known for their careful and extensive work in this area. Yet the statement has been criticized on the basis of a study of 150 patients who underwent minor gynecologic procedures during which thiopental and nitrous oxide were used primarily, although some patients received enflurane, halothane, or fentanyl as well.[38]

The patients were divided into two groups: One group received 25 mg of hydroxyzine hydrochloride intramuscularly as premedication and the other received the same dose of hydroxyzine plus 0.2 mg glycopyrrolate intramuscularly (time interval between injection and induction not stated). The patients were evaluated on a double-blind basis as having "satisfactory" or "unsatisfactory" premedication. Of the

group that received no glycopyrrolate, 35.9% were judged unsatisfactory, as compared with 19.4% of the group that had received the anticholinergic agent. The difference was statistically significant. When the results were broken down further, the difference was significant only in the group that had not undergone intubation (13.6% unsatisfactory with glycopyrrolate versus 27.4% without). The incidence of "unsatisfactory" was much higher among the patients who had been intubated (42.9% after glycopyrrolate versus 66.7% without the anticholinergic agent), but the difference between the groups with or without premedication was not significant. The authors concluded that the dose had been insufficient for intubation. No information on the effects of the drug on cardiovascular functions was given.

The most recent report we have found was not based on a controlled, randomized procedure. Eleven anesthetists were asked to report the following on patients who had been anesthetized during a period of one year: (1) whether "secretions constituted a problem during or after anesthesia, if anticholinergic premedication was omitted;" (2) the nature of the problem if there had been one; and (3) whether an anticholinergic drug was given and with what result.[39] Answers for 404 patients were evaluated, 244 of whom had not received an anticholinergic drug for premedication, and 160 of whom had been given either 0.6 mg atropine or 0.4 mg scopolamine intramuscularly one hour before the induction of anesthesia. The trachea was intubated in 56% of the patients with premedication and in 85% of those without. Among the patients not premedicated with an anticholinergic agent, there were 13% who had "problem secretions," as opposed to 3.75% of the premedicated patients. Of the patients reported to have had troublesome secretions, 16% were given atropine during the operation "with success." Hence, only in 2% of the nonpremedicated group did the amount of secretions prompt the anesthetist to administer an anticholinergic agent. The authors concluded that this incidence of troublesome secretions did not warrant the routine administration of anticholinergic drugs before general anesthesia.

This study can also be criticized, and it seems appropriate to pursue this question more vigorously. Yet we are still impressed by the results just quoted, for they seem to be based on sound reasoning and valid observations, even though they were the product of experiments not conducted under double-blind conditions.

What are the risks and benefits of premedication with an antimuscarinic anticholinergic agent with regard to secretions? The benefit is a lower incidence of secretions in amounts considered sufficiently serious to warrant action in the form of the intraoperative injection of an anticholinergic drug. Secretions are serious if they hinder ventilation, and deterioration of blood gases (when it is possible to determine their levels rapidly) is the best evidence of this. The risks are secondary to inhibition of secretions with the potential for inspissation of mucus, breakdown of ciliary function, and possibly obstruction of small airways.[40,41] It would be of interest to compare postanesthetic pulmonary complications with and without anticholinergic medication. In this connection, it may be remembered that anticholinergic drugs have been all but abandoned in the routine treatment of bronchial asthma.[31]

The second important question concerns the possible risks and benefits resulting from the cardiac effects of antimuscarinic drugs. Given the complex physiology of the parasympathetic cardiac innervation and the equally complex pharmacology of antimuscarinic agents, the answer is not easy.

Until recently, no studies had evaluated the preventive use of anticholinergic drugs with respect to cardiac functions as thoroughly as those that evaluated the effects of these drugs on secretions. Observations showed a high incidence of both arrhythmias and tachycardia when atropine was given

during anesthesia. These studies indicated that the effects of anticholinergic drugs were most severe (a) under conditions when sympathetic tone could be assumed to be high, and (b) in the presence of a general anesthetic agent known to sensitize the heart towards catecholamines. This was the case on the one hand with light levels of anesthesia, especially during painful surgical procedures such as oral surgery, and on the other with agents such as diethyl ether, cyclopropane, and halothane.[42-44]

One recent study was designed as a double-blind procedure to investigate the effect of atropine on the bradycardia seen with a second dose of succinylcholine injected five minutes after the first dose under halothane-nitrous oxide anesthesia, a situation associated with strong vagal activity.[45] Two episodes of extreme bradycardia prompted the investigators to break the code (these had occurred in patients who had not received atropine) and to continue without the group that had not received atropine. However, preoperative atropine blocked the vagal manifestations only when present in such concentrations that extreme tachycardia was a by-product. The investigators felt that this was too high a price to pay.

Another team of investigators compared groups that were given atropine and groups that were not with random allocations also under halothane-nitrous oxide anesthesia.[46] There was no significant difference in the incidence of arrhythmias between the two groups when the patients had not undergone intubation, although the arrhythmias in one group were clustered during and after the injection of atropine. With endotracheal intubation, the incidence of arrhythmias was higher in the atropine group and was associated mainly with the intubation.

These observations, involving systematic and lengthy ECG (electrocardiogram) monitoring, did show that the incidence of cardiac arrhythmias under the conditions chosen was high, but the authors made the point that arrhythmias, even those of ventricular origin, rarely progress to ventricular fibrillation. This corresponds to common experience, but it is not proven. The authors again emphasized the price of anticholinergic medication in the form of tachycardia and suggested that this consequence could cause myocardial damage, especially in the presence of coronary artery disease.

In this discussion we have paid little attention to the fact that the conditions predisposing to arrhythmias are well known: a high level of sympathetic/adrenergic activity, the presence of a general anesthetic known to sensitize the heart, and the presence of hypercapnia and hypoxia.[54] Whereas the studies discussed were conducted under circumstances that are probably common today, there were no special efforts made to reduce the foregoing factors. It is known that the incidence of arrhythmias, even when atropine is injected during the anesthesia, is lower with thiopental-nitrous oxide anesthesia, neurolept anesthesia, and enflurane.[42,47] It is further possible to reduce sympathetic/adrenergic influences by the use of *beta*-adrenergic blocking drugs. No systematic explorations of the effects of anticholinergic agents under such conditions have been presented.

It seems significant that the majority of investigators who have done experimental work on these questions, who have considered the problems carefully, and who may be assumed to have a degree of expertise, have advised against the *routine* use of anticholinergic drugs for premedication. They conclude that an anticholinergic drug may be given during anesthesia when there is a specific indication for it, such as in the presence of bradycardia or when situations known to cause vagal reflex activity can be anticipated (for example, with a second dose of succinylcholine), and in patients known to be prone to bradycardic arrhythmias. In these patients it is, of course, important to avoid the special risk factors discussed and to give the anticholinergic drug under conditions associated with a low incidence of arrhythmias.

Anticholinesterase agents

The situation is different when an anticholinesterase drug has to be given to improve neuromuscular transmission. The most severe arrhythmias ever reported occurred in patients during cyclopropane anesthesia when 0.8 mg of atropine was given after severe bradycardia, and marked inhibition of AV (atrioventricular)-conduction occurred following deliberate injection of 0.8 to 2.0 mg neostigmine.[48] Intermittent AV block was reported in one subject without anesthesia during another series when neostigmine was given prior to atropine.[49]

Soon after the introduction of curare into clinical medicine, several sudden deaths were reported following the injection of neostigmine-atropine.[50-52] These catastrophic events were attributed to the simultaneous injection of the two drugs.[53] In retrospect, the patients were probably underventilated at the time when the mixture of anticholinesterase-anticholinergic was given. The role of hypercapnia and hypoxia in the pathogenesis of cardiac arrhythmias was not appreciated until later, and methods for monitoring blood gases did not become more widely available until later. It has since been shown many times that the simultaneous injection of anticholinesterase and anticholinergic drug leads first to transient tachycardia and only much later to bradycardia.[54-61]

This does not mean that the common practice of giving a fixed dose combination of anticholinesterase-anticholinergic is endorsed. On the contrary, the practice contradicts pharmacologic rationale, and the issue should not be decided on a statistical basis. The rate of onset and the ultimate magnitude of cholinergic (muscarinic) effects depend on the magnitude of existing parasympathetic tone, as does the dose of the anticholinergic drug required. If for any reason the patient's vagal tone is exceptionally high during the injection of the anticholinesterase drug, a severe bradycardia may develop. If such a possibility is anticipated, the anticholinergic drug should be given prior to the enzyme inhibitor.

The consequences of the changes produced by both types of cholinergic drugs are well known in principle: bradycardia and slowing or block of AV-conduction may permit the emergence of secondary, ectopic pacemakers and hence cardiac arrhythmias.[62] An effective dose of an antimuscarinic agent can certainly block any reflex or drug-induced bradycardia (for example, from succinylcholine, halothane, narcotic analgesic, or anticholinesterase drugs), but only in doses that cause marked tachycardia.[30,63] The bradycardic effect of the atropine-like drugs themselves cannot be forgotten. On the other hand, tachycardia and the increase in cardiac output and, at times arterial blood pressure, represent an additional load on the heart, and increase the myocardial oxygen requirement.[64] This situation is hazardous in patients with coronary artery disease or with mitral stenosis. Furthermore, the resulting shift toward sympathetic/adrenergic prevalence may increase the probability of cardiac arrhythmias, and is especially dangerous in the presence of anesthetic agents known to sensitize the myocardium to catecholamines.[54]

Additional reasons for the conservative use of anticholinergic antimuscarinic drugs emerge from recent observations of a potentially beneficial effect of vagal activity on the heart and the evidence that parasympathetic activity regulates the release of sympathetic transmitter.[7-22]

We conclude that there is not sufficient evidence at this time to permit a full evaluation of the risks and benefits of the use of antimuscarinic, anticholinergic drugs for preanesthetic medication. With regard to secretions, such premedication is at least not mandatory, but the cardiac consequences are less clear-cut. The intravenous administration of an anticholinergic drug during anesthesia, which may become necessary, is definitely hazardous with anesthetic agents like cyclopropane and under

light anesthesia during painful procedures, somewhat less hazardous with halothane, and considerably less during thiopental-nitrous oxide or neurolept anesthesia. A higher dose of atropine, given rapidly intravenously, seems to be less hazardous than a smaller one.[47]

The other effects of the antimuscarinic drugs—on body temperature, on pupillary constriction and hence intraocular pressure, and on micturition—are minor by comparison.[30-32,66,67] Atropine in clinical doses does not prevent the effects of neostigmine on intestinal motility.[65]

THE SO-CALLED CENTRAL ANTICHOLINERGIC SYNDROME

Of the many putative neurotransmitters in the mammalian central nervous system, acetylcholine (ACh) is the best documented. It is its muscarinic and not its nicotinic activity that is involved. Evidence for this conclusion is based importantly on the effects of pharmacologic agents.[3,68] All anticholinesterase agents and antimuscarinic antagonists of ACh that pass the blood-brain barrier affect central nervous system functions. Recently, biochemical studies have shown abundant acetylcholine receptors of the muscarinic type in the mammalian brain.[69]

It has long been known that atropine and scopolamine, as well as plants and plant extracts containing the belladonna alkaloids (see Table 9–1), can cause a typical CNS syndrome, which has been termed the "central anticholinergic syndrome."[70] Symptoms range from sedation, stupor, and unconsciousness to anxiety, restlessness, hyperactivity, disorientation, delirium, hallucinations, loss of recent memory, dysarthria, and, ultimately, convulsions, and respiratory depression.[71] The difference between the effects of small doses of atropine and of scopolamine is well known.[30,31] Small doses of the latter (0.3 to 0.5 mg) given subcutaneously, but not orally, usually cause profound sedation, whereas atropine, in

Table 9–1
Anticholinergic antimuscarinic agents

Belladonna alkaloids	atropine scopolamine homatropine cyclopentolate
Anticholinergic drugs for Parkinsonism	benztropine (Cogentin) biperiden (Akineton) ethopropazine (Parsidol) procyclidine (Kemadrin) trihexyphenidyl (Artane)
Some over-the-counter drugs	Asthma-Dor Compoz Sleep Eze Sominex
Plants containing anti-cholinergic alkaloids	Bittersweet *(Solanum dulcamara)* Deadly nightshade *(Atropa belladonna)* Potato leaves and sprouts *(Solanum tuberosum)* Jimson weed *(Datura stramonium)*
So-called antispasmodics (quaternary anticholinergics)	Methantheline (Banthine) Propantheline (Probanthine)

doses up to 1 mg, has few CNS effects, other than the vagal stimulation discussed. It is old clinical knowledge that the condition of the patient at the time when the drug is given can make a difference: patients who have suffered head trauma, or are in pain, or are in a state of excitement are likely to respond to scopolamine with delirium and violent motor activity. Atropine in doses as high as 200 mg has been used in psychiatry for "coma therapy" in physically healthy patients, although much smaller doses have been reported to have been fatal, especially in children.[72] Therefore, care must be used with this agent.

Physostigmine, which is a tertiary amine, completely reverses even the delirium produced by a large dose of atropine, whereas it is known that neostigmine and the other quaternary ammonium anticholinesterase agents have little or no CNS effect.[73] This is logical if one considers the different lipid solubilities of the tertiary and quaternary compounds.

Anesthesia potentiates the CNS effects of the anticholinergic drugs. In one series of 1,727 patients, premedicated with up to 0.5 mg scopolamine and anesthetized with different anesthetics, 11.2% were diagnosed to have a "postoperative reaction" attributed to scopolamine.[74] Of these, 85.2% had prolonged somnolence, and 14.8% had delirium.

Thus there are two different types of postoperative central anticholinergic conditions, one characterized by profound and prolonged somnolence, the other by excitement, delirium, and motor violence. This situation seems analogous to that in patients without anesthesia, where "paradoxical," that is, excitatory, reactions to scopolamine may also occur. That both types of reactions respond quickly to the injection of physostigmine is evidence that both conditions are causally related to anticholinergic medication.[74] So far, there is no precise information about the conditions that may determine which type of reaction occurs.

Anticholinergic, antimuscarinic activity is not restricted to agents so classified (see Table 9–1), but is seen with many drugs from antihistaminics to tricyclic antidepressants. Such agents are also often contained in drug combinations and in over-the-counter preparations, and may be present in "street drugs." A partial listing is given in Tables 9–1 and 9–2. It has been stated that more than 600 pharmaceutic preparations contain

Table 9–2
Drugs possessing anticholinergic activity

Tricyclic antidepressants:
  Amitriptyline (Elavil)
  Desipramine (Norpramine, Pertofrane)
  Doxepin (Sinequan)
  Imipramine (Tofranyl, SK-Pramine)

Antipsychotic agents:
  Chlorpromazine
  Thioridazine (Mellaril)
  Haloperidol
  Droperidol

Antihistamine agents:
  Chlorpheniramine (Ornade)
  Diphenhydramine (Benadryl)
  Orphenidrine (Disipal)
  Promethazine (Phenergan)

Drugs not having anticholinergic activity but reported to have been antagonized by physostigmine:

  Diazepam (Valium)
  Chlordiazepoxide (Librium)
  Lorazepam
  Glutethimide (Doriden)
  Narcotic analgesics

agents with central anticholinergic activity.[71] Thus patients may be exposed to such drugs without the knowledge of the physician. After prolonged use of some such preparations, residual concentrations may remain in the body for a long time without causing clear symptoms. For the anesthesiologist this means that the remaining activity of such agents may be additive to that of anticholinergic drugs administered before or during anesthesia.

Lately, it has been reported that physostigmine has been used successfully to treat CNS depression from drugs with no known anticholinergic activity, such as diazepam.[75,76] It has also been claimed that physostigmine antagonizes the depressant effects of narcotic analgesics without reducing their analgesic activity.[77] These observations have led to the claim that physostigmine may be a nonspecific CNS stimulant or analeptic, independent of its anticholinesterase action. Although this could be so, there is no need to postulate it. An anticholinesterase agent ''potentiates'' cholinergic synaptic transmission or in-

creases neuronal activity even if no receptor antagonist is present. There is evidence, for example, that anticholinesterase agents can improve transmission in situations where the defect is due to decreased release of transmitter.[78] An indirect effect on the function of central cholinergic neuronal systems is possible with many drugs.

The indications for the use of physostigmine differ widely from institution to institution and from one anesthesiologist to the next. Risks and benefits must be weighed as always, but little information on their magnitude is available in this case.

It seems from a survey of the literature that the risks of physostigmine administration are small, as long as the recommended dose is not exceeded, the indication is strictly established, and the many contraindications are heeded. The dose is 1 or 2 mg, given slowly intravenously, with a possible second dose after 10 to 15 minutes, if the response to the first dose has been positive but insufficient. Physostigmine should only be given if there are signs of antimuscarinic medication in the periphery in addition to symptoms of the presence of a central anticholinergic syndrome. Relative contraindications and precautions are the same as for those anticholinesterase drugs that do not enter the CNS. If evidence of physostigmine overdosage is seen, the balance may be restored with a further dose of an anticholinergic drug, either scopolamine or atropine. If there are only symptoms of peripheral cholinergic preponderance, a quaternary ammonium anticholinergic (methylscopolamine, glycopyrrolate, methantheline, propantheline) should be used. The duration of action of physostigmine is shorter than that of the anticholinergic agents involved; thus it may be necessary to repeat its injection if the symptoms alleviated by the first dose should recur.

REFERENCES

1. Loewi, O.: Über humorale Übertragberkeit der Herznerven Wirkung. Arch. Ges. Physiol., *189*:239, 1921.

2. Dale, H. H.: The action of certain esters and ethers of choline, and their relation to muscarine. J. Pharmacol Exp. Ther., 6:147, 1914.
3. Koelle, G. B.: Neurohumoral transmission and the autonomic nervous system. *In* The Pharmacological Basis of Therapeutics. Edited by L. S. Goodman and A. Gilman. New York, Macmillan, 1975.
4. Haefely, W.: Electrophysiology of the adrenergic neuron. *In* Handbook of Experimental Pharmacology. Edited by H. Blaschko and E. Muscholl. Berlin, Springer-Verlag, 1972, Vol. 33.
5. Cannon, W. B.: Organization for physiological homeostasis. Physiol. Rev., 9:399, 1929.
6. Higgins, C. B., Vatner, S. F., and Braunwald, E.: Parasympathetic control of the heart. Pharmacol. Rev., 25:119, 1973.
7. Kent, K. M., et al.: Electrical stability of acutely ischemic myocardium: influences of heart rate and vagal stimulation. Circulation, 47:291, 1973.
8. Kolman, B. S., Verrier, R. L., and Lown, B.: The effect of vagus nerve stimulation upon vulnerability of the canine ventricle. Circulation, 52:578, 1975.
9. Kolman, B. S., Verrier, R. L., and Lown, B.: Effect of vagus nerve stimulation upon excitability of the canine ventricle. Am. J. Cardiol., 37:1041, 1976.
10. Rabinowitz, S. H., Verrier, R. L., and Lown, B.: Muscarinic effects of vagosympathetic trunk stimulation on the repetitive extrasystole (RE) threshold. Circulation, 53:622, 1976.
11. Lown, B., and Verrier, R. L.: Neural activity and ventricular fibrillation. N. Engl. J. Med., 294:1165, 1976.
12. Cope, R. L.: Suppressive effect of carotid sinus on premature ventricular beats in certain instances. Am. J. Cardiol., 4:314, 1959.
13. Lown, B., and Levine, S. A.: The carotid sinus: clinical value of its stimulation. Circulation, 23:776, 1961.
14. Lorentzen, D.: Pacemaker-induced ventricular tachycardia: reversion to normal sinus rhythm by carotid sinus massage. J.A.M.A., 235:282, 1976.
15. Waxman, M. B., et al.: Phenylephrine (Neosynephrine^R) terminated ventricular tachycardia. Circulation, 50:656, 1974.
16. Weiss, T., Lattin, G. M., and Engelman, K.: Vagally mediated suppression of premature ventricular contractions in man. Am. Heart J., 89:700, 1975.
17. Lown, B., et al.: Effect of a digitalis drug on ventricular premature beats. (VPBs). N. Engl. J. Med., 296:301, 1977.
18. Lown, B., et al.: Sleep and ventricular premature beats. Circulation, 48:691, 1973.
19. Löffelholz, K., and Muscholl, E.: Muscarinic inhibition of the noradrenaline release evoked by postganglionic sympathetic nerve stimulation. Naunyn Schmiedebergs Arch. Pharmacol., 265:1, 1969.
20. Levy, M. N., and Blattberg, B.: Effect of vagal stimulation on the overflow of norepinephrine into the coronary sinus during cardiac sympathetic nerve stimulation in the dog. Circ. Res., 38:81, 1976.
21. Ehinger, B., Falck, B., and Sporrong, B.: Possible axo-axonal synapses between peripheral adrenergic and cholinergic nerve terminals. Z. Zellforsch., 107:508, 1970.
22. Kent, K. M., et al.: Cholinergic innervation of the canine and human ventricular conducting system: anatomic and electrophysiological correlation. Circulation, 50:948, 1974.
23. Kharkevich, D. A.: Ganglion-Blocking and Ganglion-Stimulating Agents. Oxford, Pergamon Press, 1967.
24. Flacke, W. E.: Drug Therapy. Treatment of myasthenia gravis. N. Engl. J. Med., 288:27, 1973.
25. DeRoeth, A., Jr., et al.: Effect of phospholine iodide on blood cholinesterase levels of normal and glaucoma subjects. Am. J. Ophthalmol., 59:586, 1965.
26. Garfield, J. M., et al.: A pharmacological analysis of ganglionic actions of some general anesthetics. Anesthesiology, 29:79, 1968.
27. Trendelenburg, Y.: Some aspects of the pharmacology of autonomic ganglion cells. Ergebn. Physiol., 59:1, 1967.
28. Flacke, W. E., and Gillis, R. A.: Impulse transmission via nicotinic and muscarinic pathways in the stellate ganglion of the dog. J. Pharmacol. Exp. Ther., 163:266, 1968.
29. Innes, I. R., and Nickerson, M.: Atropine, scopolamine and related antimuscarinic drugs. *In* The Pharmacological Basis of Therapeutics. Edited by L. S. Goodman and A. Gilman. New York, Macmillan, 1975.
30. Eger, E. I., II: Atropine, scopolamine and related compounds. Anesthesiology, 23:365, 1962.
31. Andrews, I. C., and Belonsky, B.: Parasympatholytics. *In* Clinical Anesthesia. Pharmacology of Adjuvant Drugs. Vol. 10. Edited by H. L. Zander. Philadelphia, F. A. Davis, 1973.
32. Herxheimer, A.: A comparison of some atropine-like drugs in man, with particular reference to their end-organ specificity. Br. J. Pharmacol., 13:184, 1958.
33. Morton, H. J., and Thomas, E. T.: Effect of atropine on the heart rate. Lancet, 2:1313, 1958.
34. Gravenstein, J. S., Andersen, T. W., and DePadua, C. B.: Effects of atropine and scopolamine on the cardiovascular system in man. Anesthesiology, 25:123, 1964.
35. Hayes, A. H., Jr., and Katz, R. A.: Homatropine bradycardia in man. Clin. Pharmacol. Ther., 11:558, 1970.
36. Kottmeier, C. A., and Gravenstein, J. S.: The parasympathomimetic activity of atropine and atropine methylbromide. Anesthesiology, 29:1125, 1968.
37. Holt, A. T.: Premedication with atropine should not be routine. Lancet, 2:984, 1962.
38. Fabick, Y. S., and Smiler, B. G.: Is anticholinergic premedication necessary? Anesthesiology, 43:472, 1975.
39. Leighton, K. M., and Sanders, H. D.: Anticholinergic premedication. Can. Anaesth. Soc. J., 223:563, 1976.
40. Gravenstein, J. S., and Anton, A. H.: Premedication and drug interaction. Clin. Anesth., 3:199, 1969.

41. Annis, P., Landa, J., and Lichtiger, M.: Effects of atropine on velocity of tracheal mucus in anesthetized patients. Anesthesiology, *44*:74, 1976.

42. Jones, R. E., Deutsch, S., and Turndorf, H.: Effects of atropine on cardiac rhythm in conscious and anesthetized man. Anesthesiology, *22*:67, 1961.

43. Munchow, O. B., and Denson, J. S.: Modification by light cyclopropane and halothane anesthesia of the chronotropic effect of atropine in man. Anesth. Analg. (Cleve.), *44*:782, 1965.

44. Bradshaw, E. G.: Dysrhythmia associated with oral surgery. Anaesthesia, *31*:13, 1976.

45. Viby-Mogensen, J., et al.: Halothane anesthesia and suxamethonium I: The significance of preoperative atropine administration. Acta Anaesthesiol. Scand., *20*:129, 1976.

46. Eikard, B., and Sorensen, B.: Arrhythmias during halothane anesthesia I.: The influence of atropine during induction with intubation. II. The influence of atropine. Acta Anaesthesiol. Scand., *20*:296, 1976, and *21*:245, 1977.

47. Carrow, D. J., et al.: Effects of large doses of intravenous atropine on heart rate and arterial pressure of anesthetized patients. Anesth. Analg. (Cleve.), *54*:262, 1975.

48. Jacobson, E., and Adelman, M. H.: Electrocardiographic effects of intravenous administration of neostigmine and atropine during cyclopropane anesthesia. Anesthesiology, *15*:407, 1954.

49. Fielder, D. L., et al.: Cardiovascular effects of atropine and neostigmine in man. Anesthesiology, *30*:637, 1969.

50. MacIntosh, R. R.: Death following injection of neostigmine. Br. Med. J., *1*:852, 1949.

51. Clutton-Brock, J.: Death following neostigmine. Br. Med. J., *1*:1007, 1949.

52. Hill, M.: Death after neostigmine injection. Br. Med. J., *2*:601, 1949.

53. Kemp, S. W., and Morton, H. J. V.: The effect of atropine and neostigmine on the pulse rates of anaesthetized patients. Anaesthesia, *17*:170, 1962.

54. Katz, R. L., and Epstein, R. A.: The interaction of anesthetic agents and adrenergic drugs to produce cardiac arrhythmias. Anesthesiology, *29*:763, 1968.

55. Kemp, S. W., and Morton, H. J. V.: Effect of atropine and neostigmine on the pulse rates of anesthetized patients. Anaesthesia, *17*:170, 1962.

56. Baraka, A.: Safe reversal. 1. Atropine followed by neostigmine. An electrocardiographic study. 2. Atropine-neostigmine mixture. An electrocardiographic study. Br. J. Anaesth., *40*:27 and 30, 1968.

57. Hannington-Kiff, J. G.: Timing of atropine and neostigmine in the reversal of muscle relaxants. Br. Med. J., *1*:418, 1969.

58. Ovassapian, A.: Effect of administration of atropine and neostigmine in man. Anesth. Analg., *48*:219, 1969.

59. Ramamurthy, S., Shaker, M. H., and Winnie, A. P.: Glycopyrrolate as a substitute for atropine in neostigmine reversal. Can. Anaesth. Soc. J., *19*:399, 1972.

60. Ostheimer, G. W.: A comparison of glycopyrrolate and atropine during reversal of nondepolarizing neuromuscular block with neostigmine. Anesth. Analg. (Cleve.), *56*:182, 1977.

61. Miller, R. D., et al.: Comparative times to peak effect and durations of action of neostigmine and pyridostigmine. Anesthesiology, *41*:27, 1974.

62. Han, J., and Moe, G. K.: Nonuniform recovery of excitability in ventricular muscle. Circ. Res., *14*:44, 1964.

63. Roco, A. G., and Vandam, L. D.: Changes in circulation consequent to manipulation during abdominal surgery. J.A.M.A., *164*:14, 1957.

64. Knoebel, S. B., et al.: Atropine-induced cardioacceleration and myocardial blood flow in subjects with and without coronary artery disease. Am. J. Cardiol., *33*:327, 1974.

65. Wilkins, J. L., et al.: Effects of neostigmine and atropine on motor activity of ileum, colon, and rectum of anaesthetized subjects. Br. Med. J., *1*:793, 1970.

66. Schwartz, H., DeRoetth, A., Jr., and Papper, E. M.: Preanesthetic use of atropine and scopolamine in patient with glaucoma. J.A.M.A., *165*:144, 1957.

67. Effects of systemic drugs with anticholinergic properties on glaucoma. Medical Letter, *16*:28, 1974.

68. Feldberg, W.: Present views on the mode of action of acetylcholine in the central nervous system. Physiol. Rev., *25*:596, 1945.

69. Snyder, S. H., et al.: Biochemical identification of the mammalian muscarinic cholinergic receptor. Fed. Proc., *34*:1915, 1975.

70. Duvoisin, R. C., and Katz, R. L.: Reversal of central anticholinergic syndrome in man by physostigmine. J.A.M.A., *206*:1963, 1968.

71. Granacher, R. P., and Baldessarini, R. J.: The usefulness of physostigmine in neurology and psychiatry. *In* Clinical Neuropharmacology. Edited by H. L. Klawans. New York, Raven Press, 1976.

72. Forrer, G. R., and Miller, J. J.: Atropine coma: a somatic therapy in psychiatry. Am. J. Psychiatry, *115*:455, 1958.

73. Janson, P. A., Watt, B., and Hermos, J. A.: Success with physostigmine and failure with neostigmine in reversing toxicity. J.A.M.A., *237*:2632, 1977.

74. Holzgrafe, R. E., Vondrell, J. J., and Mintz, S. M.: Reversal of postoperative reactions to scopolamine with physostigmine. Anesth. Analg. (Cleve.), *52*:921, 1973.

75. Larson, G. F., Hulbert, B. J., and Wingard, D. W.: Physostigmine reversal of diazepam-induced depression. Anesth. Analg. (Cleve.), *56*:348, 1977.

76. DiLiberti, J., O'Brien, M.D., and Turner, T.: The use of physostigmine as an antidote in an accidental diazepam intoxication. J. Pediatr., *23*:106, 1975.

77. El-Naggar, M., and El-Ganzouri, A. R.: Physostigmine. Its use in the management of postoperative mental aberrations. Anesthesiology Rev., *5*:49, 1978.

78. Gillis, R. A., et al.: Actions of anticholinesterase agents upon ganglionic transmission in the dog. J. Pharmacol. Exp. Ther., *163*:277, 1968.

10

Digitalis

JOHN L. ATLEE, III
and
BEN F. RUSY

Digitalis, the fourth most frequently prescribed drug in the United States, is important from both therapeutic and toxicologic viewpoints.[1] Digoxin is the most commonly used preparation, probably because of its short plasma half-life of 31 hours (oral) and 33 hours (intravenous), which offers an advantage in achieving optimal digitalization and in managing suspected toxicity.[2] Digitoxin, which has a plasma half-life of five to seven days, is usually only used for maintenance digitalization.

The digitalis glycosides have one of the lowest therapeutic indices of all drugs used. Approximately 20% of the patients who take digitalis exhibit some type of toxic reaction.[3,4] The principal therapeutic effect of digitalis is an increase in contractile performance (positive inotropy) in patients with cardiac failure. Digitalis is also used to slow conduction (negative dromotropy) across the atrioventricular node and thus to decrease the ventricular rate in patients with atrial flutter or fibrillation. The positive inotropic effect of digitalis is directly proportional to the dose used; that is, the dose-response curve is linear.[5] A nearly toxic dose, however, may be necessary to achieve a negative dromotropic effect depending on the preexisting autonomic tone.[5]

Digitalis toxicity may be due to an actual overdosage or to other factors, including variations in a patient's susceptibility to disease and or sensitivity to other drugs taken simultaneously. The circumstances of anesthesia and operation may precipitate digitalis toxicity in an otherwise normally digitalized patient or in a patient who is being digitalized. Two case reports, based both on documented interactions and on our own experience, illustrate interactions that are likely to be of significance to the practicing anesthesiologist.

CASE REPORT

A 68-year-old man (66 kg) with intermittent claudication was scheduled for an aortofemoral bypass operation. He had a 20-year history of essential hypertension. Two years prior to admission he had been admitted to another hospital for treatment of congestive heart failure and had responded promptly to digitalis and diuretics. Present therapy included digoxin 0.25 mg O.D. and hydrochlorothiazide 25 mg b.i.d. Laboratory values on admission were normal except: BUN (blood urea nitrogen) = 22 mg%, creatinine = 1.8 mg%, Na = 132 meq/L, K = 3.4 meq/L, Cl = 92 meq/L. The serum digoxin level was 2.4 ng/ml. The ECG (electrocardiogram) showed sinus rhythm (64 beats/min) and signs of left ventricular hypertrophy. Occasional unifocal premature ventricular beats were also noted. The chest roentgenogram showed mild cardiac enlargement, but was otherwise normal. Blood pressure readings prior to the operation had ranged from 135 to 160 torr systolic and 86 to 105 torr diastolic.

Premedication consisted of scopolamine (hyoscine), 0.43 mg, and morphine, 8 mg IM (intramuscularly). The patient's blood pressure was 156/88 torr and the pulse rate 64 beats/min on arrival in the operating room. Lines were inserted for monitoring arterial (radial artery) and central venous (internal jugular) pressure. While the patient breathed oxygen, 100%, the induction of anesthesia was accomplished with intravenous morphine sulfate, 20 mg, diazepam, 10 mg, and thiopental, 250 mg. Succinylcholine, 100 mg IV (intravenously) was used to facilitate laryngoscopy for the topical application of 4% lidocaine (160 mg) to the trachea and for endotracheal intubation. During this procedure, the patient's blood pressure rose to 180/110 torr, and there were frequent multifocal ventricular premature beats. The elevated blood pressure and arrhythmias responded to thiopental, 100 mg. After a paralyzing dose of pancuronium, 6.5 mg, the patient's ventilation was controlled with nitrous oxide-oxygen ($F_{I_{O_2}}$ = 0.40). Minute volume was 8.2 liters. An additional 10 mg of morphine was given prior to the surgical incision, which was made approximately 20 minutes following the institution of controlled ventilation. The patient's blood pressure was 140/90 torr and his pulse rate was 84 beats/min immediately prior to the incision.

Soon after the surgical incision was made, the patient's blood pressure rose to 160/100 torr and frequent multifocal ventricular premature beats were noted, followed by ventricular tri- and quadrigeminy. The ventricular arrhythmias failed to respond to two intravenous boluses of lidocaine (100 mg). Ventilation with 100% oxygen was begun, with no improvement in the arrhythmia. Arterial blood gas and electrolyte determinations, performed shortly after the arrhythmias first appeared, revealed the following: pH = 7.46, P_{O_2} = 161 torr, P_{CO_2} = 25 torr, Na = 134 meq/L, and K = 2.8 meq/L. Minute ventilation was immediately reduced to 5.6 L/min. Potassium chloride (20 meq) and phenytoin (diphenylhydantoin) (100 mg, in divided doses) were then administered intravenously. Over the next 15 minutes, the premature beats became less numerous, then unifocal in origin, and finally disappeared. Nitrous oxide was reinstituted ($F_{I_{O_2}}$ = 0.40), and the surgeons continued with the operation. Arterial blood gas analysis 30 minutes later showed: pH = 7.41, P_{O_2} = 138 torr, P_{CO_2} = 38 torr, Na = 132 meq/L, and K = 3.7 meq/L. The remainder of the anesthetic course was uneventful.

CASE REPORT

A 74-year-old man (70 kg) was scheduled for a total hip arthroplasty. Significant findings on admission included a long history of hypertension complicated two years prior to admission by congestive heart failure, which had been treated with digitalis and diuretics. The patient had remained symptom-free until nine months prior to admission, when he had experienced palpitations caused by atrial fibrillation, which was electrically converted to sinus rhythm. Prophylactic therapy with quinidine was instituted to reduce the chances of recurrence.

During the initial preoperative hospital evaluation five days prior to his operation, the patient again experienced atrial fibrillation. Because of palpitations and the impending operation, it was elected to convert the arrhythmia electrically and to increase the quinidine dose (200 to 300 mg q.i.d.). These measures restored sinus rhythm. The patient was also taking digoxin (0.25 mg O.D.) and hydrochlorothiazide (25 mg b.i.d.). The day before the operation, the serum electrolytes were Na = 135 meq/L and K = 3.6 meq/L. The patient's serum digoxin level on the second day of hospitalization was 1.6 ng/ml. On the morning of the operation, the ECG showed sinus rhythm (rate = 72 beats/min) with infrequent (<2/min) monofocal premature ventricular beats. Other laboratory values were within normal limits.

Anesthesia was induced, while the patient breathed oxygen, with thiopental (total dose 350 mg IV) and succinylcholine (60 mg IV), and maintained with nitrous oxide ($F_{I_{O_2}}$ = 0.5)-halothane (0.5 = 1.5% inspired). Pancuronium, 3 mg, was used for muscle relaxation. Ventilation was controlled ($\dot{V}_E$ = 8.5 L/min).

The induction of anesthesia and the first hour of the operation were uneventful except for occasional (<6/min) premature ventricular beats. These gradually increased as the operation progressed, and by approximately two hours into the procedure the patient was found to have ventricular bigeminy (blood pressure 130/90 torr). Digoxin toxicity was considered to be a cause, and a blood sample was drawn for a digoxin serum level determination (this was later reported as 2.6 ng/ml). An arterial blood sample showed pH = 7.44, P_{O_2} =142 torr, P_{CO_2} = 30 torr, Na = 136 meq/L, and K = 3.2 meq/L. Initial therapy consisted of the reduction of the minute volume of ventilation (8.5 to 6.0 L/min), and the administration of potassium chloride (30 meq) over the next 40 minutes. During this time, the ventricular bigeminy was resolved and the ventricular premature beats became less numerous. By the end of the operation (3½ hours duration), their frequency was between six and eight beats/min. Arterial blood-gas values one hour after the initiation of therapy showed pH = 7.38, P_{O_2} = 128 torr, P_{CO_2} = 40 torr, Na = 136 meq/L, and K = 4.1 meq/L. The rest of the anesthetic and operative course was uncomplicated. After the operation, quinidine was continued, but the maintenance digoxin dose was reduced to 0.125 mg O.D. The patient experienced no further episodes of atrial fibrillation during his 2½-week hospital stay.

These case reports illustrate some problems presented by digitalis that are likely to be encountered by anesthetists, involving (1) potentiation of digitalis toxicity by *hypokalemia*, (2) *impaired renal function*, which reduces the rate at which digoxin is cleared from the plasma, (3) interactions between quinidine and digoxin that promote toxicity, and (4) the beneficial actions of *phenytoin (diphenylhydantoin)* and *potassium chloride* in reversing ventricular arrhythmias caused by digitalis intoxication.

Hypokalemia is a common cause of digitalis intoxication in otherwise normally digitalized patients. Hypokalemia is often secondary to the potassium-wasting effects of potent diuretics, including the benzothiadiazines, furosemide, and ethacrynic acid, which are commonly administered along with digitalis. Adequate potassium replacement or the use of potassium-sparing agents (spironolactone, triamterene) in patients who take potent diuretics is particularly important to digitalized patients.[6] Magnesium deficiencies attendant on diuretic-induced losses of this cation may also predispose a patient to digitalis intoxication.[6] The actual mechanism for diuretic-induced digitalis intoxication is the probable increase in myocardial binding of the digitalis glycosides in the presence of hypokalemia, and the possible interference with membrane adenosinetriphosphatase (ATPase—dependent on magnesium ions, and activated by sodium and potassium ions) in cases of hypomagnesemia.[7,8] Although the serum levels of potassium prior to the operations in the case reports (3.4 meq/L in the first, and 3.6 meq/L in the second case) were in the borderline hypokalemic range, these levels were acutely lowered to definite hypokalemic status (2.8 and 3.2 meq/L respectively) during the operations. Acute hypokalemia in these patients was most likely related to hyperventilation: the resulting respiratory alkalosis caused a shift in potassium into the cell in exchange for hydrogen ion. Edwards et al. noted approximately 0.5 meq/L reductions in serum potassium level for every 10 torr decrease in arterial P_{CO_2} in mechanically hyperventilated patients during anesthesia.[9] Metabolic alkalosis can also cause hypokalemia secondary to hydrogen ion shifts.

Impaired renal function is a major cause of digitalis intoxication with short-acting digitalis glycosides (ouabain, deslanoside, digoxin) that depend on renal excretion for their elimination.[7] The longer-acting preparations, digitoxin and digitalis leaf, are metabolized in the liver; their less active metabolites are eliminated by renal excretion.[7] Impaired renal function probably was partly responsible for the preoperative borderline toxic serum digoxin level of 2.5 ng/ml in the first patient.[10] The mildly elevated BUN and creatinine levels in this patient suggest impaired renal function. Arteriosclerosis or atherosclerosis, long-standing hypertension, and the patient's age may have been responsible for the diminished renal function. Although the digoxin serum level prior to operation was only borderline toxic, and there were no ECG manifestations of toxicity, anorexia, nausea or vomiting in this patient, the hypokalemia secondary to mechanical hyperventilation and diuretic therapy probably precipitated acute toxicity (ventricular arrhythmias) during the course of the operation.

Quinidine has recently been acknowledged to cause digitalis toxicity.[11] The serum digoxin concentration increased in 25 of 27 patients in a study (mean rise 1.4 to 3.2 ng/ml) during quinidine therapy. Anorexia, nausea, or vomiting developed in 16 of the 27 patients, and disappeared when the digoxin maintenance dose was reduced. This suggests a causal relationship between an increased level of digoxin and gastrointestinal effects. Furthermore, in seven patients ventricular arrhythmias developed or worsened after quinidine therapy began. In four patients an elevation in digoxin level was noted within 24 hours of the institution of quinidine therapy. By exclusion, these researchers concluded that the initial rise in the serum concentration of digoxin resulted from the displacement of digoxin from tissue-binding sites by quinidine. An interaction between quinidine and digoxin, brought about by the increased dose of quinidine (from 200 to 300 mg q.i.d.), may have caused the rise in serum digoxin levels between the second day of hospitalization and the day of the operation (1.6 to 2.6 ng/ml) in our second case report. The appearance of ventricular premature beats on the ECG taken on the morning of the operation was probably related to the increased serum level of digoxin. Toxicity was further compounded by the production of hypocapneic hypokalemia

during the mechanical ventilation of the patient. The quinidine-digoxin interaction requires additional study.[11] In the meantime, anesthesiologists should be alert to the possibility of this interaction, since quinidine and digitalis are occasionally used concurrently.

Phenytoin is almost exclusively the specific treatment for digitalis-induced ventricular arrhythmias, as is *potassium chloride* for digitalis toxicity related to hypokalemia.[12,14] Whereas lidocaine may also be effective in treating ventricular arrhythmias due to digitalis, it failed in the first case report patient.[12–14] Thus phenytoin and potassium chloride were administered while ventilation was decreased. It is impossible to decide which was more effective. Each was indicated under the circumstances, since ventricular tachycardia and/or fibrillation could have resulted had the arrhythmias remained untreated. The suggested dose of phenytoin is 50 to 100 mg intravenously, in repeated doses every 10 to 15 minutes until a therapeutic response is observed or until a total of 10 to 15 mg/kg has been administered.[12] For intravenous lidocaine, a loading dose of 2 to 3 mg/kg followed by a maintenance infusion of 20 to 30 mcg/kg/minute (1.0 gm lidocaine in 250 ml of normal saline), or 100 mg every three to five minutes are used.[13]

PHARMACOLOGY OF DIGITALIS

Inotropic effect: mechanism of action

Cardiac glycosides act directly on the heart to increase the force of contraction. Although the exact mechanism is unknown, the most likely subcellular system involved is Na^+, K^+-ATPase, an enzymatic ion transport system located in the cardiac cell membrane and often referred to as the sodium pump. Evidence for the involvement of this system is that Na^+, K^+-ATPase is inhibited by low concentrations of digitalis, whereas other subcellular systems are either not affected, or are affected only by high concentrations of digitalis.[15] The rationale for this proposed mechanism of action is based on the premise that the inhibition of sodium pump activity by digitalis ultimately increases the concentration of myoplasmic ionized calcium, which is, in turn, responsible for the observed increase in the force of myocardial contraction.[16-22]

During the depolarization of a cardiac contractile cell, calcium ions flow inward across the cell membrane. The associated movement of charge produces a current (the slow inward calcium current) that accounts for the plateau of the cardiac action potential.[23,24] The calcium that enters the cell in this way during each systole is not of sufficient quantity to activate contraction appreciably, but it does trigger the release of additional Ca^{2+} from intracellular storage sites and would, after many contractions, flood the cell with calcium, were it not for the existence of a mechanism for the extrusion of this divalent ion.[21,23,25,34] The extrusion mechanism involves a carrier-mediated exchange of one Ca^{2+} for 2 Na^+; these ions compete for carrier sites on both sides of the membrane. Energy for outward calcium transport comes presumably from the coupled inward transport of Na^+ that flows down a concentration gradient provided originally by Na^+, K^+-ATPase sodium pump activity. Since calcium and sodium compete with one another for transport, any intervention that increases intracellular Na^+ causes fewer sites to be occupied by Ca^{2+} for outward transport. Consequently, the myoplasmic concentrations of Ca^{2+} increase until the ion can again compete successfully for enough transport sites to insure that its outward transport matches the inward flux. The increase in myoplasmic Ca^{2+} concentration, brought about thus, results in the sequestration of increased amounts of the ion in sarcoplasmic reticular storage depots. This sequestration, in turn, leads to an augmented release of Ca^{2+} from these transport sites during depolarization and to an increase in contractile activity.[27] Digitalis inhibits the sodium pump. Associated with this is an accumulation of Na^+ by the cardiac cell that, by the mechanism described, accounts for the drug's positive inotropic effect.[16,17,26,27]

Consideration of the process of cardiac contraction and of the steps leading to its activation reveals that there are numerous ways to produce a positive inotropic effect. Some of the mechanisms proposed, including the one described for digitalis, are outlined in Table 10–1.

Table 10–1
Summary of mechanisms for positive inotropy

Subcellular Component	Proposed Mechanism for Positive Inotropy	Drugs Inducing Effect
1. Troponin	CAMP*, protein kinase-induced phosphorylation. Increased Ca^{2+} affinity[28,29]	catecholamines xanthines
2. Myosin light chains	Phosphorylation[30]	
3. Sarcoplasmic reticulum	CAMP, protein kinase-induced phosphorylation Increased storage and release of Ca^{2+} [27]	catecholamines xanthines
4. Sarcolemma	(a) CAMP, protein kinase-induced phosphorylation.[27] Increased Ca^{2+} influx (slow inward current)[23]	catecholamines xanthines
	(b) Non-CAMP dependent increased Ca^{2+}influx[31]	positive rate staircase (treppe)
	(c) Na^+, K^+-ATPase inhibition[17]	digitalis glycosides

*Cyclic adenosinemonophosphate

Cardiac electrophysiologic effects

The normal transmembrane resting potential of cardiac cells (-80 to -90 mv intracellular with respect to extracellular) depends on sodium and potassium gradients that in turn depend on the integrity of the sodium-potassium activated pump mechanism (Na^+, K^+-ATPase) previously discussed. There is general agreement that the toxic effects of digitalis on the generation and conduction of cardiac impulses result from inhibition of the pump mechanism, although the mechanism for the therapeutic and inotropic effects of digitalis is not fully understood.[1,14] Inhibition of the Na^+, K^+-ATPase pump mechanism leads to the accumulation of intracellular sodium and to a corresponding reduction in intracellular potassium.[1] This direct effect of digitalis on the heart is complicated by indirect or neurally mediated effects (see the section of this chapter entitled "Autonomic Actions").[1]

The electrical excitability of both the atrium and the ventricle in the intact dog heart is increased by lower doses of digitalis, but decreased by higher doses.[1,32] The increased excitability is largely due to the decreased diastolic intracellular negativity.[1] The atrium may be rendered inexcitable by doses that do not prevent propagated idioventricular impulses, although the specialized atrial conducting pathways are believed to be more resistant to such impulses than atrial muscle.[1] Purkinje fibers gradually become inexcitable at higher concentrations of digitalis, but ventricular muscle fibers are more resistant.[1] Thus resistance to digitalis-induced excitability increases progressively from the atria to the ventricles.[1] Similarly, conduction velocity within the atria and ventricles is increased by low, and decreased by toxic, doses of digitalis. Conduction through the atrioventricular node is slowed by both vagal and extravagal actions of digitalis (see "Autonomic Actions").[1,33,34]

Digitalis exerts different effects on the refractory periods of the various cardiac tissues.[1] It shortens the atrial refractory period and prolongs the functional refractory period of the atrioventricular node under conditions that permit reflex vagal activity. In the absence of vagal activity, digitalis prolongs the atrial refractory period and the magnitude of increase in nodal refractoriness is reduced. Digitalis shortens the ventricular refractory period (apparent in man as a reduced Q–T interval). This shortening effect is independent of vagal innervation.

The effects of digitalis on automaticity, the ability of certain cardiac cells to initiate spontaneously regenerative activity, are complex, since two different forms of automaticity are probably involved.[1,18-20] The first and better understood of the two mechanisms, namely spontaneous diastolic (phase 4) depolarization, is enhanced by digitalis, especially in the ventricles.[1] The second and only recently described mechanism, namely triggered activity or oscillatory afterpotentials, is a true toxic manifestation of digitalis and is enhanced by low levels of potassium and by high levels of calcium.[35-37]

These two mechanisms of automaticity are described in more detail in Chapter 12. Of particular interest to anesthesiologists is the ability of halothane to antagonize digitalis-enhanced phase 4 automaticity.[38] Cyclopropane enhances whereas pentobarbital has little effect on this form of automaticity.[38] Fentanyl droperidol, ketamine, diethyl ether, methoxyflurane, enflurane, and, to a lesser extent, fluroxene and isoflurane, also protect against digitalis-enhanced phase 4 automaticity.[39,40] The effects of anesthetics on automaticity due to oscillatory afterpotentials have not been reported. Toxic levels of digitalis may cause arrhythmias by their effects on both automaticity and conduction.[1] In addition to actual heart block, alterations in conduction or refractoriness are also required to bring about arrhythmias caused by reentry of excitation.[41]

Autonomic actions

Three autonomic actions of digitalis have been documented in animal studies: vagomimetic actions; sensitization of the baroreceptors; and, in large doses, sympathetic activation.[42] Therapeutic doses of digitalis enhance vagal tone, and, as a result, slow the sinus rate, slow atrioventricular conduction, decrease atrial ectopic pacemaker automaticity, and decrease the refractory period of atrial muscle.[42] Sensitization of the carotid baroreceptors by digitalis has several important therapeutic consequences:[43] (1) it may explain in part the vagomimetic actions of digitalis as outlined previously; (2) the withdrawal of cardiac sympathetic tone resulting from baroreceptor activation might contribute to the ability of digitalis to convert paroxysmal supraventricular tachycardias to sinus rhythm; and (3) it may help to explain the antiarrhythmic effect of therapeutic levels of digitalis in patients with ventricular arrhythmias that are due in part to enhanced sympathetic tone.[42] The sympathomimetic action of digitalis is understood less fully.[42,44] Low doses inhibit sympathetic discharge because of baroreceptor sensitization.[42] In animal studies, however, large doses of digitalis excite the central nervous system and result in enhanced sympathetic tone and cardiac arrhythmias.[42,45,46] The central stimulating effects of large doses of digitalis are not confined to the cardiac sympathetic nerves, but can be detected also in peripheral sympathetic and phrenic nerves.[42] The autonomic effects of digitalis have important implications for anesthesiologists. They are poorly understood, however, owing to the simultaneous use of a multiplicity of drugs that affect autonomic function.

Pharmacokinetics

The availability of reliable assays for measuring the level of digitalis in biologic fluids has contributed greatly to our understanding of the pharmacokinetics of the digitalis glycosides.[2,47-49] This knowledge is clinically valuable, as it enables the physician to manage digitalized patients more effectively and decreases the frequency of digitalis intoxication.

Digoxin, when given daily without an initial loading dose, accumulates until a steady state is reached within five to seven days.[50,51] This is because of a pattern of drug elimination that is characterized by the excretion of a percentage of the daily amount of the body stores instead of the excretion of a constant amount each day.[52] In patients with normal renal function, one-third of the total accumulated dose of digoxin is excreted daily.[52] Thus if 0.25 mg is absorbed daily, and one-third of this amount is excreted, the total accumulated dose after 24 hours will be 0.17 mg (0.28 mg at two days, 0.35 mg at three days). After seven days, an approximate steady-state level (0.47 mg) will be reached, since the amounts of drug absorbed and excreted nearly balance each other. This is reflected by a plateau in the serum digoxin levels.

When the administration of digoxin is discontinued, the serum level declines as a function of its serum half-life (digoxin = 31 to 33 hours, digitoxin = five to seven days).[2] The relation between serum half-life and steady-state drug accumulation in the body is: three half-lives = 90%, and five half-lives = 99% accumulation; thus approximately seven days (digoxin) and two to three weeks (digitoxin) are required to achieve a plateau effect.[52]

The daily fluctuation between maximum and minimum serum levels of the digitalis preparation used also depends on the half-life of the drug.[52] For example, if digoxin is given once daily, the variation will be approximately 33%; if given twice daily, it will be approximately 16%. For digitoxin given once daily, there will be a 10% variation in serum levels. This consideration is of practical importance when high doses of digitalis are required to control arrhythmias (for example, atrial fibrillation with cardiac decompensation).[52] Divided daily doses of digoxin allow one to achieve the high serum levels necessary to obtain the desired therapeutic effect, but at the same time to avoid toxicity. Little is gained, however, by administering digitoxin twice daily.

When a loading dose of digoxin is used for rapid digitalization, as is frequently the case in anesthetic practice for patients with heart failure or with supraventricular tachyarrhythmias, there is a greater associated risk of toxicity.[52,53] This risk is avoided if the loading dose is selected on the basis of the anticipated maintenance dose, and if it is given in divided doses.[52] Generally, the loading dose in patients with normal kidney function should be three times the anticipated maintenance dose.[52] Thus if the estimated maintenance digoxin dose is 0.25 mg daily, 0.75 mg given in divided doses during the first 24 hours will result in an accumulated body dose of 0.5 mg (33% excreted in the first 24 hours). This is approximately the same dose as that which accumulates in one week if 0.25 mg is given on a daily basis, as

digitalization. We suspect that this is mainly due to the unpredictability of absorption following intramuscular injections.

The major determinant of the maintenance dose of digoxin and ouabain [serum half-life 21 hours[7]] is renal function.[52] Digoxin excretion is linearly related to glomerular filtration or creatinine clearance.[6,54] Jelliffe suggests that a reasonable approximation of the percentage of daily loss of digoxin is:[55]

$$\frac{\text{creatinine clearance (ml/min)}}{5} + 14$$

Since this value may not be readily available, an estimate based on the serum creatinine level (expressed as C) can be made:[55]

$$\text{creatinine clearance (men)} = \frac{100}{\text{serum creatinine (mg/100 ml)}} - 12$$

$$\text{creatinine clearance (women)} = \frac{80}{\text{serum creatinine (mg/100 ml)}} - 7$$

These expressions can be combined thus:[6]

$$\% \text{ daily loss (men)} = 11.6 + \frac{20}{C} \qquad \% \text{ daily loss (women)} = 12.6 + \frac{16}{C}$$

discussed. If 1.5 mg in divided doses is selected as the initial loading dose, 1.0 mg will accumulate by the end of 24 hours. If this is followed by 0.25 mg maintenance doses daily, the accumulated body dose will gradually be reduced by 50% to the steady-state level of 0.5 mg. We usually digitalize patients acutely in the operating room by administering digoxin, 0.5 mg intravenously, followed in eight hours by an additional 0.5 mg intravenously. An additional 0.25 to 0.50 mg can be given at 16 hours if required.

The serum half-lives for digoxin administered orally or intravenously are similar, but the serum levels reach a plateau sooner (two to four as opposed to five to six hours) following intravenous administration.[2,48,49] Following intramuscular administration, the digoxin serum half-life is 38 hours; plateau serum levels are achieved in 10 to 12 hours.[2,48,49] The intramuscular route offers no advantage over other routes for achieving

The rate of accumulation of digoxin in the body depends on the excretion of a certain percentage of the total body stores daily, which can be calculated as suggested, for patients with impaired renal function. Thus a man with a serum creatinine level of 2.4 mg/100 ml can be expected to excrete only 20% of his daily dose of digoxin. Using calculations similar to those used earlier for the 33% excretion of a 0.25 mg maintenance dose of digoxin, it can be determined that a steady-state level for accumulated digoxin (0.95 mg) will not be reached for 15 days. The digoxin serum half-life (and total accumulated dose) will approximately double as a result of impaired renal excretion. The serum half-life will increase to a maximum of 4.4 days in the absence of renal function.[6] A suggested rule of thumb is that the dose of digoxin should be reduced by 50% when the serum creatinine level is in the range of 3 to 5 mg/100 ml, and by 75% in the absence of renal function.[52]

The frequent observation that digoxin is poorly tolerated in older patients is related both to reduced glomerular filtration with advancing age and to a decrease in muscle mass.[52,56] The major body store of digoxin is skeletal muscle, and a decrease in this reservoir results in increased serum and myocardial levels of the drug.[52] Little digoxin is accumulated in fat; therefore, the determinant of digoxin dose is lean body mass rather than total body weight.[7,52,57]

Toxicology and indications for obtaining serum levels

Cardiac toxicity can manifest itself by arrhythmias, which can assume the morphology of almost every known rhythm disturbance.[1,14] Extrasystoles, whether of ventricular or of atrial origin, are probably the most common.[1,58] Toxic amounts of digitalis may cause occasional dropped beats or complete atrioventricular dissociation.[1] Partial or complete atrioventricular block should be suspected if the ventricular rate falls below 60 beats/min.[1] The heart rate may not be slowed by digitalis, however, and an increase in rate from an accelerated lower pacemaker (for example, junctional) may be the first evidence of digitalis intoxication.[1] Tachycardias may be of atrial or of ventricular origin. Nonparoxysmal tachycardias are more common than paroxysmal tachycardias, but paroxysmal atrial tachycardia with heart block is considered to be dangerous.[1,58,59] Ventricular tachycardia, which may lead to fibrillation, calls for the immediate cessation of digitalis therapy. Ventricular fibrillation is the most common cause of death from digitalis overdosage, and is preceded by ventricular extrasystoles.[1] There are no unequivocal electrocardiographic features that can distinguish arrhythmias due to digitalis from those due to other causes.[14] Arrhythmias that combine the features of increased automaticity of ectopic pacemakers with conduction defects suggest digitalis toxicity.[14] The treatment of digitalis-induced arrhythmias includes the

withholding of digitalis and the correction of associated causes (for example, hypokalemia related to diuretics or to other causes). Potassium chloride administered intravenously to produce a serum level close to the upper limits of the normal range may suppress digitalis-caused arrhythmias.[1] Phenytoin (previously discussed) is often effective in treating both ventricular and supraventricular tachycardias caused by digitalis.[1,12-14] Lidocaine suppresses ventricular tachycardia, but is less effective than phenytoin against supraventricular arrhythmias.[1] Although propranolol (1 to 3 mg IV) is effective in treating extrasystoles and tachycardia of both ventricular and supraventricular origin, its tendency to prolong nodal conduction limits its usefulness in the presence of atrioventricular block.[1] Electrical countershock should not be used to convert digitalis-induced arrhythmias, since it may precipitate ventricular fibrillation.[1]

Other manifestations of digitalis toxicity include gastrointestinal and central nervous system effects.[1,14] Anorexia is often an early manifestation of toxicity, and was significantly correlated with serum glycoside levels in a prospective study.[60] Anorexia usually precedes nausea and vomiting.[1] The significance of nausea as an early indication of digitalis poisoning should not be discounted; it is often accompanied by increased salivation.[1] Although vomiting usually follows anorexia and nausea, it may develop in their absence, particularly when large doses of digitalis are given rapidly.[1] Diarrhea and abdominal discomfort or pain may also be symptoms of toxicity.[1] In some cases, it may be difficult to relate gastrointestinal symptoms to digitalis since these symptoms may also be caused by cardiac failure or associated illnesses.[14] Central nervous system effects include headache, fatigue, malaise, drowsiness, neuralgic pain, disorientation, aphasia, confusion, delirium, and convulsions.[1,14] Visual symptoms are not infrequent, and include scotomata, flickering, halos, and alterations in color perception.[1,14] These symptoms, when seen during the preanesthetic visit, should be considered to be valid evidence of digitalis toxicity.

The determination of digitalis serum levels is indicated when there is a suspicion of digitalis toxicity, or when there is need to know the status of digitalization.[10] A steady-state level of digoxin should be present in the serum for it to reflect accurately the myocardial level.[10,61] The most important question concerning the status of digitalization is, "Is the patient taking digitalis?"[10] The affirmative answer to this question transcends a suspicion of toxicity as an indication for obtaining a serum level.[10] A serum digoxin level of less than 0.5 ng/ml eliminates the possibility of toxicity; moreover, it is suggestive of insufficient digitalization in most clinical situations.[10] Each laboratory should establish its own limits of confidence and normal values for serum levels of digoxin. Levels between 0.5 and 2.5 ng/ml are usually considered to be therapeutic and those above 3.0 ng/ml to be definitely toxic, although there may be some overlap between 2.0 and 3.0 ng/ml.[10] Compared with adults, infants and children tolerate higher levels of digitalis without signs of toxicity; accordingly, the normal values for this age group should probably be revised upward about 1 ng/ml.[10] Whereas the determination of serum digitalis levels may be helpful in the management of toxicity, the diagnosis of toxicity is always based on clinical symptoms, owing to the range of individual variation.[62] High serum levels of digoxin without a toxic reaction are often observed in atrial arrhythmias (which can require large doses to control the ventricular response) and in renal failure with hyperkalemia.[10] Normal or low serum levels with a toxic reaction are common with hypokalemia, hypomagnesemia, recent myocardial infarction, myxedema, and hypoxia, in the presence of other radioisotopes that interfere with the digoxin assay.[10] Reduced gastrointestinal absorption of digoxin may require the administration of large oral doses to maintain optimal

digitalization.[10] This may be the case with rapid transit syndromes, hyperthyroidism, intestinal malabsorption, or the concurrent administration of cholestyramine, antacids, or kaolin with pectin.[10]

FACTORS THAT AFFECT DIGITALIS TOXICITY

Some factors have already been alluded to or discussed in the preceding two sections. However, other factors that affect digitalis toxicity are presented in alphabetical order for the convenience of the reader.

Age. Infants and children have an increased tolerance to digitalis; the range of normal serum digoxin levels should be revised upward approximately 1.0 ng/ml from the normal range for adults (<2.5 ng/ml to <3.5 ng/ml).[7,10] The reduction in glomerular filtration rate and the decrease in muscle mass with advancing age decrease the tolerance to digoxin; the former because of reduced renal excretion and the latter because skeletal muscle is the major body depository for digoxin.[52]

Anesthetics. Halothane, enflurane, diethyl ether, methoxyflurane, ketamine, fentanyl droperidol, and, to a lesser extent, isoflurane and fluroxene, protect against experimental ventricular arrhythmias in digitalized dogs.[38–40] Cyclopropane enhances and pentobarbital has little effect on similar arrhythmias in dogs.[38] Documentation of this interaction in human beings is unavailable.

Antacids. The simultaneous administration of antacids that contain magnesium trisilicate, magnesium hydroxide, or aluminum hydroxide may decrease the gastrointestinal absorption of orally administered cardiac glycosides.[63,64]

Barbiturates. Phenobarbital may increase the metabolism of digitoxin by inducing hepatic microsomal enzymes.[65–67] Digitoxin is excreted partially by enzymatic conversion to digoxin and by other breakdown products in the liver. The metabolic products are then excreted in the urine. The clinical significance of this interaction is unknown, but patients taking digitoxin and phenobarbital, as well as other enzyme-inducing drugs, should be observed for underdigitalization.

Calcium. Parenteral calcium may precipitate fatal cardiac arrhythmias in patients receiving digitalis therapy.[68] A lowering of the blood concentration of calcium in patients may help to abolish cardiac arrhythmias due to digitalis excess.[69] Additional documentation of calcium-digitalis interactions in human beings is needed. Until such evidence is available, however, parenteral calcium should be given judiciously and with careful monitoring to patients who take digitalis.[6]

Cardioversion. The attempted electrical conversion of digitalis-induced arrhythmias may precipitate ventricular fibrillation.[1] If electrical conversion cannot be avoided, one should start with low-energy discharges and gradually increase until the arrhythmia is terminated or until there is evidence of further electrical instability.[6,14]

Cholestyramine. Digitoxin undergoes enterohepatic circulation, and agents that bind the drug within the intestinal lumen should decrease its half-life.[14,70] Steroid binding resins, including cholestyramine and colestipol, have been used effectively in man for this purpose.[71–73] Although digoxin has only a minimal enterohepatic circulation, cholestyramine interferes with its initial absorption from the gut.[14,74]

Diuretics. Potassium-wasting diuretics, including furosemide, the benzothiadiazides, and ethacrynic acid may cause acute or chronic hypokalemia and thus may precipitate digitalis toxicity. Adequate potassium replacement or the use of potassium-sparing agents (spironolactone, triamterene) in patients who are given such potent diuretics is particularly important for those who take digitalis.[6]

Gastrointestinal Function. Unpredictable absorption of orally administered digitalis preparations may occur in patients with intestinal malabsorption or rapid transit syndromes.[75] Similarly, drugs that alter gastrointestinal motility also cause unpredictable absorption.[76]

Glucose Infusions. Large infusions of carbohydrate may cause an intracellular shift of potassium with a resultant decrease in serum levels of potassium.[66] The similar action of insulin to promote potassium uptake into cells is well known, and is mentioned here as a possible cause of hypokalemia and resultant digitalis toxicity.

Heparin. Animal studies indicate that digitalis preparations increase blood coagulability, whereas heparin antagonizes this response.[1] Clinical verification of these effects of digitalis on coagulation, or on their reversal by heparin, is lacking.[1]

Hypoxia. Hypoxia and disturbances of acid-base balance decrease a patient's tolerance to digitalis, and certainly contribute to problems in digitalizing patients with cor pulmonale or chronic lung disease.[6,7]

Lidocaine. This drug suppresses ventricular ectopy due to digitalis, but is less effective than phenytoin in the control of supraventricular arrhythmias.[1,6,14]

Liver Disease. Patients with hepatic insufficiency metabolize and excrete digoxin in a normal fashion.[2] Digitoxin, however, is largely metabolized by the liver to digoxin and other by-products that are then excreted by the kidney.[1,7,44] Smaller doses of digitoxin may be required in patients with hepatic dysfunction.[2]

Magnesium. Hypomagnesemia may cause digitalis toxicity.[1,2,6,7] Magnesium may abolish digitalis-induced ventricular ectopy, but is rarely used for this purpose unless hypomagnesemia is also present.[76,77] Magnesium deficiency may or may not be associated with decreased intracellular potassium or with enhanced toxicity to digitalis.[78]

Obesity. One might anticipate a greater volume of distribution in obesity. This does not occur, however, since the concentration of digoxin is low in adipose tissue.[52] Serum digoxin levels and pharmacokinetics are the same before and after the loss of large amounts of adipose tissue in obese subjects, which suggests that lean body mass rather than total body weight should be used to calculate the dose of digoxin.[7,52,57]

Phenylbutazone. This drug enhances the metabolism of digitoxin, possibly through the induction of hepatic microsomal enzymes.[67,79] The known ability of phenylbutazone to induce sodium retention should also be considered carefully in patients who take digitalis.[67]

Phenytoin (Diphenylhydantoin). Phenytoin is a specific agent for the management of ventricular arrhythmias caused by digitalis, and is frequently effective in supraventricular arrhythmias as well.[1,12-14] Phenytoin can improve sinoatrial and atrioventricular block by improving conduction prolonged by digitalis at these sites.[1,12,14,80] Although it has been reported that phenytoin may enhance digitalis-induced bradycardia or may decrease serum digitoxin levels, there is little evidence that these effects are clinically significant.[79,81]

Potassium. Hypokalemia frequently causes arrhythmias in otherwise normally digitalized patients. Hypokalemia can be caused by excessive doses of digitalis or by the potassium-wasting effects of concomitant diuretic therapy. Potassium depletion may also result from corticosteroid therapy, malnutrition, or hemodialysis.[1] The administration of potassium sufficient to bring the serum limits to the upper limits of the normal range is indicated in the treatment of digitalis arrhythmias when hypokalemia is a cause.[1] Monitoring of both potassium levels and the electrocardiogram is necessary, however, as too large or too rapid an increase in the serum level of potassium may precipitate arrhythmias, including ventricular fibrillation. Potassium is not indicated when atrioventricular block or other conduction defects are present, since it increases both the effective refractory period of the atrioventricular node and the possibility of atrioventricular block.[1,82]

Propantheline. Propantheline, which decreases gastrointestinal motility, may delay the absorption of slowly dissolving types of digoxin.[83] Since more rapidly dissolving preparations (for example, Lanoxin) are commonly used in the United States, this interaction is probably of little clinical significance here.[67]

Propranolol. This drug is useful in the treatment of some digitalis toxic arrhythmias due to supraventricular or ventricular ectopy.[1,14] It suppresses automaticity through its antiadrenergic action, whereas by virtue of its direct myocardial action it shortens the effective refractory period of atrial muscle, ventricular muscle, and Purkinje fibers, and slows the rate of depolarization and conduction velocity in these fibers.[14,84] Its tendency to increase atrioventricular nodal refractoriness limits its usefulness in situations where atrioventricular block is present.[1] Propranolol's negative inotropic effect may be deleterious in the presence of impaired myocardial function.

Quinidine. Quinidine, possibly by the displacement of digoxin from noncardiac tissue binding sites, can raise the serum levels of digoxin, thereby producing both gastrointestinal and cardiac manifestations of toxicity.[11] The clinical course, electrocardiogram, and serum levels of digoxin should be monitored closely in patients who are receiving combined therapy with digoxin and quinidine.[11] Furthermore, quinidine and procainamide carry a substantial risk of cardiac toxicity that includes the depression of conduction, the potential for eliciting ventricular arrhythmias, and decreased myocardial contractility.[14]

Renal Function. The route of excretion of digoxin and other shorter-acting digitalis preparations (ouabain, deslanoside) is primarily renal.[7] The fecal route accounts for a small fraction of the drug excreted.[52] Whereas in patients with renal failure there is a compensatory increase in fecal excretion, this is not an adequate alternative route of excretion.[85] Digitoxin and its metabolites are also excreted primarily by the kidney.[86,87] However, most of the drug is metabolized by the liver, and only 8% of the total dose is excreted in unchanged form.[52] Stool excretion of digitoxin is approximately 17% of the dose in the form of metabolites.[52] The metabolism of digitoxin is unique in that the fecal route is an alternative to the urinary route of excretion.[52] The blood levels are reported to be no higher in patients with impaired renal function who take digitoxin than in patients with normal function.[88] Patients with impaired renal function who take digoxin should be closely observed for signs of toxicity. The dose of digoxin can be adjusted based on measured or estimated creatinine clearances as discussed in this chapter under the heading "Pharmacology of Digitalis," subheading "Pharmacokinetics."

Reserpine. The likelihood of arrhythmias, particularly in patients with atrial fibrillation, may be increased by the concurrent use of cardiac glycosides and reserpine or related rauwolfia alkaloids.[67,89,90] A true causal relationship has not been established, but the possibility of serious drug-related arrhythmias should be considered when these drugs are used concomitantly.[67,90] The mechanism for this interaction is not known, but it may involve the central (neural) effects of digitalis and reserpine or the release of catecholamines by reserpine.[67,90]

Succinylcholine. Succinylcholine may cause ventricular arrhythmias in fully digitalized patients.[67,91,92] The mechanism for this interaction is not established, but it may relate to the loss of intracellular potassium.[91,93] Tubocurarine has been recommended for the treatment of such arrhythmias based on both clinical and experimental evidence.[91,93] One study did not demonstrate a statistically significant difference in the incidence of ventricular arrhythmias following succinylcholine between digitalized and nondigitalized patients.[94] Until further information is available, succinylcholine should be used cautiously in fully digitalized patients. The pos-

sibility that this interaction might be prevented by a small (defasciculating) dose of a nondepolarizing relaxant is open to investigation.

Sympathomimetics. Sympathomimetics, especially those with significant *beta*-adrenergic activity (isoproterenol, epinephrine, norepinephrine), enhance automaticity, as do toxic doses of digitalis. The concomitant use of these drugs could at least theoretically increase the patient's propensity to arrhythmias, although further clinical documentation of this interaction is needed.[67]

Thyroid Function. Thyroid disease affects digitalis sensitivity by two mechanisms.[2,6] Hyperthyroidism increases and hypothyroidism decreases the rates of renal excretion of ouabain and digoxin. In addition, the thyrotoxic heart is less sensitive to digitalis with respect to control of the ventricular rate in atrial flutter or fibrillation. The intrinsic, autonomic nervous system tone or concurrently administered drugs may be responsible for increased or diminished digitalis sensitivity in patients with disordered thyroid function.[6]

In summary, the digitalis glycosides have one of the lowest therapeutic indices of all commonly used drugs. They are indicated in the treatment of heart failure (positive inotropic action) and atrial flutter or fibrillation (negative dromotropic action). The inotropic action is a linear function of the dose administered, whereas the dromotropic action may be observed only with nearly toxic doses of digitalis. During the preoperative visit, the anesthesiologist should attempt to assess the status of digitalization with the following questions: Is the patient digitalized? Has the desired therapeutic effect been achieved? Does the patient show signs of digitalis toxicity? Intraoperatively, the anesthesiologist should know how and when to digitalize patients. For this task, a familiarity with drug and other interactions involving digitalis will be helpful.

Concerning the status of digitalization,

the need to observe the clinical effect is paramount. Serum levels of digitalis alone never establish the diagnosis of either a therapeutic or a toxic effect. A level of digitalis that is toxic for one patient may be therapeutic for another. For example, serum levels of digoxin in the lower toxic range (2.5 ng/ml for adults, 3.5 ng/ml for children) may be required for a therapeutic effect in more resistant cases of atrial flutter or fibrillation. Serum levels of digoxin below 0.5 ng/ml virtually eliminate the possibility of toxicity and usually call for more drug to achieve the desired effect. The serum levels for digitoxin are approximately ten times higher than those for digoxin.

The toxicity of digitalis is manifested by cardiac, neural, and gastrointestinal disturbances. Cardiac toxicity is most important from the anesthesiologist's standpoint and includes almost every known form of rhythm disturbance. Life-threatening arrhythmias are not uncommon. Cardiac toxic manifestations may be brought about by actual overdosage or by interactions with drugs or other factors. With the exception of succinylcholine-related arrhythmias in digitalized patients, anesthetic or adjuvant drug interactions involving digitalis that are significant to anesthesiologists have not been well documented. The anesthesiologist must recognize, however, that disturbances of acid-base or electrolyte imbalance are the most common causes of digitalis toxicity in surgical patients. Hypokalemia secondary to diuretic therapy or related to metabolic or respiratory alkalosis should be watched for in particular. Impaired renal function is also a common cause of digitalis toxicity, since it reduces the elimination of shorter-acting digitalis preparations.

Preoperatively and intraoperatively, digitalis is indicated for the treatment of heart failure and atrial flutter or fibrillation. In addition, digitalis is sometimes used as a prophylactic measure to reduce the risk of heart failure or the chance of supraventricular arrhythmias attendant on cardiac or thoracic surgical procedures. The indications for prophylactic digitalization are not well established. In considering the low therapeutic index and the potential danger of some of the toxic effects of the digitalis glycosides, it is probably better to use these drugs only for established indications.

REFERENCES

1. Moe, G. K., and Farah, A. E.: Digitalis and allied cardiac glycosides. *In* The Pharmacological Basis of Therapeutics. 5th Edition. Edited by L. S. Goodman and A. Gilman. New York, Macmillan, 1975.
2. Doherty, J. E., and Kaul, J. J.: Clinical pharmacology of digitalis glycosides. Annu. Rev. Med., *26*:159, 1975.
3. Rodensky, P. L., and Wasserman, F.: Observations on digitalis intoxication. Arch. Intern. Med., *108*:171, 1961.
4. Smith, T. W., and Haber, E.: Digitalis. (Fourth of Four Parts). N. Engl. J. Med., *285*:1125, 1973.
5. Kim, Y. I., Noble, R. J., and Zipes, D. P.: Dissociation of the inotropic effect of digitalis from its effect on atrioventricular conduction. Am. J. Cardiol., *36*:359, 1975.
6. Smith, T. W.: Digitalis glycosides. (Second of Two Parts). N. Engl. J. Med., *288*:942, 1973.
7. Smith, T. W., and Haber, E.: Digitalis. (Third of Four Parts). N. Engl. J. Med., *289*:1063, 1973.
8. Neff, M. S., et al.: Magnesium sulfate in digitalis toxicity. Am. J. Cardiol., *29*:377, 1972.
9. Edwards, R., Winnie, A. P., and Ramamurphy, S.: Acute hypocapneic hypokalemia: An iatrogenic complication. Anesth. Analg. (Cleve.), *56*:586, 1977.
10. Doherty, J. A.: How and when to use digitalis serum levels. J.A.M.A., *239*:2594, 1978.
11. Leahey, E. B., et al.: Interaction between quinidine and digoxin. J.A.M.A., *240*:533, 1978.
12. Moe, G. K., and Abildskov, J. A.: Antiarrhythmic drugs. *In* The Pharmacological Basis of Therapeutics. 5th Edition. Edited by L. S. Goodman and A. Gilman. New York, Macmillan, 1975.
13. Bigger, J. T., Jr.: Arrhythmias and antiarrhythmic drugs. Adv. Intern. Med., *18*:251, 1972.
14. Smith, T. W., and Haber, E.: Digitalis. (Fourth of Four Parts). N. Engl. J. Med., *289*:1125, 1973.
15. Schwartz, A.: Newer aspects of cardiac glycoside action. Fed. Proc., *36*:2207, 1977.
16. VanWinkle, W. G., and Schwartz, A.: Ions and Inotropy. Annu. Rev. Physiol., *38*:247, 1976.
17. Langer, G. A.: Relationship between myocardial contractility and the effects of digitalis on ionic exchange. Fed. Proc., *36*:2231, 1977.
18. Weber, A., and Murray, J. M.: Molecular control mechanisms in muscle contraction. Physiol. Rev., *53*:612, 1973.
19. Lymn, R. W., and Taylor, E. W.: Mechanism of adenosine triphosphate hydrolysis by actomyosin. Biochemistry, *10*:4617, 1971.

20. Ebashi, S.: Excitation-contraction coupling. Annu. Rev. Physiol., *38*:293, 1976.
21. Fabiato, A., and Fabiato, F.: Calcium release from the sarcoplasmic reticulum. Circ. Res., *40*:119, 1977.
22. Weber, A., and Winicur, S.: The role of calcium in the superprecipitation of actomyosin. J. Biol. Chem., *236*:3198, 1961.
23. Reuter, H.: Exchange of calcium ions in the mammalian myocardium. Circ. Res., *34*:599, 1974.
24. Reuter, H.: Divalent ions as charge carriers in excitable membranes. Prog. Biophys. Mol. Biol., *26*:1, 1973.
25. Langer, G. A.: Ion fluxes in cardiac excitation and contraction and their relation to myocardial contractility. Physiol. Rev., *48*:708, 1968.
26. Solaro, R. J., et al.: Calcium requirements for cardiac myofibrillar activation. Circ. Res., *34*:525, 1974.
27. Dhalla, N. S., Ziegelhoffer, A., and Harrow, J. A. C.: Regulatory role of membrane systems in heart function. Can. J. Physiol. Pharmacol., *55*:1211, 1977.
28. Reddy, Y. S., et al.: Phosphorylation of cardiac native tropomyosin and troponin. J. Mol. Cell Cardiol., *5*:461, 1973.
29. Solaro, R. J., Moir, A. J., and Perry, S. V.: Phosphorylation of troponin I and inotropic effect of adrenalin. Nature, *262*:615, 1976.
30. Reddy, Y. S., Pitts, B. J., and Schwartz, A.: Cyclic-AMP dependent and independent protein kinase phosphorylation of canine cardiac myosin light chains. J. Mol. Cell Cardiol., *9*:501, 1977.
31. Endoh, M., et al.: Frequency dependence of cyclic AMP in mammalian myocardium. Nature, *261*:716, 1976.
32. Mendez, D., and Mendez, R.: The action of cardiac glycosides on the excitability and conduction velocity of the mammalian atrium. J. Pharmacol. Exp. Ther., *121*:402, 1957.
33. Watanabe, Y., and Dreifus, L. S.: Electrophysiologic effects of digitalis on A–V transmission. Am. J. Physiol., *211*:1461, 1966.
34. Watanabe, Y., and Dreifus, L. S.: Interactions of lantoside-C and potassium on atrioventricular conduction in rabbits. Circ. Res., *27*:931, 1970.
35. Ferrier, G. R.: Digitalis arrhythmias: Role of oscillatory afterpotentials. Prog. Cardiovasc. Dis., *19*:459, 1977.
36. Cranefield, P. F.: Action potentials, afterpotentials, and arrhythmias. Circ. Res., *41*:415, 1977.
37. Tsien, R. W.: Ionic mechanisms of pacemaker activity in cardiac Purkinje fibers. Fed. Proc., *37*:2127, 1978.
38. Morrow, D. H., and Townley, N. T.: Anesthesia and digitalis toxicity: An experimental study. Anesth. Analg. (Cleve.), *43*:510, 1964.
39. Ivankovich, A. D., et al.: The effects of ketamine and Innovar[R] anesthesia on digitalis tolerance in dogs. Anesth. Analg. (Cleve.), *54*:106, 1975.
40. Ivankovich, A. D., et al.: The effect of enflurane, isoflurane, fluroxene, methoxyflurane, and diethyl ether anesthesia on ouabain tolerance in the dog. Anesth. Analg. (Cleve.), *55*:360, 1976.
41. Moe, G. K.: Evidence for re-entry as a mechanism of cardiac arrhythmias. Rev. Physiol. Biochem. Pharmacol., *72*:55, 1975.
42. Gillis, R. A., Pearle, D. L., and Levitt, B.: Digitalis: A neuroexcitatory drug. Circulation, *52*:739, 1975.
43. Quest, J. A., and Billis, R. A.: Carotid sinus reflex changes produced by digitalis. J. Pharmacol. Exp. Ther., *177*:650, 1971.
44. Smith, T. W., and Haber, E.: Digitalis. (First of Four Parts). N. Engl. J. Med., *289*:945, 1973.
45. McLain, P. L.: Effects of cardiac glycosides on spontaneous efferent activity in vagus and sympathetic nerves of cats. Int. J. Neuropharmacol., *8*:379, 1969.
46. Gillis, R. A.: Cardiac sympathetic nerve activity: Changes induced by ouabain and propranolol. Science, *166*:508, 1969.
47. Butler, V. P., Jr.: Assays of digitalis in the blood. Prog. Cardiovasc. Dis., *14*:571, 1972.
48. Doherty, J. E.: The clinical pharmacology of digitalis glycosides: a review. Am. J. Med. Sci., *225*:382, 1968.
49. Doherty, J. E.: Digitalis glycosides. Pharmacokinetics and their clinical implications. Ann. Intern. Med., *79*:229, 1973.
50. Marcus, F. I., et al.: Administration of tritiated digoxin with and without a loading dose. Circulation, *34*:865, 1966.
51. Marcus, F. I., et al.: The metabolic fate of tritiated digoxin in the dog: A comparison of digitalis administration with and without a loading dose. J. Pharmacol. Exp. Ther., *156*:548, 1967.
52. Marcus, F. I.: Digitalis pharmacokinetics and metabolism. Am. J. Med., *58*:452, 1975.
53. Ogilvie, R. F., and Ruedy, J.: An educational program in digitalis therapy. J.A.M.A., *222*:50, 1972.
54. Bloom, P. M., Nelp, W. B., and Truell, S. H.: Relationship of the excretion of tritiated digoxin to renal function. Am. J. Med. Sci., *251*:133, 1966.
55. Jelliffe, R. W.: Factors to consider in planning digoxin therapy. J. Chronic Dis., *24*:407, 1971.
56. Ewy, G. A., et al.: Digoxin metabolism in the elderly. Circulation, *39*:449, 1969.
57. Ewy, G. A., et al.: Digoxin metabolism in obesity. Circulation, *44*:810, 1971.
58. Rios, J. C., Dziok, C. A., and Ali, N. A.: Digitalis-induced arrhythmias: Recognition and management. *In* Arrhythmias. Guest edited by L. S. Dreifus. Philadelphia, F. A. Davis, 1970.
59. Lown, B., Wyatt, N. F., and Levine, H. D.: Paroxysmal atrial tachycardia with block. Circulation, *21*:129, 1960.
60. Beller, G. A., et al.: Digitalis intoxication: Prospective clinical study with serum level correlations. N. Engl. J. Med., *284*:989, 1971.
61. Doherty, J. A.: Digitalis serum level: Practical value. *In* Controversy in Cardiology. Edited by E. Cheung. New York, Springer-Verlag, 1976.
62. Noble, R. J., et al.: Limitations of serum digitalis levels. *In* Complex Electrocardiography 2. Edited by C. Fisch. Philadelphia, F. A. Davis, 1974.
63. Brown, D. D., and Juhl, R. P.: Decreased bioavailability of digoxin due to antacids and kaolin-pectin. N. Engl. J. Med., *295*:1034, 1976.
64. Khalil, S. A. H.: The uptake of digoxin and digitoxin

by some antacids. J. Pharm. Pharmacol., *26*:961, 1974.

65. Jelliffe, R. W., and Blankenhorn, D. H.: Effect of phenobarbital on digitoxin metabolism. Clin. Res., *14*:160, 1966.

66. Hansten, P. D.: Drug Interactions. Philadelphia, Lea & Febiger, 1975.

67. Solomon, H. M., and Abrams, W. B.: Interactions between digitoxin and other drugs in man. Am. Heart J., *83*:277, 1972.

68. Bower, J. O., and Mengle, H. A. K.: The additive effects of calcium and digitalis. J.A.M.A., *106*:1151, 1936.

69. Jick, S. and Karsh, R.: The effect of calcium chelation on cardiac arrhythmias and conduction disturbances. Am. J. Cardiol., *4*:287, 1959.

70. Okita, G. T., et al.: Metabolic fate of radioactive digitoxin in human subjects. J. Pharmacol. Exp. Ther., *115*:371, 1955.

71. Caldwell, H. J., and Greenberger, N. J.: Interruption of the enterophepatic circulation of digitoxin by cholestyramine. I. Protection against lethal digitoxin intoxication. J. Clin. Invest., *50*:2626, 1971.

72. Caldwell, J. H., and Bush, C. A.: Interruption of the enterohepatic circulation of digitoxin by cholestyramine. II. Effect on metabolic disposition of tritium-labeled digitoxin and cardiac systolic intervals in man. J. Clin. Invest., *50*:2638, 1971.

73. Bazzano, G., and Bazzano, G. S.: Digitalis intoxication: treatment with a new steroid-binding resin. J.A.M.A., *220*:828, 1972.

74. Doherty, J. E., et al.: Tritiated digoxin. XIV. Enterohepatic circulation, absorption, and excretion studies in human volunteers. Circulation, *42*:867, 1970.

75. Heizer, W. D., Smith, T. W., and Goldfinger, S. E.: Absorption of digoxin in patients with malabsorption syndromes. N. Engl. J. Med., *285*: 257, 1971.

76. Sodeman, W. A.: Diagnosis and treatment of digitalis toxicity. N. Engl. J. Med., *273*:35, 93, 1965.

77. Peach, M. J.: Cations: calcium, magnesium, barium, lithium, and ammonium. *In* The Pharmacological Basis of Therapeutics. 5th Edition. Edited by L. S. Goodman and A. Gilman. New York, Macmillan, 1975.

78. Seller, R. H., et al.: Digitalis toxicity and hypomagnesemia. Am. Heart J., *79*:57, 1970.

79. Solomon, H. M., et al.: Interactions between digitoxin and other drugs *in vitro* and *in vivo*. Ann. N.Y. Acad. Sci., *179*:362, 1971.

80. Helfant, R. H., Scherlag, B. J., and Damato, A. N.: The electrophysiological properties of diphenylhydantoin sodium as compared to procainamide in the normal and digitalis/intoxicated heart. Circulation, *36*:108, 1967.

81. Viukari, N. M.A., and Aho, K.: Digoxin-phenytoin interaction. Br. Med. J., *2*:51, 1970.

82. Fisch, C., et al: Potassium and the monophasic action potential, electrocardiogram, conduction and arrhythmias. Prog. Cardiovasc. Dis., *8*:387, 1966.

83. Manninen, V., et al.: Altered absorption of digoxin in patients given propantheline and metoclopramide. Lancet, *1*:398, 1973.

84. Davis, L. D., and Temte, J. V.: Effects of propranolol on the transmembrane potentials of ventricular muscle and Purkinje fibers of the dog. Circ. Res., *22*:661, 1968.

85. Marcus, F. I., et al.: The metabolism of tritiated digoxin in renal insufficiency in dogs and man. J. Pharmacol. Exp. Ther., *152*:372, 1966.

86. Lukas, D. S.: The pharmacokinetics and metabolism of digitoxin in men. *In* Symposium on Digitalis. Edited by O. Storstein. Oslo, Norway, Gyldendal Norsk Forlay, 1973.

87. Beermann, B., Hellstrom, K., and Rosen, K.: Fate of orally administered ³H digitoxin in man with special reference to the absorption. Circulation, *43*:852, 1971.

88. Rasmussen, K., et al.: Digitoxin kinetics in patients with impaired renal function. Clin. Pharmacol. Ther., *13*:6, 1971.

89. Lown, B., et al.: Effect of digitalis in patients receiving reserpine. Circulation, *24*:1185, 1961.

90. Ascione, F. J.: Digitalis-reserpine. *In* Evaluations of Drug Interactions. 2nd Edition. Washington, D.C., American Pharmaceutical Association, 1976.

91. Dowdy, E. G., and Fabian, L. W.: Ventricular arrhythmias induced by succinylcholine in digitalized patients. Anesth. Analg. (Cleve.), *42*:501, 1963.

92. Smith, R. B., and Petrusack, J.: Succinylcholine, digitalis and hypercalcemia: A case report. Anesth. Analg. (Cleve.), *51*:202, 1972.

93. Dowdy, E. G., Duggar, P. N., and Fabian, L. W.: Effect of neuromuscular blocking agents on isolated digitalized mammalian hearts. Anesth. Analg. (Cleve.), *44*:608, 1965.

94. Perez, H. R.: Cardiac arrhythmias after succinylcholine. Anesth. Analg. (Cleve.), *49*:33, 1970.

Chapter 11

Diuretics

ROBERT G. MERIN
and
R. DENNIS BASTRON

CASE REPORT

A 44-year-old man was admitted to the emergency department of a hospital with a complaint of vomiting blood. His past medical history included more than 15 years of alcohol abuse, documented hepatic cirrhosis for ten years, recurrent ascites and edema, and congestive heart failure of undetermined cause. Current medications included furosemide, 20 mg t.i.d., and digoxin, 0.25 mg q.d. The patient had been feeling poorly for several days and had been drinking heavily with little food or other fluid intake. However, he had taken his medications. Shortly after his arrival in the Emergency Room he vomited a large quantity of blood and lost consciousness. An anesthesiologist was summoned for resuscitation and intubated the trachea with considerable difficulty because of blood in the mouth and resistance by a semicomatose patient. Immediately after endotracheal intubation, the pulse became irregular and then absent. An electrocardiogram showed ventricular fibrillation. There was considerable difficulty in restoring an adequate rhythm. A serum potassium level was reported as 2.5 meq/L. By means of judicious intravenous injection of potassium, volume replacement, alkalization, and ventilation, cardiac output was restored. The serum digoxin concentration was subsequently reported as 1.8 ng/ml.

Fortunately, the anesthesiologist is not often faced with such a patient. Most of us are aware of the hazards of hypokalemia in a patient taking potent diuretic drugs, and would not anesthetize this patient without knowing the level of serum potassium. Here, however, the combination of an emergency endotracheal intubation, hypokalemia (both from cirrhosis and from diuretic therapy), and digitalis produced ventricular irritability and fibrillation. Although other drug interactions that involve the use of diuretics may not be so dramatic, there is a potential for serious interaction between diuretics and other drugs administered to patients. We frequently anesthetize patients who are taking diuretic agents for the treatment of salt and water retention and for hypertension, and less frequently for disorders such as diabetes insipidus and hypercalcemia.[1-5] Moreover, we administer diuretic agents to surgical patients to reduce brain size or intracranial pressure;[6] to treat acute fluid overload;[2] and to prevent or to diagnose the cause of oliguria.[7-9] In order to understand the basis for interactions between diuretics and other drugs, it is necessary to understand the way in which the body and the kidney regulate water and electrolyte balance and to have a basic knowledge of the pharmacology of diuretic drugs.

OSMOTIC PRESSURE AND DISTRIBUTION OF WATER

Osmostic pressure depends solely on the number of particles in solution, not on their size or molecular weight. One gram molecular weight of a nondissociating compound is equivalent to one osmole. If the compound dissociates into two molecules (for example, NaCl), one gram molecular weight equals two osmoles. Body solutions average around 0.3 osmoles (300 milliosmoles) per kilogram of water.

Perhaps osmotic pressure is easier to understand if we consider the forces that regulate the movement of water across membranes. Passive movement of ions across membranes can be accomplished by establishing concentration gradients. Thus, if a 0.1 molar sodium chloride solution is separated from another 0.1 molar sodium chloride solution by a permeable membrane, the concentration (escaping tendency) of sodium from each solution will be equal, and no net exchange will occur. If, however, the solution on one side of the membrane is 1 molar, and the other side remains 0.1 molar, the sodium activity or escaping tendency in the concentrated solution will cause net flux of sodium into the more dilute solution (less

activity) until the concentration gradient is abolished.

Pure water has a greater activity or escaping tendency for water than does a solution; that is, in a solution, water molecules are diluted and have less molecular activity. Movement of water across a membrane depends on two factors: water "activity" and hydrostatic pressure. If the water level is higher on one side of a membrane separating two chambers, the higher hydrostatic pressure will provide a driving force (gradient) down which water will flow until hydrostatic pressure is equal on both sides of the membrane and the gradient is abolished. At this point, the concentration and, therefore, the tendency of water molecules to escape is equal on both sides of the membrane. Assuming that the membrane is freely permeable to water but not to substance "X," if substance X is added to one side of the membrane, water activity on that side will decrease. This creates a gradient that will cause a net transfer of water into the chamber containing X. The flow of water will continue until the tendency of water molecules to escape into the solution "X-water" (osmotic pressure) is balanced by the hydrostatic pressure gradient. At this point net transfer of water will again be zero (Fig. 11–1). If the membrane is freely permeable to water and to solute "Y", there will be concentration gradients for both water and Y that will rapidly disappear as Y equalizes on both sides of the membrane. In this instance, although solution Y has the colligative property of osmotic pressure, no actual pressure gradient exists across the membrane, and no net flux of water occurs.

Various water compartments in the body are separated by membranes that are freely permeable to water but are less permeable to certain compounds. These compounds are osmotically active and, along with hydrostatic pressure, determine the volume of each compartment. For example, intravascular water is separated from interstitial water by capillary endothelium. The capillary endothelium is readily permeable to small molecules (for example, water, sodium chloride, and mannitol) but is less permeable to larger molecules such as albumin. Albumin exerts osmotic pressure and draws water from interstitial fluid into the

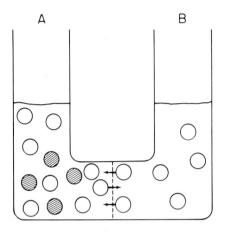

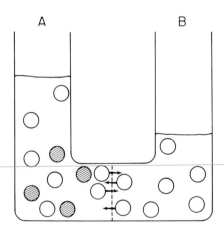

Fig. 11–1. Chambers A and B are separated by a membrane that is permeable to water but not to certain compounds. A nondiffusible compound, "X", (shaded circles) is added to chamber A. This decreases ("dilutes") the water (open circles) activity of A, i.e., it increases the osmotic pressure of A, causing a gradient for the water-escaping tendency from B to A. Thus, the net flux of water is from B to A (top figure). This continues until the escaping tendency for water from B to A is balanced by the hydrostatic pressure gradient tending to move water from A to B (bottom figure). Therefore, the oncotic pressure of a solution is equal to the hydrostatic pressure required to stop osmotic transfer of a solvent into a solution through a semipermeable membrane.

vascular bed. Interstitial water is separated from intracellular water by cell membranes that are relatively impermeable to such molecules as sodium and mannitol. Sodium and mannitol exert osmotic pressure in the extracellular space and draw intracellular water into that space. Some molecules, such as water, carbon dioxide, and hydrogen ion, easily pass through all membranes and therefore do not exert any osmotic pressures.

RENAL REGULATION OF WATER AND ELECTROLYTES

Although it is well known that juxtamedullary nephrons are essential to the formation of concentrated urine, the influence of shifts of blood flow between the cortex or medulla on salt metabolism is less certain.[10–12] Moreover, the primary actions of diuretics are on tubular function, even though some changes in renal blood flow may also occur. Therefore, this discussion focuses on diuretic actions on renal tubules (Fig. 11–2). Additionally, whereas simplified descriptions of tubular functions may not be accurate, they are useful functional models.

Urine formation begins with ultrafiltration of plasma by the glomeruli. Approximately 20% of total plasma flow is filtered and enters Bowman's capsule (capsula glomeruli) and the renal tubule. In the adult, this amounts to about 180 liters a day and contains large amounts of NaCl, $NaHCO_3$ and other essential compounds that must be reabsorbed, as well as various waste products that must be eliminated from the body.

Modification of the glomerular filtrate begins in the proximal convoluted tubule where approximately 60 to 80% of the filtrate is reabsorbed. The major fraction is reabsorbed down-gradients generated by active sodium transport. Sodium reabsorption in proximal tubules is isosmotic; that is, no concentration of urine occurs. The reabsorptive mechanism is designed to transport large volumes of salt and water against small gradients.

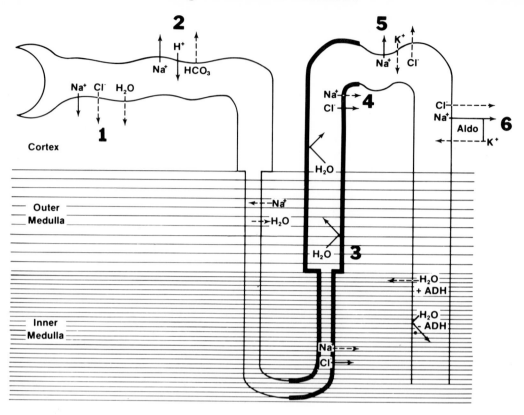

Fig. 11–2. Schematic representation of the major transport processes in the nephron. Solid arrows indicate active transport; dashed arrows indicate passive transport. Low permeability is shown as reflected arrows.

Sodium is actively transported out of proximal tubule cells into intercellular spaces (Fig. 11–3). This transport creates an electrical gradient that causes sodium to move from tubular fluid into the cell. Moreover, osmotic and electrochemical gradients are generated, causing water and chloride to move from tubular fluid to the intercellular space. Sodium chloride (followed by water) then diffuses either back into tubular fluid or into peritubular capillaries and is "reabsorbed." As in all other capillary beds, the amount of fluid that enters peritubular capillaries is influenced by Starling's forces. Therefore, an increase in capillary oncotic pressure favors reabsorption, whereas increased capillary hydrostatic pressure results in greater back-diffusion and less reabsorption.[13,14] Changes

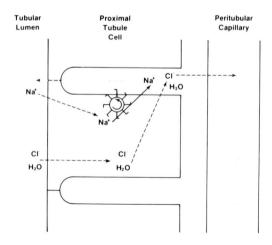

Fig. 11–3. Schematic representation of proximal tubule salt and water reabsorption.

in oncotic pressure can occur with changes in filtration fraction and in systemic oncotic pressure.[15,16] Peritubular capillary hydrostatic pressure increases with renal perfusion pressure.[17] This may be partly responsible for the well-known phenomenon of pressure natriuresis.[18,19]

Another transport process in the proximal convoluted tubule results in the secretion of hydrogen ions and in the reabsorption of sodium bicarbonate ($NaHCO_3$). This mechanism depends on carbonic anhydrase in the brush (luminal) border (Fig. 11–4) and is designed to transport large amounts against small gradients. Sodium is actively pumped out of the cell into peritubular fluid. This creates a gradient that causes sodium to diffuse passively from tubular fluid into the cell. Intracellular hydrogen ions are actively transported into the tubular lumen.[20] The hydrogen combines with bicarbonate to form carbonic acid, which, in the presence of luminal carbonic anhydrase, is rapidly dehydrated to form carbon dioxide and water. The carbon dioxide diffuses into the cell where it rehydrates, in the presence of intracellular carbonic anhydrase, to form carbonic acid. This compound then dissociates into hydrogen ion, which is transported into the lumen, and bicarbonate, which diffuses

down an electrochemical gradient into peritubular fluid.

The majority of phosphate reabsorption also occurs in proximal convoluted tubules. This is why phosphaturia has been used as an indicator of proximal tubular inhibition.[21]

Only a small portion of the filtered fluid enters the descending limb of Henle's loop. At this point the tubular fluid is still isosmotic, although its composition is considerably modified. The descending limb is permeable to water and relatively impermeable to salt.[22] Consequently, as the tubule descends into the hypertonic medullary tissue, water leaves the tubule to maintain osmotic equilibrium between tubular fluid and the interstitium. The thin ascending limb of Henle's loop is relatively impermeable to water but permeable to salt.[23] Sodium chloride passively diffuses from lumen to interstitium down a concentration gradient. This helps to maintain the high medullary interstitial osmolality and causes the concentration of tubular fluid to decrease gradually.

The thick portion of the ascending limb remains almost impermeable to water.[24,25] Chloride is actively transported out of the tubule followed passively by sodium.[24,25] Since water does not follow, this causes further reduction in tubular fluid osmolality until the fluid becomes hypotonic compared to both plasma and interstitium. The medullary portion contributes the active force for maintaining hypertonicity of medullary interstitium and therefore is the concentrating segment of the nephron. The cortical segment, which pumps chloride (and sodium), but not water, into the isotonic cortical interstitium, is the major diluting segment of the nephron.[26] (The difference in tonicity between hypertonic medullary interstitium and isotonic cortical interstitium is related to differences in blood-flow rates, the anatomic pattern of medullary circulation, and the recycling of urea. These factors are important in the concentrating mechanism but are not germane to this discussion.)

The distal convoluted tubule is also rela-

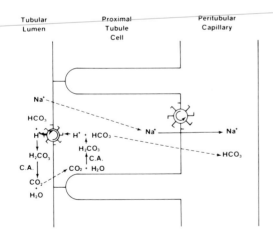

Fig. 11–4. Schematic representation of hydrogen ion secretion and bicarbonate reabsorption in the proximal tubule.

tively impermeable to water.[27] Sodium is actively reabsorbed and potassium is passively secreted. The amount of potassium secretion is loosely related to distal sodium delivery; that is, urinary potassium secretion increases with increased distal sodium delivery and reabsorption.[28] Tubular fluid then enters the collecting duct where further sodium reabsorption and potassium secretion can occur. This process is modulated by mineralocorticoids.[27] Collecting-duct epithelium is permeable to water in the presence of antidiuretic hormone and relatively impermeable in its absence.[29] When water permeability is increased, osmotic equilibrium is attained between tubular fluid and the hypertonic medullary interstitium, and small volumes of concentrated urine are produced. In the absence of antidiuretic hormone, tubular fluid remains hypotonic and large volumes of dilute urine result.

There are other hormonal interactions besides those of antidiuretic hormone involved in the renal regulation of water and salt.[30] The stimulus for the release of the mineralocorticoid, aldosterone, on the distal tubule and collecting duct (increasing sodium reabsorption and potassium secretion) may be either direct or indirect. Catecholamines and antidiuretic hormone stimulate aldosterone secretion by the adrenal cortex. The major physiologic regulator of aldosterone secretion appears to be the renin-angiotensin system. Conditions associated with decreased fluid volumes or sodium content stimulate renin secretion. Renin is converted to a decapeptide, angiotensin I, that is subsequently converted to an octapeptide, angiotensin II. Angiotensin II is not only a potent vasoconstrictor, but also a potent stimulator of aldosterone secretion by the adrenal cortex. Aldosterone then increases sodium reabsorption by the distal tubule that results in volume expansion and decreased renin production. There is also an interplay between the renin-angiotensin system and the antidiuretic hormone system.[31] Prostaglandins may also be involved in renal salt and water

homeostasis.[32] Prostaglandins E and possibly A are synthesized in the renal medulla and produce efferent arteriolar vasodilation, particularly in the inner cortical nephrons. This results in an increased glomerular filtration rate. A concomitant, but less well understood, effect on tubular mechanisms increases free water and osmolar clearance. Opposing this effect, sodium restriction in man increases plasma prostaglandin A, aldosterone, and plasma renin activity. Infusion of prostaglandin A also increases plasma renin activity and aldosterone. Thus, it appears that prostaglandins affect the regulation of salt and water homeostasis by the kidney.

SITES OF ACTION OF DIURETICS

Various methods have been employed to localize the sites of action of diuretics. These include clearances of sodium, chloride, bicarbonate, phosphate, and water; stop-flow techniques; and micropuncture, including the recently developed methods to perfuse isolated segments of renal tubules.[33] For an analysis of these methods the interested reader should consult the review by Goldberg.[34]

Osmotic diuretics

Mannitol, a six-carbon sugar, is the prototype of osmotic diuretics and the most commonly used osmotic diuretic in clinical practice. It is distributed primarily in plasma and interstitial fluid. The initial effect of intravenous administration of mannitol is increased plasma osmolality. Intravascular and interstitial volumes then increase and intracellular volume decreases. The effects of mannitol in the kidney are complex. Increased blood volume may temporarily increase renal plasma flow. Moreover, mannitol may decrease resistance in the afferent arterioles, thereby increasing plasma flow and glomerular filtration.[35] In poorly perfused kidneys, this action on the afferent arteriole may be related to the suppression of renin release.[3] In addition, mannitol diuresis results in significant decreases in medullary interstitial osmolality, possibly secondary to increased medullary blood flow.[37,38]

Renal tubular effects of mannitol are related to its poor reabsorption. Under usual circumstances, sodium is actively reabsorbed by the proximal tubule, and water and chloride follow passively. The sodium transport mechanism is capable of transporting large amounts of sodium but can do so only against a small electrochemical gradient. The presence of a nonreabsorbable compound such as mannitol decreases water reabsorption (Fig. 11–5). Since sodium reabsorption continues in excess of water reabsorption, tubular sodium concentration decreases, eventually to a level where net transport of sodium is zero.[39] Net sodium transport is also decreased in the proximal convoluted tubule secondary to decreased oncotic pressure in peritubular capillaries.[40]

An even greater effect of hypertonic mannitol on salt transport occurs in the loop of Henle. This results from a combination of the intratubular osmotic effect and the washout of the high medullary interstitial osmolality.[41] Decreased salt and water reabsorption by the loop of Henle is probably the major component of the action of mannitol and other osmotic diuretics.

Other clinically useful osmotic diuretics include urea and glycerol. Anesthesiologists should also be aware that glucose in the urine (that is, filtered glucose load that exceeds glucose reabsorptive capacity) can produce an osmotic diuresis. Moreover, contrast material used for angiography may cause osmotic diuresis if given in high doses or if injected directly into a renal artery.[39]

Osmotic diuretics are used most com-

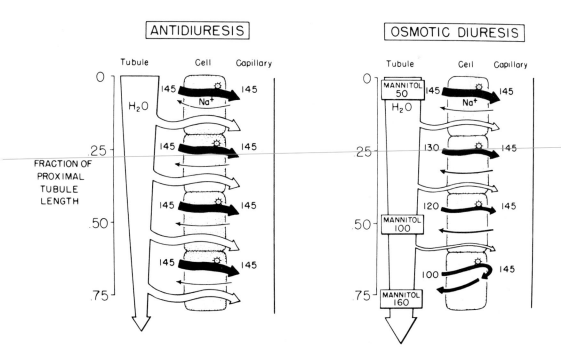

Fig. 11–5. Schematic representation of sodium and water reabsorption in the proximal tubule during antidiuresis and osmotic diuresis. During antidiuresis, the concentration of sodium in the tubular fluid does not change; during osmotic diuresis, the presence of mannitol in the filtrate (50 mmoles per liter) reduces water reabsorption. Thus tubular-fluid sodium concentration falls progressively as sodium reabsorption proceeds. (From Gennari, F. J., and Kassier, J. P.: Osmotic diuresis. N. Engl. J. Med., *291*:715, 1974.)

monly to "protect" the kidneys against acute renal failure (for example, in transfusion reactions or in high renal risk surgical patients), to evaluate the cause of oliguria, and to reduce intracranial pressure.[6-9] Mannitol may be useful in the treatment of myocardial ischemia by decreasing cellular edema.[42]

One predictable side effect of osmotic diuretics is increased extracellular fluid volume, which may be disastrous in patients with impending pulmonary edema. If large doses of osmotic diuretics are administered to a patient who is unable to excrete them, severe plasma hyperosmolality may ensue. If a brisk diuresis does occur, it may cause severe electrolyte disturbances and loss of water.

Acid-forming salts

Ammonium chloride is the most commonly used acidifying salt. The administration of ammonium chloride results in hyperchloremic metabolic acidosis. With increased chloride delivery to the tubules, less chloride is reabsorbed and therefore less is excreted along with an equivalent amount of cation (sodium and potassium) and water. Over a period of one or two days, renal compensatory processes against acidosis result in the excretion of chloride with ammonium ion, and the diuretic effect is lost. Thus the usefulness of acidifying salts as sole diuretics is limited. They are used most commonly to compensate for alkalosis produced by other diuretics. Severe acidosis may occur in patients whose renal function is impaired. The use of ammonium chloride is contraindicated in patients with hepatic failure.[43]

Carbonic anhydrase inhibitors

Acetazolamide produces noncompetitive inhibition of carbonic anhydrase. Renal effects of acetazolamide include decreased glomerular filtration rate and urinary loss of bicarbonate, phosphate, and potassium

that results in hypokalemic metabolic acidosis.[44-46] As acidosis becomes more pronounced, the effectiveness of acetazolamide is diminished. Phosphaturia and fractional excretion of bicarbonate exceeding 20% of the filtered load suggest that the primary site of action is the proximal tubule,[29] although distal delivery of excess bicarbonate is responsible for urinary potassium loss.[47] In high doses, acetazolamide may cause drowsiness and paresthesias and may disorient patients with cirrhosis.[43]

Acetazolamide is used to reduce intraocular pressure, to alkalinize the urine, and to treat edema, periodic paralysis, and convulsive disorders.[43] Sulfamylon, used to treat burns, is also a carbonic anhydrase inhibitor.[48]

Mercurial diuretics

Mercurial diuretics are the oldest potent diuretics. They appear to affect proximal tubular transport mechanisms, but their major action is to interfere with chloride transport in the thick ascending limb of the loop of Henle.[49] Distal tubular effects are variable; if potassium secretion is high (for example, in a potassium-loaded patient), it is reduced, whereas in cases of potassium depletion where excretion is initially low, potassium losses are augmented.[50,51] With the repeated administration of mercurial diuretics, a hypochloremic alkalosis eventually develops. When this occurs, these agents become less effective.[52]

Mercurial diuretics are used primarily to treat edema. General side effects, related to chloride loss in excess of sodium loss, are fluid deficits and metabolic alkalosis. Toxic effects include mercury poisoning, bone marrow depression, and, rarely, fatal arrhythmias.[43]

Thiazides

Thiazides appear to decrease glomerular filtration rate even in the absence of decreased blood volume.[34] These drugs are secreted by proximal tubules as organic acids.[53] Probenecid, a competitive inhibitor of organic acid transport, can block the effect of minimal doses of thiazides but not that of large doses.[34] This suggests that the tubular fluid concentration of drug is an important determinant of activity. The proximal tubular effects of thiazides are variable and related to the degree of carbonic anhydrase inhibition caused by different compounds.[54] The main site of action is in the cortical diluting segment, where chloride transport is inhibited.[55,56] This inhibition results in diluting effects and in increased distal delivery of salt and water. Increased distal delivery of sodium augments potassium secretion.

Thus the consequences of prolonged thiazide administration include increased urinary losses of water, sodium, chloride, potassium, and some loss of bicarbonate. These losses can cause hypochloremic, hypokalemic metabolic alkalosis. In addition, thiazide administration may cause hyperuricemia, bone marrow depression, and dermatitis with photosensitivity.[43] Thiazide diuretics are used to treat edema, hypertension, and diabetes insipidus.[2]

Loop diuretics

Ethacrynic acid and furosemide are the most potent diuretics available. Although chemically different, their actions are similar, except that furosemide is a mild inhibitor of carbonic anhydrase. Both drugs are protein-bound and are secreted into the proximal tubules by organic acid transport.[57,58] In low doses, furosemide inhibits proximal reabsorption of bicarbonate.[59] In high doses, both drugs appear to decrease proximal reabsorption of sodium.

The major effect of these agents is to inhibit active chloride transport along the length of the ascending limb of the loop of Henle.[60,61] Far smaller concentrations are effective on the luminal side of the tubular membrane than on the capillary side. Consequently, any interference in tubular secre-

tion of the drugs could affect the diuretic response. Tubular action interferes with both concentrating and diluting capacities and results in the excretion of an almost isotonic urine. Recent evidence suggests that the action of furosemide and ethacrynic acid may be involved with renal prostaglandins. Administration of the potent inhibitor of prostaglandin synthesis, indomethacin, has resulted in an inhibited increase in renal blood flow produced by both drugs.[62,63] Consequently, the increase may be a result of prostaglandin effect on renal arterioles. Indomethacin also decreases the natriuretic effect of furosemide in man.[64,65] Since this effect was not seen in dogs, the interaction is not certain. The increased distal delivery of salt and water increases potassium secretion.[66,67]

These renal effects may result in the contraction of extracellular fluid volume, and hypochloremic, hypokalemic metabolic alkalosis. Other effects include hyperuricemia, deafness, and hepatic dysfunction.[68,69] These drugs are used primarily to treat fluid retention and oliguria.

Ethacrynic acid and furosemide can cause severe electrolyte disturbances if replacement therapy is not carefully carried out.

Potassium-sparing diuretics

Included in this group of distally acting drugs are spironolactone, triamterene, and amiloride. Although the effect of these drugs is mild natriuresis and decreased potassium excretion, each agent acts differently.[34] Spironolactone is an aldosterone antagonist and is effective only when aldosterone is present and affects potassium secretion.[70] Triamterene and amiloride block potassium secretion unrelated to aldosterone.[71,72]

Potassium-sparing diuretics are used as a second drug, along with more proximal-acting diuretics, in treating refractory edema with potassium loss. Hyperkalemia may result from the use of these diuretics.

Figure 11–6 provides a summary of the site of various diuretics.

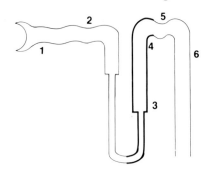

Diuretic	Site					
	1	2	3	4	5	6
Mannitol	(+)		+	(+)	(+)	
Acetazolamide		+			(+)	
Mercurial Diuretics	(+)		+	(+)		(+)
Thiazide Diuretics		(+)		+	(+)	
Ethacrynic acid	(+)		+	(+)	(+)	
Furosemide	(+)	(+)	+	(+)	(+)	
Spironolactone						+
Triamterene					+	
Amiloride					+	

+ = major   (+) = minor actions

Fig. 11–6. Sites of action of diuretics.

DIURETIC-DRUG INTERACTION

Drug interaction with diuretics can be divided into two categories: the first group is related to the desired effect of the diuretic therapy, that is, the increased excretion of salt and water. The potent diuretics interfere with normal salt and water regulation. Consequently, patients may develop both volume and electrolyte abnormalities that may change pharmacologic response to other drugs. The second group of drug interactions involves specific and subtle effects of the diuretic drugs. In most cases undesirable side effects are involved, although sometimes the combination may be advantageous (for example, in antihypertensive therapy).

Interactions from the deranged salt and water regulation

Digitalis. The following case report illustrates the interaction between digitalis and diuretics in combination with a high intake of potassium.

CASE REPORT

A 75-year-old man was admitted to a hospital emergency department with an incarcerated left inguinal hernia. In addition to a painful inguinal mass, he also complained of shortness of breath and reported episodes of fainting. The patient was known to have chronic rheumatic valvular disease involving the aortic and mitral valves. He had been seen regularly as an outpatient and had been in stable condition and adequately compensated until the day of admission. He had been treated with a low-sodium diet, digoxin, and spironolactone (Aldactone), 100 mg daily. On admission, the patient appeared lethargic and weak. His breathing was labored. His systemic arterial blood pressure was 90 torr systolic and his radial pulse was faint and regular at a rate of 12 to 15 beats per minute. The patient's jugular venous pressure was moderately elevated and basilar crepitant rales were heard bilaterally. The cardiac apical impulse was displaced to the left anterior axillary line and down to the sixth intercostal space. Murmurs of aortic and mitral regurgitation were heard. The patient's extremities were free of edema. There was a firm tender mass in the left inguinal region, bowel sounds were hypoactive, and the abdomen was soft but slightly tender. The electrocardiogram taken on admission demonstrated atrial arrest with an idioventricular rhythm at a rate of 12 per minute. Laboratory determinations were as follows: Serum potassium, 7.8 meq/L; serum sodium, 119 meq/L; BUN, 57 mg/100 ml; creatinine, 1.8 mg/100 ml. A transvenous right ventricular endocardial pacing electrode was inserted immediately after the electrocardiogram was taken and capture was effected at a pacemaker output of 0.6 milliamperes. Immediate improvement in the patient's hemodynamic and clinical status was observed as soon as his heart rate was restored to 70 beats per minute. After premedication with diazepam (Valium), 10 mg, the patient was taken to the operating room, where a hyperbaric spinal anaesthetic was administered using tetracaine, 10 mg. After an analgesic level to the sixth thoracic dermatome was achieved, an uneventful herniorrhaphy was accomplished. The patient was taken to the surgical intensive care unit for hyperkalemia where a potassium-exchange resin lowered his serum potassium level to normal value within 24 hours. The patient's heart then resumed its previous rhythm, which had been a chronic atrial tachycardia and AV dissociation with a junctional rhythm and a ventricular rate of 70 beats per minute. The patient's sudden clinical deterioration and the development of severe hyperkalemia were puzzling until his wife told us that he had been liberally using a commercially available salt substitute for several days prior to admission. This salt substitute was composed predominately of potassium salts, particularly potassium chloride.

In the case report that introduced this chapter, the combination of cirrhosis, diuretics, alcoholism, and digitalis produced cardiovascular collapse as a result of *hypo*kalemia. Here the combination of diuretics, digitalis, and high potassium intake resulted in cardiovascular collapse due to *hyper*kalemia. The latter case emphasizes the importance of knowing what type of diuretic the patient is taking. The potassium-sparing diuretics are used to prevent hypokalemia and, hence, digitalis toxicity in patients who take both digitalis and diuretics. However, digitalis may prevent skeletal muscle from serving as the normal sink for potassium. Tissue hypoxia from congestive heart failure may actually mobilize potassium from body stores. Thus it is possible, particularly with an increased potassium intake, that the effect on serum potassium opposite from that desired may occur.[73] In this case a temporary transvenous pacemaker produced an acceptable cardiovascular system for the emergency operation. However, this may not always be the case.

CASE REPORT

A 76-year-old woman was admitted to the hospital with the chief complaints of weakness and syncope. One year before, she had been subjected to the insertion of a permanent demand pacemaker because of "sick sinus" syndrome and second degree AV block. During the next year, the patient developed shortness of breath and orthopnea, and she was placed on furosemide 10 mg t.i.d. with supplemental enteric-coated potassium chloride. Her symptoms of congestive heart failure progressed over the next several months and she was placed on digoxin. Shortly after this, five days prior to hospital admission, her diuretic therapy was changed to Dyazide (hydro-chlorothiazide and triamterene). The patient continued to take potassium chloride. On examination, her pulse was found to be slow and she complained of weakness. An electrocardiogram showed regular pacemaker spikes at a constant rate, but most of the impulses failed to stimulate the ventricles that were contracting independently at a rate of approximately 30 beats per minute. Her serum potassium level was 6.9 meq/L; sodium level, 135 meq/L; chloride level 101 meq/L; and BUN 135 mg/100 ml. The patient was admitted to the medical intensive care unit where the hyperkalemia was treated with sodium bicarbonate, glucose, and insulin. Triamterene was discontinued. Within 48 hours, the serum potassium concentration had declined to 4.6 meq/L. Pacemaker capture was maintained after the drug therapy was discontinued; the atrial rhythm reverted to fibrillation with marked atrioventricular block.[74]

Thus there are times when the effect of hyperkalemia on normal cardiac rhythm may not respond to artificial pacing because of a change in the pacing threshold. This is a particular problem in the case of a permanently implanted pacemaker where current strength cannot be adjusted. These three case reports indicate that the interaction of diuretics and digitalis may produce severe alterations in cardiac function from more than one mechanism. Careful attention to electrolyte status, especially potassium, is mandatory in these patients. The problem must be corrected before anesthesia and operation are performed, if abnormalities are detected.

Anesthetics. Evidence for the interactions between anesthetics and diuretics is theoretical and anecdotal. Certainly, patients whose fluid volume has been depleted by overzealous diuretic therapy will be prime candidates for cardiovascular collapse when potent anesthetics that cardiodepress, vasodilate, and adrenergically block are administered. Similarly, substantial sympathetic blockade from a regional anesthetic will be poorly tolerated. Although there is experimental evidence to suggest that some general anesthetics protect the heart from the arrhythmias of digitalis intoxication, there have been no clinical reports.[75,76] Most anesthesiologists can recall a case with cardiac complications (hypotension, arrhythmia), when a patient with unknown hypokalemia was anesthetized. As documented with digitalis, the other extreme can be just as dangerous, since hyperkalemia can also result in cardiovascular collapse.[77] The obvious conclusion is that one should carefully assess the state of hydration and electrolyte balance in patients who take diuretics on a regular basis before administering an anesthetic. Judicious correction of an imbalance of either condition may require considerable time, particularly in a patient with a compromised cardiovascular system.

Neuromuscular Blocking Drugs. As in the case of anesthetics, the fluid-depleted patient may respond with exaggerated hypotension to a large dose of d-tubocurare. However, the important interactions between neuromuscular blocking drugs and diuretics involve the potassium ion again. Theoretically, the hypokalemic patient may have reduced skeletal muscle function.[78] Consequently, great care is advised in administering neuromuscular blocking drugs to these patients. The patient with hyperkalemia may be an even greater risk. The administration of succinylcholine to patients with renal failure and a high serum potassium has been associated with dangerous arrhythmias and with cardiac arrest.[79] Because of this, the risk to the patient who is receiving the potassium-sparing diuretics (spironolactone and triamterene) and whose potassium intake is above normal may be especially high. Again, it is the responsibility of the anesthesiologist to ascertain the fluid and electrolyte (particularly potassium) status of patients taking diuretics before giving a neuromuscular blocking drug. In hyperkalemic patients, succinylcholine is best avoided. In patients with hypokalemia, nondepolarizing neuromuscular blockers should be carefully titrated.

Specific interactions: beneficial effects

Diuretic-Antihypertensive Drugs. Because the thiazides are mildly antihypertensive,

probably by means of direct vasodilating activity, smaller doses of more potent antihypertensives such as reserpine, guanethidine, *alpha*-methyldopa, minoxidil, and clonidine are often effective.[80] Conversely, the usual doses of these drugs may cause unwanted hypotension. The decrease in intravascular volume produced by potent diuretics may trigger reflex tachycardia, which can be effectively prevented by small doses of the *beta*-adrenergic blocking drug propranolol.[81]

Specific interactions: modification of dose effect

Furosemide-Anticonvulsant Therapy. The diuretic response to oral and intravenous furosemide is blunted in patients with seizure disorders who are taking phenytoin (diphenylhydantoin) and phenobarbital.[82] This may be due to the stimulation of membrane transport of sodium by these drugs.

Furosemide-Indomethacin. The prostaglandin synthetase inhibitor, indomethacin, appears to decrease the diuretic response of patients to furosemide.[65,66] This decrease is probably related to the role of the intrarenal prostaglandins in sodium and water regulation discussed previously.

Spironolactone-Acetylsalicylic Acid (Aspirin). Aspirin decreases the diuretic response to spironolactone by a mechanism that is unknown at this time.[83]

Furosemide-d-Tubocurarine. Furosemide given after d-tubocurarine enhanced the neuromuscular blockade produced in three patients with chronic renal failure.[84] *In-vitro* and intact animal experiments suggest that the interaction may be at the motor-nerve terminal, but the significance for patients with normal renal function is not established (see Chap. 17).

Diuretics-Lithium. The loop diuretics (furosemide and ethacrynic acid) decrease the tubular reabsorption of sodium and conversely increase the tubular reabsorption of lithium.[85] Consequently, serum levels of lithium increase and acute toxicity may be produced if the dosage is not reduced (see Chap. 13).

Spironolactone-Digitalis. Spironolactone appears to decrease the serum half-life of digitoxin and to increase the excretion of its metabolites, probably through enzyme induction.[86] On the other hand, spironolactone has been shown to decrease renal excretion and to increase the plasma levels of digoxin.[87] Furosemide does not affect the pharmacokinetics of digoxin in man.[88]

Ethacrynic Acid-Warfarin. Both enhancement of and interference with the anticoagulant effect of warfarin have been reported with ethacrynic acid.[89,90] Therefore, careful monitoring of the clotting status of a patient is necessary when diuretics and Coumadin are administered concurrently.

Thiazide Diuretics—Chlorpropamide. The thiazide diuretics possess a weak diabetogenic action (most potent in the hypotensive agent diazoxide, which is not a diuretic). Consequently, diabetes, particularly in those patients who control the disease by diet alone or by oral hypoglycemic drugs, may be exacerbated by the initiation of diuretic therapy.[91]

Thiazide Diuretics—Probenecid. Thiazide diuretics cause the retention of uric acid and can cause a flare-up of gouty arthritis even in patients taking probenecid.[92] In addition, the effects of anesthesia and an operation may also decrease uric acid excretion.[93] Consequently, patients with gout must be carefully followed if diuretics and anesthetics are being used.

Specific interactions: toxic effects

Ethacrynic Acid and Aminoglycoside Antibiotics. Both ethacrynic acid and aminoglycoside antibiotics can cause deafness with prolonged high-dose therapy. The combination in lower doses of each drug has also resulted in this complication.[94] This is particularly likely to happen to patients with renal failure.

Furosemide-Cephalosporin. The renal toxicity of cephalosporin may be enhanced by simultaneous furosemide administration.[95]

CLINICAL IMPLICATIONS OF DIURETIC-DRUG INTERACTIONS

Deranged salt and water regulation

Clearly, the interactions most important for the anesthesiologist between diuretics and other drugs involve the predictable effect of diuresis on salt and water homeostasis.

The state of the circulating blood volume of all patients who take diuretics regularly and who are scheduled for anesthesia and operations should be carefully evaluated. Although isotopic measurements are ideal, obviously, this is impractical. Clinically, the most important signs are the response of the blood pressure and heart rate to maneuvers that decrease venous return, such as rapid change from the supine to the upright position or a Valsalva maneuver. A decrease in blood pressure of more than 15% and/or an increase in heart rate of more than 25% should arouse suspicion. A decrease in skin turgor or in ocular tension is a good indicator in children, but if present, indicates significant hypovolemia.[96] "Furrowing" of the tongue also suggests a decrease in extracellular fluid volume. A valuable sign of adequate circulating blood volume is an increase in the volume of urine with a fluid challenge. Laboratory indications of hemoconcentration (increased hematocrit, BUN, sodium, chloride) may corroborate the suspicion of hypovolemia. Low central or pulmonary artery occluded ("wedge") pressure are valuable confirmatory signs.

In patients without significant cardiac or renal disease, fluid deficits can usually be easily corrected overnight by the infusion of electrolyte solutions appropriate to the patient's status. However, most patients who take diuretics on a regular basis will have cardiac or renal disease. For elective surgery, a day or two of careful replacement, using blood and *urinary* electrolyte measurements as a guide, may be necessary. Urinary electrolyte measurement indicates the kidney's response to the body deficit (or surplus) and helps to guide replacement therapy. Patients who are scheduled for emergency operations will need faster correction. This may be safely accomplished by careful monitoring of blood pressure, heart rate, urine output, and at least central venous pressure, but preferably pulmonary artery occluded pressure. For both anesthetic and neuromuscular blocking drug use, an adequate circulating blood volume is essential.

A second important aspect of the derangement of homeostasis is the state of body potassium.

CASE REPORT

A 46-year-old obese woman was admitted to the hospital with a history of fat intolerance and episodic cramping epigastric pain. An oral cholecystogram showed poor visualization and small radiolucent stones. She had been taking "water pills" for several years because of ankle edema, but was told that her heart was "O.K." She was admitted for cholecystectomy and possible common duct exploration. At the time of the preanesthetic visit, no blood had been taken for electrolyte determination. Aside from obesity (weight–84 kg, height–160 cm) and mild hypertension, the patient's history and physical examination were unremarkable. Properly, the anesthesiologist insisted on knowing the serum electrolyte concentration. On arrival in the operating room the next morning, he was informed that the electrolytes were: Na 132 meq/L, Cl 98 meq/L, K 2.8 meq/L, CO_2 23 meq/L. An SMA–12 was within normal limits. The surgeon was anxious to proceed with the operation and cited possible common duct obstruction as the reason.

Hypokalemia is more common than hyperkalemia in chronic diuretic therapy. Although hypokalemia can cause renal concentrating defects, its effects on nerve and muscle activity are more important to the anesthesiologist. These include: paralytic ileus, severe weakness or flaccid paralysis, hypotension, atrial and ventricular dysrhythmias, and potentiation of digitalis toxicity.[97] Serum potassium levels are not reliable indicators of total body potassium. Nevertheless, serum potassium concentration is the only clinical indicator of potassium stores. It has been claimed that a serum potassium concentration of 3 meq/L implies a 200 to 400 meq deficit and that below 3 meq/L, each 1 meq/L decrease in serum potassium indicates an additional 200 to 400 meq loss.[98,99] Therefore, in the patient discussed in this last case report, one should suspect a potassium deficit of at least 200 meq. There is little scientific basis for setting a lowest acceptable level of serum potassium. We believe that it is reasonable, however, until proven otherwise, to suggest a minimum level of 3.0 meq/L in patients who are not digitalized and of 3.5 meq/L in patients who are.

Elective operations and anesthesia should be delayed until acceptable potassium levels are attained by oral potassium chloride replacement and/or by the addition of potassium-sparing diuretics to the therapeutic regimen. In the case of an emergency operation, intravenous potassium chloride can be administered. In our patient, the operation was not an emergency. Without evidence of bile duct obstruction (normal SMA-12), it is prudent to proceed cautiously with potassium replacement. The rate of replacement should not exceed 40 meq/hr, and the concentration should not exceed 40 meq/L unless continuous electrocardiographic monitoring is performed. Hyperkalemia can result if the potassium-containing solution is infused too rapidly or if potassium chloride is added to solutions in flexible plastic bags without careful mixing.[100,101] Consequently, at least five hours of intravenous potassium therapy would be necessary to bring the patient back in balance. One must be careful to avoid respiratory or metabolic alkalosis in hypokalemic patients, so as to prevent the intracellular movement of potassium and the further decrease in extracellular potassium. Glucose, insulin, and bicarbonate solutions, even if they contain potassium, can drive potassium intracellularly and can potentiate hypokalemia. Therefore these solutions must be administered with caution.[102] This potentiation can be especially hazardous if the patient is digitalized.

Hyperkalemia can cause ascending muscular weakness, myocardial conduction defects, ventricular dysrhythmias, and ileus.[103] Elective operations and anesthesia should not be performed on a patient who is hyperkalemic, but rather should be delayed until normal serum potassium levels can be obtained by appropriate means. In a patient with normal renal function, this can usually be accomplished by decreasing the potassium intake and/or by withholding potassium-sparing diuretics. In patients with renal failure, it may be necessary to use ion exchange resins, peritoneal- or hemodialysis, or some of the regimens outlined in the next paragraph.

Hyperkalemic patients admitted to a hospital for an emergency operation must be treated more aggressively. Serum potassium levels can be lowered by the intravenous administration of 10% calcium gluconate, 20 or 30 ml; by the correction of any existing metabolic acidosis with sodium bicarbonate; or by the administration of a combination of regular insulin, 15 units, with glucose, 50 grams. There is insufficient information pertaining to a safe upper limit for serum potassium levels. A review of anesthetics in 33 patients with chronic renal failure described cardiac arrests in two patients in whom preoperative potassium levels had been greater than 5.5 meq/L.[77] On this basis, 5.5 meq/L serum potassium was recommended as the highest acceptable level. One should remember that acidosis, depolarizing muscle relaxants, and certain sympathomimetic amines can increase serum potassium slightly.[79,104]

Untoward effects of digitalis, anesthetics, and neuromuscular blocking drugs are minimized by careful attention to potassium balance in patients who take diuretic drugs.

Types of interactions

In general, the awareness that there are drug interactions between diuretics and the drugs mentioned under this category is the most important factor. Puzzling preoperative symptoms in patients (for example, disorientation from lithium toxicity) can be explained. Poor control of diabetes or gout might be anticipated. Patients who take anticoagulants should be carefully evaluated prior to anesthesia and operation regardless of the drugs that they take, but poor control is more understandable in patients taking diuretics. The hypertensive patient who is subject to combined drug therapy may be more sensitive to cardiodepressant anesthetics. It is important to be certain that these patients are adequately hydrated.

Some specific interactions are important in the intraoperative management of patients. Larger doses of a diuretic may be necessary for acute effects in patients taking anticonvulsant or anti-inflammatory (aspirin, indomethacin) agents. Careful attention to the degree of neuromuscular blockade is necessary when diuretics are given, at least in patients with renal failure. Finally, the toxicity of aminoglycoside antibiotics may be increased, and perhaps another drug should be substituted if the patient is receiving or needs to receive a diuretic.

As in most phases of the practice of anesthesiology, knowledge of the pharmacology and physiology involved in each case will allow physicians to provide optimal management of their patients.

REFERENCES

1. Frazier, H. S., and Yager, H.: The clinical use of diuretics. N. Engl. J. Med., *288*:246, 455, 1973.
2. Gifford, R. W.: A guide to the practical use of diuretics. J.A.M.A., *235*:1890, 1976.
3. Martinez-Maldonado, M., Eknoyan, G., and Suki, W. N.: Diuretics in nonedematous states. Arch. Intern. Med., *131*:797, 1973.
4. Early, L. E., and Orloff, J.: The mechanism of antidiuresis associated with the administration of hydrochlorothiazide to patients with vasopressin-resistant diabetes insipidus. J. Clin. Invest., *41*:1988, 1962.
5. Suki, W. N., et al.: Acute treatment of hypercalcemia with furosemide. N. Engl. J. Med., *283*:836, 1970.
6. Michenfelder, J. C., Gronert, G. A., and Rehder, K.: Neuroanesthesia. Anesthesiology, *30*:65, 1969.

7. Barry, K. G., et al.: Mannitol infusion II: The prevention of acute renal failure during resection of an aneurysm of the abdominal aorta. N. Engl. J. Med., *264*:967, 1961.

8. Barry, K. G.: Post-traumatic renal shutdown in humans: its prevention and treatment by the intravenous infusion of mannitol. Milit. Med., *128*:224, 1963.

9. Franklin, S. S., and Maxwell, M. H.: Acute renal failure. *In* Clinical Disorders of Fluid and Electrolyte Metabolism. Edited by M. H. Maxwell and C. R. Kleeman. New York, McGraw-Hill, 1972.

10. O'Dell, R., and Schmidt-Nielsen, B.: Concentrating ability and kidney structure. Fed. Proc., *19*:366, 1960.

11. Barger, A. C.: Renal hemodynamic factors in congestive heart failure. Ann. N.Y. Acad. Sci., *139*:276, 1966.

12. Stein, J. H.: The renal circulation. *In* The Kidney. Edited by B. M. Brenner and F. C. Rector, Jr. Philadelphia, W. B. Saunders, 1976.

13. Daugharty, T. M., et al.: Interrelationship of physical factors affecting sodium reabsorption in the dog. Am. J. Physiol., *215*:1442, 1968.

14. Grandchamp, A., and Boulpaep, E. L.: Pressure control of sodium reabsorption and intracellular backflux across proximal kidney tubule. J. Clin. Invest., *54*:69, 1974.

15. Brenner, B. M., et al.: Quantitative importance of changes in postglomerular colloid osmotic pressure in mediating glomerulotubular balance in the rat. J. Clin. Invest., *52*:190, 1973.

16. Martino, J. A., and Earley, L. E.: Demonstration of role of physical factors as determinants of natriuretic response to volume expansion. J. Clin. Invest., *46*:1963, 1967.

17. DiBona, G. F., Kaloyanides, G. J., and Bastron, R. D.: Effect of increased perfusion pressure on proximal tubular re-absorption in an isolated kidney. Proc. Soc. Exp. Biol. Med., *143*:830, 1973.

18. Starling, E. H., and Verney, E. B.: The secretion of urine as studied in the isolated kidney. Proc. R. Soc. Lond. [Biol.], 97:321, 1925.

19. Martino, J. A., and Earley, L. E.: Relationship between intrarenal hydrostatic pressure and hemodynamically induced changes in sodium excretion. Circ. Res., 23:371, 1968.

20. Rector, F. C., Jr., Carter, N. W., and Seldin, D. W.: The mechanism of bicarbonate reabsorption in the proximal and distal tubules of the kidney. J. Clin. Invest., 44:278, 1965.

21. Strickler, J. C., et al.: Micropuncture study in inorganic phosphate excretion in the rat. J. Clin. Invest., *43*:1596, 1964.

22. Kokko, J. P.: Sodium chloride and water transport in the descending limb of Henle. J. Clin. Invest., *49*:1838, 1970.

23. Imai, M., and Kokko, J. P.: Sodium chloride, urea and water transport in thin ascending limb of Henle. Generation of osmotic gradients by passive diffusion of solutes. J. Clin. Invest., *53*:393, 1974.

24. Burg, M. B., et al.: Furosemide effect on isolated perfused tubules. Am. J. Physiol., *225*:119, 1973.

25. Rocha, A. S., and Kokko, J. P.: Sodium chloride and water transport in the medullary thick ascending limb of Henle. Evidence for active chloride transport. J. Clin. Invest., *52*:612, 1973.

26. Burg, M. B.: Renal chloride transport and diuretics (Editorial). Circulation, *53*:587, 1976.

27. Gross, J. B., Imai, M., and Kokko, J. P.: A functional comparison of the cortical collecting tubule and the distal convoluted tubule. J. Clin. Invest., *55*:1284, 1975.

28. Giesbisch, G.: Functional organization of proximal and distal tubular electrolyte transport. Nephron, 6:260, 1969.

29. Gottschalk, C. W.: Micropuncture studies of tubular function in the mammalian kidney. Physiologist, *4*:35, 1961.

30. Papper, S.: Sodium and water: an overview. Am. J. Med. Sci., *272*:43, 1976.

31. Schrier, R. W., and Berl, T.: Nonosmolar factors affecting renal water excretion. N. Engl. J. Med., *292*:81, 1975.

32. Lee, J. B., Patek, R. V., and Mookerjee, B. K.: Renal prostaglandins and the regulation of blood pressure and sodium and water homeostasis. Am. J. Med., *60*:798, 1976.

33. Burg, M. B., et al.: Preparation and study of fragments of single rabbit nephrons. Am. J. Physiol., *210*:1293, 1966.

34. Goldberg, M.: The renal physiology of diuretics. *In* Renal Physiology. Handbook of Physiology, Section 8. Edited by J. Orloff and R. W. Berliner. Washington, D.C., American Physiological Society, 1973.

35. Flores, J., et al.: The role of cell swelling in ischemic renal damage and the protective effect of hypertonic solute. J. Clin. Invest., *51*:118, 1972.

36. Morris, C. R., et al.: Restoration and maintenance of glomerular filtration by mannitol during hypoperfusion of the kidney. J. Clin. Invest., *51*:1555, 1972.

37. Goldberg, M., and Ramirez, M. A.: Effects of saline and mannitol diuresis on the renal concentrating mechanisms in dogs: alterations in renal tissue solutes and water. Clin. Sci., *32*:475, 1967.

38. Thurau, K.: Renal hemodynamics. Am. J. Med. *36*:698, 1964.

39. Gennari, F. J., and Kassirer, J. P.: Osmotic diuresis. N. Engl. J. Med., *291*:714, 1974.

40. Blantz, R. C.: Effect of mannitol on glomerular ultrafiltration in the hydropenic rat. J. Clin. Invest., *54*:1135, 1974.

41. Seely, J. F., and Dirks, J. H.: Micropuncture study of hypertonic mannitol diuresis in the proximal and distal tubule of dog kidney. J. Clin. Invest., *48*:2330, 1969.

42. Willerson, J. T., et al.: Influence of hypertonic mannitol on ventricular performance and coronary blood flow in patients. Circulation, *51*:1095, 1975.

43. Mudge, G. H.: Drugs affecting renal function and electrolyte metabolism. *In* The Pharmacological Basis of Therapeutics. Edited by L. S. Goodman and A. Gilman. New York, Macmillan, 1975.

44. Rosin, J. M., et al.: Acetazolamide in studying sodium reabsorption in diluting segment. Am. J. Physiol., 219:1731, 1970.

45. Maren, T.H.: Pharmacological and renal effects of Diamox (6063), new carbonic anhydrase inhibitor. Trans. N.Y. Acad. Sci., *15*:53, 1953.
46. Maren, T.H.: Carbonic anhydrase: chemistry, physiology and inhibition. Physiol. Rev., *46*:597, 1967.
47. Malnic, G., Klose, R.M., and Giebisch, G.: Micropuncture study of distal tubular potassium and sodium transfer in rat kidney. Am. J. Physiol., *211*:529, 1966.
48. White, M. G., and Asch, M. J.: Acid-base effects of topical mafenide acetate in the burned patient. N. Engl. J. Med., *284*:1281, 1971.
49. Burg, M. B., and Green, N. L.: Effect of mersalyl on the thick ascending limb of Henle's loop. Kidney Int., *4*:245, 1973.
50. Goldstein, M. H., et al.: Effect of meralluride on solute and water excretion in hydrated man: comments on site of action. J. Clin. Invest., *40*:731, 1961.
51. Orloff, J., and Davidson, D. G.: The mechanism of potassium secretion in the chicken. J. Clin. Invest., *38*:21, 1959.
52. Levy, R. I., Weiner, I. M., and Mudge, G. H.: The effects of acid-base balance on diuresis produced by organic and inorganic mercurials. J. Clin. Invest., *37*:1016, 1958.
53. Kessler, R. H., Hierholzer, H., and Guard, K. S.: Localization of action of chlorothiazide in the nephron of the dog. Am. J. Physiol., *46*:1346, 1959.
54. Holzgreve, H.: The pattern of inhibition of proximal tubular reabsorption by diuretics. *In* Renal Transport and Diuretics. Edited by K. Thurae and H. Jahrmarker. Heidelberg, Springer/Verlag, 1969.
55. Earley, L. E., Kahn, M., and Orloff, J.: The effects of infusions of chlorothiazide on urinary dilution and concentration in the dog. J. Clin. Invest., *40*:857, 1961.
56. Suki, W., Rector, F. C., Jr., and Seldin, D. W.: The site of action of furosemide and other sulfonamide diuretics in the dog. J. Clin. Invest., *44*:1458, 1965.
57. Beyer, H. K., et al.: Renotropic characteristics of ethacrynic acid: a phenoxyacetic saluretic-diuretic agent. J. Pharmacol. Exp. Ther., *147*:1, 1965.
58. Hook, J. B., and Williamson, H. E.: Influence of probenecid and alterations of acid-base balance on the saluretic activity of furosemide. J. Pharmacol. Exp. Ther., *149*:404, 1965.
59. Puschett, E. B., and Goldberg, M.: The acute effects of furosemide on acid and electrolyte excretion in man. J. Lab. Clin. Med., *71*:666, 1968.
60. Burg, M., et al.: Furosemide effect on isolated perfused tubules. Am. J. Physiol., *225*:119, 1973.
61. Burg, M., and Green, N.: Effect of ethacrynic acid on the thick ascending limb of Henle's loop. Kidney Int., *4*:301, 1973.
62. Williamson, H. E., et al.: Inhibition of ethacrynic acid induced increase in renal blood flow by indomethecin. Prostaglandins, *8*:297, 1974.
63. Williamson, H. E., et al.: Furosemide induced release of prostaglandin E to increase renal blood flow. Proc. Soc. Exp. Biol. Med., 150, 1975.
64. Frolich, J., et al.: Effect of indomethacin on furosemide stimulated renin and sodium excretion. Circulation (Suppl. 2), *52*:75, 1975.
65. Patak, R., et al.: Antagonism of the effects of furosemide by indomethacin in normal and hypertensive man. Prostaglandins, *10*:649, 1975.
66. Bailie, M. D., Crosslan, K., and Hook, J. B.: Natriuretic effects of furosemide after inhibition of prostaglandin synthetase. J. Pharmacol. Exp. Ther., *199*:469, 1976.
67. Durate, C. G., Chomety, F., and Giebisch, G.: Effect of amiloride, ouabain and furosemide on distal tubular function in the rat. Am. J. Physiol., *221*:632, 1971.
68. Quick, C. A., and Hoppe, W.: Permanent deafness associated with furosemide administration. Ann. Otol. Rhinol. Laryngol. *84*:94, 1975.
69. Mitchell, J. R., et al.: Hepatic necrosis caused by furosemide. Nature, *251*:508, 1974.
70. Liddle, G. W.: Aldosterone antagonists and triamterene. Ann. N.Y. Acad. Sci., *139*:466, 1966.
71. Baba, W. I., et al.: Pharmacological effects in animals and normal human subjects of the diuretic amiloride hydrochloride. Clin. Pharmacol. Ther., *9*:318, 1968.
72. Baba, W. I., Tudhope, G. R., and Wilson, G. M.: Site and mechanism of action of the diuretic triamterene. Clin. Sci., *27*:181, 1964.
73. Sobel, B. E.: Valvular heart disease, hyperkalemia and death. Am. J. Med., *62*:743, 1977.
74. O'Rielly, M. V., Murnaghan, D. P., and Williams, M. B.: Transvenous pacemaker failure induced by hyperkalemia. J.A.M.A., *228*:336, 1974.
75. Morrow, D. H., Knapp, D. E., and Logic, J. R.: Anesthesia and digitalis toxicity V: Effect of the vagus on ouabain-induced ventricular automaticity during halothane. Anesth. Analg. (Cleve.), *49*:23, 1970.
76. Logic, J. R., and Morrow, D. H.: Effect of halothane on ventricular automaticity. Anesthesiology, *36*:107, 1972.
77. Hampers, C. L., et al.: Major surgery in patients on maintenance hemodialysis. Am. J. Surg., *115*:747, 1968.
78. Feldman, S. A.: Muscle Relaxants. London, W. B. Saunders, 1973.
79. Koide, M., and Waud, B. E.: Serum potassium concentration after succinylcholine in patients with renal failure. Anesthesiology, *36*:142, 1972.
80. Ascione, F. J.: Guanethidine-hydrochorothiazide. *In* Evaluation of Drug Interactions. 2nd Edition. Washington, D.C., American Pharmaceutical Association, 1976.
81. Lorimer, A. R., et al.: Beta-adrenoreceptor blockade in hypertension. Am. J. Med., *60*:877, 1976.
82. Ahmad, S.: Renal insensitivity to furosemide caused by chronic anti-convulsant therapy. Br. Med. J., *3*:657, 1975.
83. Ascione. F. J.: Spironolactone-aspirin. *In* Evaluations of Drug Interactions. 2nd Edition. Washington, D. C., American Pharmaceutical Association, 1976.

84. Miller, R. D., Sohn, Y. J., and Matteo, R. S.: Enhancement of d-tubocurarine neuromuscular blockade by diuretics in man. Anesthesiology, *45*:442, 1976.

85. Ascione, F. J.: Lithium carbonate-chlorothiazide. *In* Evaluations of Drug Interactions. 2nd Edition. Washington, D.C., American Pharmaceutical Association, 1976.

86. Wirth, K. E., et al.: Metabolism of digitoxin in man and its modification by spironolactone. Eur. J. Clin. Pharmacol., *9*:345, 1976.

87. Steiness, E.: Renal tubular secretion of digoxin. Circulation, *50*:103, 1974.

88. Malcolm, A. D., et al.: Digoxin kinetics during furosemide administration. Clin. Pharmacol. Ther., *21*:567, 1977.

89. Koch-Weser, J., and Sellers, E. M.: Drug interactions with coumarin anticoagulants. Part I. N. Engl. J. Med., *285*:487, 1971.

90. Koch-Weser, J., and Sellers, E. M.: Drug interactions with coumarin anticoagulants. Part II. N. Engl. J. Med., *285*:547, 1971.

91. Ascione, F. J.: Chlorpropamide-hydrochlorothiazide. *In* Evaluations of Drug Interactions. 2nd Edition. Washington, D. C., American Pharmaceutical Association, 1976.

92. Ascione, F. J.: Probenecid-chlorothiazide. *In* Evaluations of Drug Interactions. 2nd Edition. Washington, D. C., American Pharmaceutical Association, 1976.

93. Samuelson, P. N., et al.: Toxicity following methoxyflurane anaesthesia. IV. The role of obesity and the effect of low dose anaesthesia on fluoride metabolism and renal function. Can. Anaesth. Soc. J., *23*:465, 1976.

94. Ascione, F. J.: Kanamycin-ethacrynic acid. *In* Evaluations of Drug Interactions. 2nd Edition. Washington, D.C., American Pharmaceutical Association, 1976.

95. Dodds, M. G., and Foorb, R. D.: Enhancement by potent diuretics of renal tubular necrosis induced by cephaloridine. Br. J. Pharmacol., *49*:277, 1970.

96. Berry, F. A.: Pediatric fluid and electrolyte therapy. Regional Refresher Courses in Anesthesiology, *3*:1, 1975.

97. Lindeman, R. D.: Hypokalemia: causes, consequences and correction. N. Engl. J. Med., *272*:5, 1976.

98. Hutch, E. J., Squires, R. D., and Elkington, J. R.: Experimental potassium depletion in normal human subjects. II. Renal and hormonal factors in the development of extracellular alkalosis during depletion. J. Clin. Invest., *38*:1149, 1959.

99. Schribner, B. H., and Burnell, J. M.: Interpretation of the serum potassium concentration. Metabolism, *5*:468, 1956.

100. Chambers, D. G.: Dangers of rapid infusion of potassium. Med. J. Aust., *2*:945, 1973.

101. Williams, R. H. P.: Potassium overdosage: A potential hazard of non-rigid parenteral fluid containers. Br. Med. J., *1*:714, 1973.

102. Kunin, A. S., Surawicz, B., and Sims, E. A. H.: Decrease in serum potassium concentrations and appearance of cardiac arrhythmias during infusion of potassium with glucose in potassium-depleted patients. N. Engl. J. Med., *266*:228, 1962.

103. Whang, R.: Hyperkalemia: Diagnosis and treatment. Am. J. Med. Sci., *272*:19, 1976.

104. Smith, N.T., and Corbascio, A. N.: The use and misuse of pressor agents. Anesthesiology, *33*:58, 1970.

12

Antiarrhythmic Agents

JOHN L. ATLEE, III

Anesthesiologists are increasingly required to administer anesthesia to patients receiving antiarrhythmic therapy. Moreover, in patients with possible concurrent cardiovascular, pulmonary, renal, or metabolic disease, the development of arrhythmias during anesthesia is likely. Indeed, cardiac arrhythmias have been reported to occur in as many as 61.7% of anesthetized patients.[1] The majority of these arrhythmias, however, are not sufficiently serious to require antiarrhythmic drugs or electrical therapy. Arrhythmias require treatment only when (1) they cannot be corrected promptly by removing the precipitating cause, (2) hemodynamic function or myocardial oxygen supply are seriously compromised, and (3) the nature of the disturbance predisposes the patient to more serious rhythm disturbances such as ventricular tachycardia or fibrillation. Whether a patient to be anesthetized is receiving antiarrhythmic drug therapy, or whether this therapy is required during the course of anesthesia, the potential for an adverse drug interaction exists. This is not surprising, since anesthetics and adjuvant drugs have such profound and, at the same time, diverse effects on cardiac function.

Three types of adverse anesthetic-antiarrhythmic drug interactions are likely to be encountered clinically:

1. Hemodynamic effects: The cardiovascular side effects of antiarrhythmic drugs, which are usually depressant, augment that depression from anesthetics.
2. Altered antiarrhythmic effects: The expected antiarrhythmic action of a specific drug is altered by anesthetics

or adjuvant drugs with the abolition of response or by precipitation of a more serious cardiac irregularity.

3. Extracardiac effects: Antiarrhythmic drugs possess pharmacologic actions that may modify those of anesthetics or adjuncts; for example, potentiation of neuromuscular blockade.

ELECTROPHYSIOLOGY OF CARDIAC ARRHYTHMIAS

Cardiac arrhythmias result from abnormalities in impulse initiation, propagation, or both.[2] Impulse initiation, or automaticity, is a property of specialized fibers located within the sinoatrial node, the atrioventricular node, and the His-Purkinje system. These fibers differ from ordinary atrial and ventricular muscle fibers in their ability to undergo spontaneous, diastolic depolarization. Characteristic cardiac action potentials for different heart fibers are schematically shown in Figure 12–1. A resting ventricular muscle fiber (Panel A) normally has transmembrane potential of approximately -90 millivolts inside with respect to outside. On arrival of a propagated action potential or on application of an external electrical stimulus, the fiber is rapidly depolarized (phase 0). The transmembrane potential polarity is reversed, becoming approximately +30 millivolts inside because of the rapid influx of sodium ions accompanied by a slower inward movement of calcium ions. Subsequently, the fiber repolarizes, rapidly at first (phase 1), then more gradually (phase 2 or plateau), and once again rapidly (phase 3). Repolarization is associated with an outward movement of potassium ions that restores the negative intracellular potential. Active extrusion of sodium ions from within the cell against an electrochemical gradient takes place during the quiescent phase (phase 4) before the arrival of the next stimulus or propagated impulse.

The events outlined in the previous paragraph are different from those that occur in a Purkinje fiber that exhibits automaticity

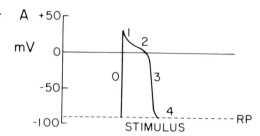

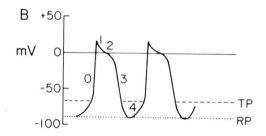

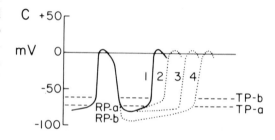

Fig. 12–1. Schematic diagrams of action potentials recorded from ventricular muscle (Panel A), Purkinje (Panel B), and SA nodal (Panel C) fibers. RP=resting transmembrane potential level. TP = threshold potential. See text for discussion.

(Fig. 12–1, Panel B). These fibers, as well as those found within the sinus or atrioventricular nodes (Fig. 12–1, Panel C), can undergo spontaneous, diastolic (phase 4) depolarization. When phase 4 depolarization reaches a critical level of threshold potential, rapid (phase 0) depolarization follows. The remaining electrophysiologic events are similar to those outlined for a ventricular muscle fiber. Different fiber types (Fig. 12–1, Panels A, B, and C) vary with respect to the amount of overshoot or final positivity reached during phase 0. A critical level of overshoot must occur for the action potential to be propagated. The ionic mechanisms responsible for spontaneous phase 4 depolarization are not completely understood. They probably vary according to fiber type; for example, those for Purkinje fibers differ from those for sinus node fibers.[3] Normal pacemaker activity is believed to be governed by the time-dependent decay of a transmembrane potassium current designated I_{K_2} with a concomitant loss in transmembrane potential due to a background inward flux of sodium.[3,4]

The rate at which pacemaker cells discharge is determined by the slope of phase 4 depolarization and by the values of transmembrane resting and threshold potential (Fig. 12–1, Panel C). The normal rate of discharge (condition 1) is slowed by raising the threshold potential (TP-a to TP-b, condi-

tion 2), by decreasing the slope of phase 4 (condition 3), or by lowering the resting membrane potential (RP-a to RP-b, condition 4). Epinephrine augments automaticity by increasing the slope of phase 4; however, this is accompanied by a small increase in resting membrane potential that limits this effect.[3] Acetylcholine, on the other hand, decreases automaticity by simultaneously increasing (hyperpolarizing) the resting membrane potential and reducing the rate of phase 4 depolarization.[3] Halothane slows the heart by reducing spontaneous phase 4 depolarization and by increasing the threshold potential.[5]

A second type of automaticity, which differs from spontaneous phase 4 depolariza-

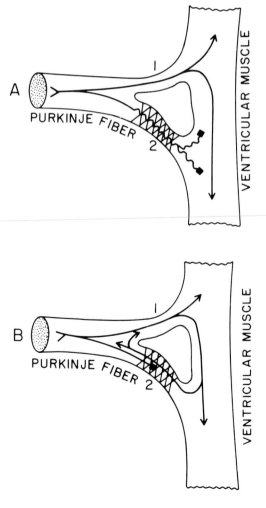

Fig. 12–2. Schematic representation of branching Purkinje fiber terminating on a ventricular muscle fiber; model for reentry of excitation. Reentry is prevented in Panel A, but permitted in Panel B. In Panels A and B, the impulse arriving from above conducts normally through branch 1 and excites the ventricular muscle fiber. The impulse in branch 2, however, fails to conduct normally. This may happen when the fibers are subject to hypoxia, stretch, catecholamines, digitalis excess, electrolyte imbalances, or possibly, anesthetics. In Panel A, the impulse *propagates slowly* through branch 2 to excite the ventricular fiber, which is now refractory following previous excitation by the impulse conducted through branch 1. In Panel A, reentry is not possible because the impulse traveling through branch 1 cannot be conducted antidromically through branch 2, and the impulse traveling orthodromically and slowly through branch 2 cannot excite the ventricular fiber. Reentry of excitation is possible in Panel B where the orthodromically conducted impulse is *blocked* in branch 2. The impulse conducted through branch 1 excites the ventricular fiber and returns antidromically through branch 2, which is no longer absolutely refractory. The impulse traveling back through branch 2 excites the more proximal portions of the Purkinje fiber and returns via branch 1 to reexcite the ventricular fiber resulting in a return extrasystole. If the reentry circuit is maintained, a series of extrasystoles or tachycardia results. Reentry is abolished if another impulse from above reaches branch 1 before the return extrasystole coming back up branch 2. Whereas the reentrant circuit discussed above involves the ventricular muscle-Purkinje fiber junction, the potential for reentry exists anywhere in the heart.

tion, involves oscillations in the diastolic transmembrane potential of specialized conducting tissues. These are referred to as oscillatory afterpotentials (OAP).[6,7] If these are large enough to reach threshold, they can induce extrasystoles or even tachycardias. Oscillatory afterpotentials are mentioned here because they are the probable mechanism for many arrhythmias induced by toxic doses of digitalis.[8] The interested reader is referred to two reviews on the subject.[8,9]

Altered impulse propagation or conduction is the other possible arrhythmia mechanism, which is necessary for arrhythmias caused by reentry of excitation.[2] Reentry occurs when there is an imbalance between conduction and refractoriness in cardiac tissues. Reentry is illustrated schematically in Figure 12–2. With the exception of occasional premature extrasystoles and parasystole, almost all clinical arrhythmias have at some time been ascribed to reentry of excitation.[10]

The mechanism invoked as the cause for a particular arrhythmia, be it phase 4 automaticity, oscillatory afterpotentials, or reentry of excitation, will determine the type of therapy employed. Unfortunately, the mechanism at work in the anesthetic and nonanesthetic environments may not be the same. Anesthetic-related arrhythmias have usually been ascribed to abnormal pacemaker activity; that is, the dominant (sinus node) pacemaker is suppressed with the emergence of latent pacemakers within the atrioventricular junctional tissues or below.[5,11,12] This applies particularly to ventricular arrhythmias caused by catecholamine sensitization. This mechanism, however, has been challenged by the proponents of reentry.[13–15] It is certain that anesthetic agents have effects on specialized atrioventricular conduction.[16,17] These effects may be related causally to reentry of excitation.[17] Furthermore, anesthetic effects on conduction are altered by those of adjuvant drugs, including antiarrhythmics, used during anesthesia.[18–21]

In summary, although much is known about the electrophysiology of cardiac arrhythmias and the drugs used to treat these disturbances in the nonanesthetic setting, comparable information is lacking for anesthetic-related arrhythmias. More knowledge of how anesthetic agents and adjuvant drugs cause arrhythmias, as well as of potential adverse interactions between anesthetic and antiarrhythmic drugs, is required. This is because rational treatment for any arrhythmia demands that one take a causal approach based on sound physiologic and pharmacologic concepts.

CLASSIFICATION OF ANTIARRHYTHMIC DRUG ACTIONS

The currently accepted classification of antiarrhythmic drugs is based on their known electrophysiologic actions.[22,23] This classification of antiarrhythmic drugs is summarized in Table 12–1 along with an outline of their principal electrophysiologic actions.[23–25] Only the first three classes (groups 1A, 1B and 2) of these drugs are currently approved for use in the United States.

Group 1A. The dominant electrophysiologic properties of quinidine and procainamide are related to their ability to block the rapid inward flux of sodium ions during phase 0 depolarization.[23] This causes a reduced level of membrane responsiveness.[26] The upstroke velocity (rate of rise or dV/dt) and the overshoot of phase 0 of the action potential are decreased for cardiac fibers excited at any given level of transmembrane potential. Thus the curve relating dV/dt to level of transmembrane potential is shifted to the right. A reduced level of membrane responsiveness results in slowed conduction. In addition to their effects on membrane responsiveness, quinidine and procainamide reduce the slope of spontaneous phase 4 depolarization.[23] Therefore, this class of drugs has important effects both on conduction and on automaticity. The noncardiac effects of these drugs are discussed later in this chapter.

Table 12–1
*Classification of Antiarrhythmic Drugs and
Summary of Principal Electrophysiologic Actions*

Action	Quinidine Procainamide (Group 1A)	Lidocaine Phenytoin (Group 1B)	Propranolol (Group 2)	Bretylium (Group 3)	Verapamil (Group 4)
Automaticity (phase 4)					
sinus node	N.C.[1]	N.C.	↓	N.C.[2]	↓[3]
latent pacemakers	↓	↓	↓	N.C.[2]	↓
Membrane Responsiveness (phase 0)	↓	N.C. or ↓[4]	↓	N.C.	N.C.
Action Potential Duration (phases 1 to 3)	↑	↓	↓	↑	↑[3]
Conduction					
AV node	↓[5]	N.C. or ↑	↓	N.C.	↓
Purkinje fibers	↓	N.C. or ↑	↓	N.C.	N.C. or ↑[3]

1. N.C. = no change; ↑ = increase; ↓ = decrease.
2. Early effect ↑ due to release of catecholamines.[24]
3. Refer to Cranefield.[25]
4. Effect dependent on extracellular K+ concentration and drug level.[23]
5. Quinidine has an anticholinergic action which tends to offset this direct effect.[24]

Group 1B. Lidocaine and phenytoin (diphenylhydantoin) share many electrophysiologic properties with quinidine and procainamide. These drugs, however, have little effect on membrane responsiveness.[23] The improvement in atrioventricular conduction occasionally seen clinically with these drugs is not related to this small effect on membrane responsiveness.[23] These drugs further depress specialized atrioventricular conduction in conjunction with halothane.[19] Furthermore, in conjunction with halothane and lidocaine, His-Purkinje and ventricular conduction are heart rate-dependent, an effect of lidocaine that may relate to its effectiveness in the treatment of ventricular arrhythmias during halothane anesthesia.

Group 2. Propranolol is the only *beta*-adrenergic blocker currently approved for clinical use in the United States. It depresses both automaticity and conduction; however, the latter effect depends largely on the degree of underlying sympathetic tone.[24] Propranolol has both *beta*-adrenergic blocking and, at higher dose levels, membrane-depressant actions that contribute to its overall effectiveness as an antiarrhythmic drug.[23]

Group 3. Bretylium tosylate, the prototype of this class of experimental drugs, has recently been approved for clinical use in the United States. It prolongs the action potential duration in both ventricular and Purkinje fibers but has no electrophysiologic effects on atrial muscle.[27,28] Thus it is effective in treating ventricular, but not supraventricular, arrhythmias.[23]

Group 4. Verapamil, the prototype of this class of drugs, is a specific inhibitor of the slow response, which is a response probably carried by a slow, inward current of calcium (and possibly also of sodium) and which is initiated during phase 0 of the action potential when the level of potential reaches approximately −60 mv.[25] The slow response is probably critical to the initiation of many forms of clinically observed arrhythmic activity; thus a specific inhibitor of this response is of theoretical interest to investigators.[25] Verapamil is a clinically effective antiarrhythmic agent currently used in

Europe, although it is not yet available in the United States. This drug exerts a negative inotropic effect by blocking calcium entry into the cell following membrane activation.[25] If verapamil or drugs with a similar action become available, it appears that extreme caution will be required when used in anesthetized patients (myocardial depression; ventricular standstill).

The following two case reports, the first from this institution and the second extracted from the literature, involve the hemodynamic effects, antiarrhythmic actions, or extracardiac effects of antiarrhythmic drugs and anesthetic agents.[29]

INTERACTIONS INVOLVING HEMODYNAMIC AND ANTIARRHYTHMIC EFFECTS

CASE REPORT

A 62-year-old man underwent elective four-vessel coronary revascularization. His medical history included five years of episodic anginal attacks, which were relieved by nitroglycerin and rest, and a 15-pack-per-year history of smoking. No other coronary risk factors, such as obesity or hypertension, were evident.

Two weeks prior to hospital admission the patient had had an episode of severe anginal pain, associated with dizziness and diaphoresis, for which he was admitted to the coronary care unit. The initial diagnosis of acute myocardial infarction was not substantiated. He underwent cardiac catheterization on the fifth hospital day. His systemic, pulmonary, and right- and left-sided filling pressures were normal, as was his cardiac index. The patient had diffuse, high grade, occlusive disease involving both the left and right coronary arteries and their major branches. The proximal left anterior descending artery, the distal portions of which filled from collaterals, was 100% occluded. An operation was scheduled for the following week.

Digoxin (250 µg/day, orally) was started three days prior to the operation with nitroglycerin continued sublingually as needed. The patient's blood chemistries and serum electrolytes were all normal the day before the operation. Premedication consisted of scopolamine (hyoscine), 0.43 mg, and morphine, 10 mg IM (intramuscularly).

When the patient arrived in the operating room, his arterial blood pressure (Riva-Rocci) was 126/70 torr and his heart rate was 83 beats/min. The ECG (II) showed sinus rhythm (Fig. 12–3A). Peripheral and central venous catheters were placed and percutaneous radial artery cannulation was performed to monitor direct arterial pressure and to sample blood gases and electrolytes. Anesthesia was induced with thiopental (250 mg, IV [intravenously]) followed by halothane (0.5 to 2.0%, inspired) and nitrous oxide (50%). Following anesthetic induction, pancuronium (8 mg, IV) was given. A supraventricular tachycardia (150 to 160 beats/min, Fig. 12–3B) appeared within three minutes. This was associated with a decrease in arterial pressure to 80/50 torr. Arterial blood gases drawn at this time revealed: $P_{O_2} = 220$ torr, $P_{CO_2} = 33$ torr, pH = 7.40, serum K+ = 3.4 meq/L (preoperative value = 4.6 meq/L). Halothane was discontinued and edrophonium was administered (10 mg, IV), but it failed to abolish the tachycardia (Fig. 12–3C). Lidocaine (200 mg, IV) was administered next, also without success (Fig. 12–3D), and this in turn was followed by propranolol (1.5 mg IV, divided doses over two minutes). Five minutes after the administration of propranolol, the patient's ventricular rate had slowed substantially (Fig. 12–3E), and he appeared to be experiencing atrial flutter with varying degrees of atrioventricular block. His arterial blood pressure was 150/80 torr. Approximately 15 minutes after the administration of pancuronium, the patient still was not sufficiently relaxed to allow endotracheal intubation. Peripheral nerve stimulation demonstrated well-sustained tetanus without post-tetanic facilitation or twitch suppression. Halothane was reinstituted, and a second dose of pancuronium (8 mg, IV) was administered. The patient then appeared to be relaxed, and his trachea was intubated successfully. However, the tachycardia reappeared (Fig. 12–3F), accompanied by a decrease in arterial blood pressure. Sinus rhythm (Fig. 12–3G) was restored within 15 minutes after an additional dose of propranolol (0.5 mg, IV). This rhythm persisted for the next 2½ hours, during which time the patient's blood pressure was stable (range 120 to 140 torr systolic). Two minutes after the second dose of pancuronium, the patient's serum potassium was 2.6 meq/L, and ten minutes later it was 4.1 meq/L. Concomitant arterial blood gas analyses revealed a mild, compensated metabolic acidosis (pH = 7.41, $P_{CO_2} = 33$ and 35 torr) at both sampling intervals. A third dose of pancuronium (7 mg, IV) immediately before cardiopulmonary bypass resulted in a junctional bradycardia (Fig. 12–3H). This lasted approximately two minutes and was accompanied by a small, transient decrease (0.5 meq/L) in serum potassium level. The remainder of the patient's surgical and anesthetic course was uneventful, as was his postoperative course. He was discharged from the hospital on the fourteenth postoperative day.

This case illustrates the dilemma faced by the clinician when confronted with a serious cardiac arrhythmia. Several possible drug interactions could have caused the hemodynamic alterations and rhythm disturbances encountered. Digitalis, halothane, and pancuronium could have caused the arrhythmias. The prophylactic administration of digitalis has been recommended in patients who undergo aortocoronary bypass operations to reduce the incidence of perioperative arrhythmias.[30] That this practice does reduce the incidence and severity of intraoperative arrhythmias, however, has not been established. Our studies suggest that therapeutic serum levels of digoxin may protect against experimental atrial arrhythmias in halothane-anesthetized dogs.[31] Furthermore, similar experimental atrial arrhythmias were more easily induced in dogs anesthetized with halothane than enflurane.[17] An apparent relation between alterations in conduction produced by anesthesia and the incidence of arrhythmias suggested a reentrant mechanism for these arrhythmias. Several reports taken together indicate that both supraventricular and ventricular arrhythmias are more likely when halothane and pancuronium are used in association than with other volatile anesthesics. Since this association is not proven, it awaits further clinical verification.[32–34]

Acute hypokalemia in the patient in our case report appeared to be temporally related to the administration of pancuronium. However, the administration of pancuronium or of other nondepolarizing muscle relaxants is not believed to be associated with significant acute alterations in serum potassium. Regardless of cause, the hypokalemia noted in this patient could have precipitated digitalis toxicity in an otherwise nontoxic patient. Acute hypocapnia produced by mechanical ventilation may be associated with a concomitant fall in serum potassium level, although this did not appear to be so in our patient. It is well known that acutely induced hypokalemia potentiates digitalis toxicity. Hypokalemia also augments the neuromuscular effects of pancuronium.[35,36] Whether it alters the cardiac

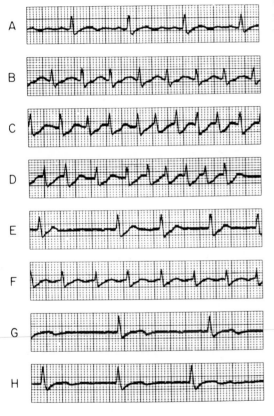

Fig. 12–3.   ECG (II) recordings (25 mm/sec) from patient described in first case report. Panel A—sinus rhythm prior to induction of anesthesia. Panel B—supraventricular tachycardia following first dose of pancuronium. Panel C—supraventricular tachycardia after edrophonium 10 mg, IV. Panel D—supraventricular tachycardia after lidocaine 200 mg, IV. Panel E—atrial flutter, varying degrees of atrioventricular block, after propranolol 1.5 mg, IV. Panel F—supraventricular tachycardia following second dose of pancuronium. Panel G—sinus bradycardia prior to third dose of pancuronium. Panel H—junctional bradycardia following third dose of pancuronium.

electrophysiologic effects of pancuronium or of halothane is unknown.

The treatment of the supraventricular tachycardia in this patient deserves comment. Because of his coronary atherosclerosis, carotid massage was not attempted, since this maneuver might have caused embolization of atherosclerotic plaques. Maneuvers that increase parasympathetic tone, such as anticholinesterase therapy, or *alpha*-adrenergic vasopressors, have been recommended.[37,38] Vasopressors were not chosen for this patient because of the potential danger of hypertension with a tachycardia. In addition to contractile force development, heart rate and blood pressure are major determinants of oxygen consumption. This patient's oxygen supply appeared to be seriously compromised. Because the patient did not respond to edrophonium, a longer acting anticholinesterase drug (for example, neostigmine) was not given. Despite the lack of effect in our case, edrophonium is often effective in treating supraventricular tachycardia. It alters the refractoriness of supraventricular conducting pathways under parasympathetic control. Presumably, this makes conduction more homogeneous and reduces the likelihood of reentry. Whatever the reason for the lack of an edrophonium effect in our patient (it could be argued that an additional 10 mg should have been given), the choice of this drug was logical. A substantial increase in blood pressure without a concomitant reduction in heart rate would have been dangerous to this patient, since he had advanced coronary artery disease.

Intravenous lidocaine was also ineffective. I have noted occasionally that sinus rhythm is restored after the administration of lidocaine (2 to 3 mg/kg body weight, IV) in apparent cases of supraventricular tachycardia during halothane or enflurane anesthesia. Whereas lidocaine is generally considered to be ineffective in supraventricular arrhythmias, its beneficial effect during anesthesia may relate to an action of lidocaine that promotes less temporal dispersion of refractoriness in reentry loops responsible for supraventricular arrhythmias. Its effects on supraventricular excitability during inhalation anesthesia have not been tested. It is also possible that the apparent effectiveness of lidocaine in treating some supraventricular tachycardias is spurious. Supraventricular tachycardia associated with aberrant ventricular conduction is easily mistaken for ventricular tachycardia, and lidocaine is the drug preferred in the treatment of the latter. I do not advocate the use of lidocaine as a first choice for the treatment of supraventricular tachycardias. Indeed, it may cause alarming ventricular acceleration during atrial flutter, and has been reported to cause SA nodal arrest when used with quinidine.[39,40] However, when a supposed supraventricular tachycardia associated with aberrant ventricular conduction fails to convert following cholinergic interventions, the possibility that the arrhythmia is of ventricular origin must be considered. Lidocaine may be tried under these circumstances.

Propranolol has been recommended for the treatment of supraventricular tachyarrhythmias.[36] It was used in the patient in our case report to prolong atrioventricular nodal conduction and thereby to slow the ventricular response to the supraventricular tachycardia. In addition to reducing myocardial oxygen demand, the slower ventricular rate can improve hemodynamics by allowing an improvement in ventricular filling as well as an increase in coronary blood flow due to an increase in diastolic minute time. Such an effect can also be expected from digitalis, which slows atrioventricular nodal conduction as well. In this patient, however, one cannot be certain that the arrhythmia was not the direct result of acute digitalis intoxication brought about by sudden changes in the serum potassium level. The use of additional digitalis, therefore, seemed inadvisable under the circumstances. Propranolol had the desired effect of reducing the ventricular rate (Fig. 12–3*E*), and of restoring blood pressure to more acceptable levels (systolic range 120 to 140 torr). Furthermore, this intervention revealed the underlying mechanism, namely atrial flutter, as evidenced by the small, regular undulations in the baseline (Fig. 12–3*E*). The additional dose of propranolol (0.5 mg) used to treat the episode of supraventricular tachycardia (Fig. 12–3*F*) after the second dose of pancuronium also slowed the ventricular rate and shortly thereafter it restored sinus rhythm (Fig. 12–3*G*). This response could be attributed to a direct membrane-stabilizing effect of propranolol, or to the hemodynamic improvement and return of serum potassium to more physiologic levels.

It has been reported that succinylcholine is effective in abolishing supraventricular arrhythmias during anesthesia.[41] In retrospect this might have been the best treatment after the first attack of tachycardia. Succinylcholine would have controlled the tachycardia either by a direct myocardial or postganglionic sympathetic stimulating effect, or by simultaneously increasing the serum potassium level and providing adequate muscle relaxation for endotracheal intubation.[42–44] As for the use of additional pancuronium, it can be argued that this was improper and that d-tubocurarine, an agent less likely to precipitate tachycardia, should have been administered.[34]

The case report illustrates the complexities of treating arrhythmias during anesthesia. These complexities arise because we are poorly informed of the type of interactions involved. In arrhythmic patients, there is little assurance that the remedy will not be worse than the disease.

INTERACTIONS INVOLVING EXTRACARDIAC EFFECTS

The main interactions of this kind involve the well-known potentiation of a nondepolarizing neuromuscular blockade by antiarrhythmic drugs. A clinical example is quinidine. The following case report was extracted from the literature:[29]

CASE REPORT

A 71-year-old man was scheduled for a cholecystectomy following an episode of acute cholecystitis. He had had a myocardial infarction ten years before. Three weeks prior to admission, an operation under general anesthesia for a hip fracture was performed without problems. The patient was taking oral quinidine (200 mg, q.i.d.) for ventricular premature beats, which included runs of quadrigeminy and trigeminy noted on a preoperative ECG. Sinus rhythm had been restored by quinidine therapy by the time of the operation.

Anesthesia was induced with cyclopropane and maintained with nitrous oxide supplemented by meperidine (160 mg) and by tubocurarine (36 mg). Several episodes of intraoperative hypotension responded well to the administration of intravenous fluids and plasma protein fraction. Ephedrine sulfate (total dose 100 mg IV and 45 mg IM) was also administered. At the conclusion of a 160-minute procedure, the neuromuscular block was reversed with atropine, 1.4 mg, and neostigmine, 3.5 mg.

The patient's condition for the first hour in the recovery room was stable. He then received 300 mg of quinidine IM. Shortly thereafter (approximately 20 minutes), the patient appeared mildly cyanotic and was breathing shallowly. Oxygen therapy by mask was started and the patient received an additional 1.0 mg of neostigmine and 0.4 mg of atropine. He did not respond and his condition further deteriorated to apnea. Nasal tracheal intubation was performed and controlled ventilation with oxygen was started. The patient's condition worsened, complicated by severe hypotension and ventricular arrhythmias. The former did not respond to fluids and ephedrine. An acceptable level of blood pressure (100 torr systolic) was achieved with a metaraminol drip. Neuromuscular function failed to improve in response to edrophonium 10 mg, IV. Controlled ventilation was continued for approximately six hours, at which time the patient was able to breathe spontaneously and the endotracheal tube was removed. Arrhythmias were still present at this time, but neuromuscular function was normal.

The following morning the patient was mildly cyanotic and dyspneic. The nasotracheal tube was reinserted and intermittent positive pressure breathing (IPPB) was started, with resultant clinical improvement. An ECG at this time showed normal sinus rhythm with ST–T wave changes probably due either to quinidine or to residual myocardial ischemia. The remainder of the patient's post-operative course was uneventful.

This patient probably became recurarized after receiving quinidine in the recovery room. Quinidine and other antiarrhythmic drugs currently approved for use in the

United States, which include lidocaine, procainamide, phenytoin, and propranolol, enhance the neuromuscular block produced by d-tubocurarine.[45,46]

The interaction between neuromuscular blocking and antiarrhythmic drugs may become manifest under another circumstance. It is not unusual for the clinician to administer a small, "defasciculating" dose of pancuronium or of d-tubocurarine prior to the administration of succinylcholine. This is a common practice in minor or outpatient surgical procedures requiring endotracheal intubation such as dental extractions and laparoscopies. Many of these patients have negative medical histories, but still frequently have diastolic pressures between 85 and 95 torr and systolic pressures between 130 and 140 torr. Endotracheal intubation following the induction of anesthesia (thiopental, succinylcholine) in these borderline-hypertensive patients is frequently associated with hypertension, where systolic pressures in some cases reach 200 torr or more. Hypertension of this magnitude is often associated with ventricular arrhythmias, including multifocal extrasystoles. Based on experimental evidence gathered by C. Prys-Roberts et al., I administer a small dose of intravenous propranolol (1.0 to 2.0 mg) ten minutes prior to the induction of anesthesia in borderline hypertensive patients.[47] This effectively obtunds the hypertensive response to laryngoscopy and surgical stimulation. On at least two occasions, however, I have seen patients become weak and acutely dyspneic following a "defasciculating" dose of pancuronium (1.0 mg) given five minutes after the propranolol. The same response has been observed with "defasciculating" doses of d-tubocurarine. The most reasonable explanation for this occurrence is the potentiation of pancuronium neuromuscular block by propranolol.

ANTIARRHYTHMIC DRUGS

Those drug actions of interest to anesthesiologists, aside from the cardiac elec-

trophysiologic effects discussed earlier, with the greatest potential for causing interactions are discussed for each antiarrhythmic agent in this section.

Quinidine

Quinidine depresses myocardial automaticity, conduction, and contractility. Large doses may reduce arterial pressure by causing peripheral vasodilation.[24] In addition, quinidine has an anticholinergic action that opposes its direct depression of conduction.[24] This is a disadvantage when quinidine is used to treat supraventricular tachyarrhythmias: it enhances the conductivity of the atrioventricular node and prolongs the atrial effective refractory period. Unfortunately, these effects are contrary to what is needed to treat paroxysmal supraventricular tachycardia. Quinidine is most effective in the treatment of atrial flutter or fibrillation and of other supraventricular arrhythmias. It has rarely been used in the long-term treatment of ventricular arrhythmias since the advent of other drugs that are both less toxic and at least as effective (for example, procainamide, phenytoin). Quinidine and propranolol administered together in reduced doses appear to be more effective than high doses of either drug alone in converting supraventricular tachyarrhythmias to sinus rhythm.[48,49]

Anesthetists must be cautious in their approach to patients who take quinidine, not only because of quinidine's neuromuscular blocking actions mentioned earlier, but also because of its depressant effects on the circulation. Thus quinidine administered parenterally to patients who are deeply anesthetized with halothane or enflurane might cause additional circulatory depression. More appropriate and effective measures are available for the treatment of cardiac arrhythmias including, in addition to drugs, direct current (DC) cardioversion in more refractory cases.

Procainamide

Procainamide has actions similar to those of quinidine. Following intravenous administration, its cardiac depressant and vas-odilating properties may be dangerous to the patient whose circulation is already com-promised. Both procainamide and quinidine should not be administered to patients with advanced atrioventricular conduction block, and should be administered only cau-tiously to patients with partial block.[24] In patients who have a complete block with dependence on a junctional or idioventricu-lar pacemaker, procainamide may suppress the pacemaker and cause asystole. Fur-thermore, an incomplete block can progress to a complete one with consequent asystole. Anesthetics may enhance this adverse ef-fect.[17,18] The problem of producing asystole, however, is less serious today because most patients with significant atrioventricular conduction block benefit from pacemaker therapy. Finally, procainamide or quinidine may be used in conjunction with ventricular pacing in patients with the sick sinus syn-drome clinically manifested as the brady-cardia-tachycardia syndrome.[50] These drugs may be used when retrograde activation of the atria during ventricular pacing fails to effectively suppress ectopic atrial rhythms.

Lidocaine

Lidocaine is an effective, safe, and rapidly acting drug for the treatment of ventricular arrhythmias and is well suited for in-traoperative use. It is the drug preferred for most ventricular arrhythmias that occur dur-ing anesthesia, except perhaps for those caused by digitalis excess where phenytoin is indicated (see the section on phenytoin). Lidocaine is not recommended for the treatment of supraventricular arrhythmias, except when aberrant conduction is present and when confusion exists as to the diag-nosis of ventricular tachycardia (see discus-sion following first case report).[24] This drug has accelerated the ventricular response during atrial flutter and has caused sinus arrest when used in conjunction with quini-dine.[39,40] I noted earlier, in relation to the first case report, that lidocaine frequently restores sinus rhythm in apparent cases of

supraventricular tachycardia during anesthesia with either enflurane or halothane. This beneficial effect could be spurious, or it could be attributed to an undiagnosed ven-tricular tachycardia. Furthermore, lidocaine may have different cardiac electrophysi-ologic effects in the presence of potent vol-atile anesthetic agents that are responsible for its apparent effectiveness in some cases of supraventricular tachycardia.[19] Until more information is available, however, lidocaine should be used cautiously in the treatment of supraventricular tachyar-rhythmias during anesthesia. Cholinergic maneuvers, propranolol, or digitalis are pre-ferred to lidocaine. Finally, lidocaine may cause seizures. To achieve a therapeutic (antiarrhythmic) effect and to avoid sei-zures, the initial intravenous dose of lidocaine should not exceed 2 to 3 mg/kg body weight. A maintenance infusion of lidocaine (1.0 gm in 250 ml normal saline solution) can be administered at the rate of 20 to 30 mcg/kg body weight per minute.

Phenytoin (Diphenylhydantoin)

Phenytoin, or diphenylhydantoin, shares many of the cardiac electrophysiologic properties of lidocaine.[24] It is unique, how-ever, in its ability to antagonize ventricular arrhythmias caused by digitalis intoxication. Lidocaine is not as effective as phenytoin in this regard.[24] Procainamide is also effective against ventricular arrhythmias. It differs from phenytoin in that atrioventricular con-duction is further impaired by procain-amide, whereas phenytoin improves con-duction.[51] Phenytoin can depress the sinus node.[24] It should be used with caution when administered intravenously, particularly in connection with potent inhalation agents that also depress the sinus node.[5,11] For these reasons, phenytoin is not recom-mended for the treatment of ventricular ar-rhythmias that are not caused by digitalis. Lidocaine is a more rapidly acting and effec-tive drug for this purpose. Phenytoin is of little use in treating atrial flutter or fibrilla-tion, but it is effective in some cases of paroxysmal supraventricular tachycardia, particularly when associated with digitalis toxicity.[52] Therapeutic levels of phenytoin can be attained by the slow administration of 50 to 100 mg doses IV every 10 to 15 minutes until a therapeutic response is observed or until a maximum dose of 10 to 15 mg/kg of body weight has been given.[52-54]

Propranolol

The principal use of propranolol in treating cardiac arrhythmias is to control the ventricular rate in cases of supraventricular tachycardia. Its *beta*-blocking as opposed to quinidine-like action causes prolongation of the atrioventricular nodal refractory period. The *beta*-blocking action of propranolol sets it apart from other antiarrhythmic drugs that usually increase atrioventricular conduction and accelerate the ventricular rate.[24] Its main drawback in anesthetic practice resides in its myocardial depressant effects, which may be augmented by the presence of anesthetic agents. Thus propranolol should be given in small doses (that is, up to 3.0 mg IV in 0.5-mg increments). Many investigators recommended the concomitant administration of digitalis.[24] The desired effect is slowing of the ventricular rate sufficient to improve the cardiac output. Extreme caution should be exercised in the presence of atrioventricular block. Finally, based on experimental evidence, propranolol is expected to augment the slowing of conduction produced by halothane or enflurane.[18]

In conclusion, cardiac arrhythmias occur frequently during anesthesia and thus concern the anesthetist. They warrant treatment when impaired hemodynamics compromise tissue perfusion, when there is an unfavorable ratio between myocardial oxygen supply and demand, or when the arrhythmia is likely to predispose the patient to ventricular tachycardia or fibrillation. Treatment in most cases simply involves the removal of the precipitating cause, which frequently is hypoxia, inadequate ventilation, or an electrolyte imbalance. In many patients, however, the precipitating cause is not readily apparent; or, as in the case of digitalis intoxication, it is not easily removed. Antiarrhythmic agents themselves, when used improperly, may cause or further aggravate existing arrhythmias. Increasing evidence suggests that anesthetic agents may alter the pharmacologic properties of commonly used antiarrhythmic agents. Further research is needed to elucidate the mechanisms and frequency of anesthetic-antiarrhythmic drug interactions. In the meantime, a cautious approach to the problem is advised. An increased understanding on the part of clinicians of arrhythmia mechanisms and of the pharmacology of antiarrhythmic drugs could decrease the incidence of adverse interactions or could direct their proper management. In addition, careful monitoring and selection of drugs, or the use of smaller doses, are recommended.

REFERENCES

1. Kuner, J., et al.: Cardiac arrhythmias during anesthesia. Dis. Chest, *52*:580, 1967.
2. Cranefield, P. F., Wit, A. L., and Hoffman, B. F.: Genesis of cardiac arrhythmias. Circulation, *47*:190, 1973.
3. Noble, D.: The Initiation of the Heartbeat. Oxford, Clarendon Press, 1975.
4. Noble, D., and Tsien, R. W.: The kinetics and rectifier properties of the slow potassium current in cardiac Purkinje fibers. J. Physiol. (Lond.), *195*:185, 1968.
5. Reynolds, A. K., Chiz, J. F., and Pasquet, A. F.: Halothane and methoxyflurane: A comparison of their effects on cardiac pacemaker fibers. Anesthesiology, *33*:602, 1970.
6. Ferrier, G. R., Saunders, J. H., and Mendez, C.: A cellular mechanism for the generation of ventricular arrhythmias by acetylstrophanthidin. Circ. Res., *32*:600, 1973.
7. Hashimoto, K., and Moe, G. K.: Transient depolarizations induced by acetylstrophanthidin in specialized tissue of dog atrium and ventricle. Circ. Res., *32*:618, 1973.
8. Ferrier, G. R.: Digitalis arrhythmias: Role of oscillatory afterpotentials. Prog. Cardiovasc. Dis., *19*:459, 1977.
9. Cranefield, P. F.: Action potentials, afterpotentials and arrhythmias. Circ. Res., *41*:415, 1977.
10. Moe, G. K.: Evidence for reentry as a mechanism of cardiac arrhythmias. Rev. Physiol. Biochem. Pharmacol., *72*:55, 1975.
11. Reynolds, A. K., Chiz, J. F., and Pasquet, A. F.: Pacemaker migration and sinus node arrest with

methoxyflurane and halothane. Can. Anaesth. Soc. J., *18*:137, 1971.

12. Reynolds, A. K., Chiz, J. F., and Tanikella, T. K.: On the mechanism of coupling in adrenaline-induced bigeminy in sensitized hearts. Can. J. Physiol. Pharmacol., *53*:1158, 1975.

13. Sasyniuk, B. I., and Dresel, P. E.: Mechanism and site of origin of bigeminal rhythms in cyclopropane-sensitized dogs. Am. J. Physiol., *220*:1857, 1971.

14. Zink, J., Sasyniuk, B. I., and Dresel, P. E.: Halothane-epinephrine-induced cardiac arrhythmias and the role of heart rate. Anesthesiology, *43*:548, 1975.

15. Hashimoto, K., et al.: Effects of halothane on automaticity and contractile force of isolated blood-perfused canine ventricular tissue. Anesthesiology, *42*:15, 1975.

16. Atlee, J. L., and Alexander, S. C.: Halothane effects on conductivity of the AV node and His-Purkinje system in the dog. Anesth. Analg. (Cleve.), *56*:378, 1977.

17. Atlee, J. L., et al.: Supraventricular excitability in dogs during anesthesia with halothane and enflurane. Anesthesiology, *49*:407, 1978.

18. Atlee, J. L., and Rusy, B. F.: Halothane depression of A–V conduction studied by electrograms of the bundle of His in dogs. Anesthesiology, *36*:112, 1972.

19. Atlee, J. L., Homer, L. D., and Tobey, R. E.: Diphenylhydantoin and lidocaine modification of A–V conduction in halothane anesthetized dogs. Anesthesiology, *43*:49, 1975.

20. Morrow, D. H., Logic, J. R., and Haley, J. V.: Anti-arrhythmic anesthetic action 1: The effect of halothane on canine intracardiac impulse conduction during sinus rhythm. Anesth. Analg. (Cleve.), *56*:187, 1977.

21. Geha, D. G., et al.: Pancuronium bromide enhances atrioventricular conduction in halothane-anesthetized dogs. Anesthesiology, *46*:342, 1977.

22. Vaughan Williams. E. M.: Classification of antiarrhythmic drugs. *In* Symposium on Cardiac Arrhythmias. Edited by E. Sandoe, E. Flenstedt-Jensen, and K. H. Olesen. Södertälje, Sweden, A. B. Astra, 1970.

23. Singh, B. N., and Hauswirth, O.: Comparative mechanisms of action of antiarrhythmic drugs. Am. Heart J., *87*:367, 1974.

24. Moe, G. K., and Abildskov, J. A.: Antiarrhythmic drugs. *In* The Pharmacological Basis of Therapeutics. 5th Edition. Edited by L. S. Goodman and A. Gilman. New York, Macmillan, 1975.

25. Cranefield, P. F.: The Conduction of the Cardiac Impulse. Mount Kisco, New York, Futura, 1975.

26. Weidmann, S.: The effect of the cardiac membrane potential on the rapid availability of the sodium-carrying system. J. Physiol. (Lond.), *127*:213, 1955.

27. Bigger, J. T., and Jaffe, C. C.: The effect of bretylium tosylate on the electrophysiological properties of ventricular muscle and Purkinje fibers. Am. J. Cardiol., *27*:82, 1971.

28. Papp, J. G., and Vaughan Williams, E. M.: The effect on intracellular atrial potentials of bretylium

in relation to its local anesthetic potency. Br. J. Pharmacol., *35*:352, 1969.

29. Way, W. L., Katzung, B. G., and Larson, C. P., Jr.: Recurarization with quinidine. J.A.M.A., *200*:163, 1967.

30. Johnson, L. W., et al.: Prophylactic digitalization for coronary artery bypass surgery. Circulation, *53*:819, 1976.

31. Atlee, J. L.: Effect of serum digoxin levels on an experimental atrial arrhythmia in halothane anesthetized dogs. Fed. Proc., *37*:729, 1978.

32. Basta, J. W., and Lichtiger, M.: Comparison of metocurine and pancuronium—myocardial tension-time index during endotracheal intubation. Anesthesiology, *46*:366, 1977.

33. Miller, R. D., et al.: Pancuronium-induced tachycardia in relation to alveolar halothane, dose of pancuronium, and prior atropine. Anesthesiology, *42*:352, 1975.

34. Stoelting, R. K.: The hemodynamic effects of pancuronium and d-tubocurarine in anesthetized patients. Anesthesiology, *36*:612, 1972.

35. Edwards, R., Winnie, A. P., and Ramamurthy, S.: Acute hypocapneic hypokalemia: An iatrogenic anesthetic complication. Anesth. Analg. (Cleve.), *56*:786, 1977.

36. Miller, R. D., and Roderick, L.: Diuretic-induced hypokalemia, pancuronium neuromuscular blockade and its antagonism by neostigmine. Br. J. Anaesth., *50*:541, 1978.

37. Warner, H.: Therapy of common arrhythmias. Med. Clin. North Am., *58*:995, 1974.

38. Sprague, D. H., and Mandel, S. D.: Paroxysmal supraventricular tachycardia during anesthesia. Anesthesiology, *46*:75, 1977.

39. Marriott, H. J. L., and Bieza, C. F.: Alarming ventricular acceleration after lidocaine administration. Chest, *61*:682, 1972.

40. Jeresaty, R. M., Kahn, A. H., and Landry, A. B., Jr.: Sinoatrial arrest due to lidocaine in a patient receiving quinidine. Chest, *61*:683, 1972.

41. Galindo, A., Wyte, S. R., and Wetherhold, J. W.: Junctional rhythm induced by halothane anesthesia—Treatment with succinylcholine. Anesthesiology, *37*:261, 1971.

42. Galindo, A., and Davis, T. B.: Succinylcholine and cardiac excitability. Anesthesiology, *23*:32, 1962.

43. Dowdy, E. G., and Fabian, L. W.: Ventricular arrhythmias induced by succinylcholine in digitalized patients. Anesth. Analg. (Cleve.), *42*:501, 1963.

44. Birch, A. A. B., Mitchell, G. D., and Playford, G. A.: Changes in serum potassium response to succinylcholine following trauma. J.A.M.A., *210*:490, 1969.

45. Miller, R. D., Way, W. L., and Katzung, B. G.: The potentiation of neuromuscular blocking agents by quinidine. Anesthesiology, *28*:1036, 1967.

46. Harrah, M. D., Way, W. L., and Katzung, B. G.: The interaction of d-tubocurarine with antiarrhythmic drugs. Anesthesiology, *33*:406, 1970.

47. Prys-Roberts, C., et al.: Studies of anaesthesia in relation to hypertension V: Adrenergic *beta*-receptor blockade. Br. J. Anaesth., *45*:671, 1973.

48. Stern, S.: Conversion of chronic atrial fibrillation to

sinus rhythm with combined propranolol and quinidine treatment. Am. Heart J., *74*:170, 1967.

49. Fors, W. J., Vanderark, C. R., and Reynolds, E. W., Jr.: Evaluation of propranolol and quinidine in the treatment of quinidine-resistant arrhythmias. Am. J. Cardiol., *27*:190, 1971.

50. Scarpa, W. J.: The sick sinus syndrome. Am. Heart J., *92*:648, 1976.

51. Helfant, R. H., Scherlag, B. J., and Damato, A. N.: The electrophysiological properties of diphenylhydantoin sodium as compared to procainamide in the normal and digitalis-intoxicated heart. Circulation, *36*:108, 1967.

52. Bigger, J. T.: Arrhythmias and anti-arrhythmic drugs. Adv. Intern. Med., *18*:251, 1972.

53. Lang, T. W., et al.: The use of diphenylhydantoin for the treatment of digitalis toxicity. Arch. Intern. Med., *116*:573, 1965.

54. Bigger, J. T., Jr., Schmidt, D. H., and Kutt, H.: Relationship between plasma level of diphenylhydantoin sodium and its cardiac antiarrhythmic effects. Circulation, *38*:363, 1968.

Chapter **13**

Psychotropic Agents

ESTHER C. JANOWSKY
S. CRAIG RISCH
and
DAVID S. JANOWSKY

Psychotropic drugs are important in the treatment of schizophrenia, mania, and severe depression and play an essential role in the practice of medicine. Psychotropic drugs, often given in combination and/or with nonpsychiatric drugs, in general profoundly affect central and peripheral neurotransmitter and ionic mechanisms. Hence, prior intake of these drugs is an important consideration in the management of the surgical patient. The drugs reviewed in this chapter include: (1) antidepressants (tricyclic antidepressants and monoamine oxidase inhibitors), (2) dopamine blocking antipsychotic drugs (phenothiazines, thioxanthenes, and butryophenones), (3) the catecholamine-depleting antipsychotic agent, reserpine, and (4) the antimanic agent, lithium. In addition, (5) the anesthetic implications of anticholinergic agents, used to antagonize the extrapyramidal side effects of the antipsychotic drugs, will be considered. Generally, each group of drugs will be discussed under the headings of psychiatric indications, proposed psychobiologic mechanism of action, effects on various anesthetic agents and the mechanism of these effects, and clinical implications and management of these effects.

ANTIPSYCHOTIC DRUGS (TABLE 13–1)

Phenothiazines, thioxanthenes, and butyrophenones are widely used to treat psychotic symptoms in patients affected with schizophrenia, mania, and organic brain syndromes associated with psychosis. All antipsychotic drugs elevate serum

177

Table 13–1
Some Interactions Between Phenothiazines and Butyrophenones and Drugs Used in Anesthesia

Phenothiazine Butyrophenone	Interaction
Inhalation Drugs	↓ arterial blood pressure (halothane, enflurane)
Narcotics	↑, ↓ analgesia ↑ respiratory depression ↑ sedation
Barbiturates	↑ sleep time
Anticholinergics	↑ peripheral activity ↑ central activity
Sympathomimetics	↓ *alpha*-adrenergic activity

prolactin and block dopaminergic receptors.[1] However, antipsychotic drugs differ from one another in their central and peripheral antiadrenergic and anticholinergic properties, and thus in their side effects. Chlorpromazine and thioridazine possess anticholinergic and antiadrenergic actions, and therefore their predominant side effects are hypotension, sedation, and anticholinergic symptoms. Obvious antidopaminergic effects, such as extrapyramidal symptoms, occur less frequently. Conversely, haloperidol, fluphenazine, trifluoperazine, and butaperazine induce few autonomic actions, and their predominant side effects are antidopaminergic-extrapyramidal.[2]

The most popular current psychobiologic theory attributes the effect of antipsychotic drugs to their dopamine blocking properties.[1] In fact, phenothiazines and butyrophenones effectively block dopamine receptors, a characteristic not found in related compounds devoid of antipsychotic properties.

Antipsychotic agents have been important in anesthetic practice since the 1950's, with the introduction in Europe of the "lytic cocktail," that is, a mixture of chlorpromazine, meperidine, and promethazine.[3] This combination never gained popularity in the United States, and later it became obsolete abroad because of hypotension, ex-

trapyramidal signs, and prolonged somnolence.[4] However, in the last decade, a form of neuroleptanesthesia has again become popular, with the use of droperidol, which is a butyrophenone cogener of haloperidol, combined with fentanyl citrate, a synthetic opiate.[5–9]

Effects on narcotic analgesics

Generally, the antipsychotic drugs exert additive and/or synergistic effects in combination with narcotic analgesics.[10–12] The depth of meperidine, morphine, and other narcotic-induced analgesia is increased in the presence of some phenothiazine antipsychotic agents, although this effect may simply be additive rather than synergistic.[10] Among phenothiazines, promethazine appears to be antianalgesic, and others, such as perphenazine, prochlorperazine, fluphenazine, and trifluoperazine, appear to possess slight antianalgesic properties.[13] In rodents and in man, the respiratory-depressant effects of narcotic analgesics are enhanced by the presence of antipsychotic agents, probably through a synergistic interaction.[12] There is an additive sedative-hypnotic effect when meperidine is combined with promethazine.[10] Similarly, narcotic and antipsychotic drug-induced hypotension may combine to cause dramatic hypotensive episodes.[13] The mechanisms of action by which antipsychotic drugs potentiate the effects of narcotic analgesics is uncertain.

Antipsychotic compounds enhance the effects of narcotic analgesics used in anesthetic practice.[7,8] Innovar, a combination of the butyrophenone, droperidol, and the narcotic drug, fentanyl, may be effective partly because of the synergism of its components' properties.[5] However, the anesthesiologist must realize that antipsychotic drugs generally decrease narcotic requirements, and that significant respiratory depression and hypotension can occur in patients who are given therapeutic doses of a narcotic and who are concurrently receiving antipsychotic drugs.[11,12,14]

Interactions with central nervous system depressants

In animal experiments, antipsychotic drugs increase barbiturate and sedative/hypnotic-induced sleep time, and deepen barbiturate coma. Thus antipsychotic drugs, such as chlorpromazine and trifluoperazine, decrease the narcosis threshold and increase respiratory depression in the presence of central nervous system (CNS) depressants.[15-19] The few clinical reports available in man confirm these animal findings.[4,20,21] The mechanism for this interaction is uncertain at present. In patients who take antipsychotic drugs and to whom a barbiturate is administered either as a premedicant for electroconvulsant treatment or as part of a general anesthetic induction, caution is necessary in view of this drug interaction. In one study of 50 patients, chlorpromazine prolonged thiopental sleep time and reduced the thiopental requirement by 60%.[20] Thus lower doses of sedative hypnotics, or barbiturates, are probably indicated when a patient has received antipsychotic medications.

Sympathomimetic drug interactions

Since antipsychotic drugs exert central and peripheral antiadrenergic and antidopaminergic effects, their potential interactions with various pressor agents are relevant.[2] Antipsychotic agents usually block the pressor effects of norepinephrine and related *alpha*-adrenergic stimulating drugs. However, it has been shown in dogs that pretreatment with chlorpromazine can slightly enhance the pressor response to norepinephrine, which effect is attributed to the depression of baroreceptor reflexes.[22] Conversely, antipsychotic drugs, especially chlorpromazine and thioridazine, can intensify the effects of other drugs on *beta*-adrenergic receptors. This selective blockade of *alpha*-adrenergic receptors can lead to a *beta*-adrenergic preponderance by agents, such as epinephrine, that usually exert both *alpha*- and *beta*-adrenergic effects, thus causing vasodilation and subsequent hypotension. The combination of epinephrine and chlorpromazine predictably causes hypotension in animals.[22] If paradoxical *beta*-adrenergic activation occurs in individuals receiving antipsychotic drugs, treatment with the *beta*-adrenergic blocking agent, propranolol, is indicated.

Dopamine is currently used as a vasoactive agent in anesthesia. Phenothiazines and butyrophenones are especially active in blocking dopamine receptors. Thus, theoretically, dopamine pressor action may be attenuated in the presence of these drugs. However, this hypothesis is not yet substantiated.[2,23]

Anticholinergic drug interactions

Antipsychotic drugs, especially chlorpromazine and thioridazine, possess inherent anticholinergic effects that can be additive with other anticholinergic drugs, such as the antiparkinsonian agents or those anticholinergic agents used for preanesthetic medication. Since side effects from anticholinergic agents increase with age, the risk of such side effects during or after anesthesia in patients subject to antipsychotic drug therapy is greatest in the elderly. Patients who take antipsychotic drugs, especially in combination with an antiparkinsonian agent, in addition to atropine or to scopolamine, may develop peripheral anticholinergic effects, such as adynamic ileus, glaucoma, and urinary retention, as well as central anticholinergic effects, such as confusion, fever, delirium, and agitation.[24-26]

The use of noncentrally acting preanesthetic anticholinergic drugs, such as methscopolamine or glycopyrrolate, may reduce the risk of these complications.[27]

Interactions with inhalation anesthetics

In addition to the interactions already discussed, the halogenated anesthetics, enflurane and isoflurane, given in combination with antipsychotic agents including chlorpromazine, may cause hypotensive episodes.[28,29] Similarly, a combination of halothane and droperidol may increase the incidence of hypotension.[6] The mechanism by which antipsychotic drugs augment the effects of halogenated general anesthetics is not known. The adrenergic blocking effects, along with ganglionic blockade and myocardial depression, may be contributory.[20,28,29] Hypotension that is caused by a combination of inhalation anesthetics and antipsychotic agents may be treated with moderate doses of *alpha*-adrenergic vasopressors, such as norepinephrine or phenylephrine. Since this type of hypotension is often associated with hypovolemia, the replacement of fluids and/or blood is indicated.

Additional antipsychotic anesthetic interactions

Several other interactions may occur when antipsychotic drugs are used in anesthesia. Promethazine and antipsychotic drugs enhance one another's side effects.[32] Furthermore, there has been at least one report of prolonged apnea following succinylcholine administration in a patient treated with promazine, possibly due to the inhibition of plasma cholinesterase activity.[33] In addition, antipsychotic drugs intensify the effects of *alpha*-adrenergic blocking agents, such as phentolamine, and this increases a patent's tendency to develop hypotension. Furthermore, phenothiazine antipsychotic drugs, particularly thioridazine, may have some direct myocardial-depressant effects, not unlike quinidine. Concurrent use of phenothiazine antipsychotic drugs and quinidine may lead to additive myocardial depression, and this combination should probably be avoided.

Several papers have discussed the cardiovascular complications occurring in young patients who take phenothiazine medication on a regular basis.[34-36] These complications include sudden death, cardiac dysrhythmias, disturbances of conduction, and electrocardiographic changes suggestive of infarction. Biopsy and autopsy specimens of cardiac tissue may show areas of focal myocardial necrosis similar to those found after the administration of catecholamines to animals. The mechanism that produces these abnormalities is not clear and the reversibility of the lesions after discontinuance of the drug is questionable. The butyrophenones do not seem to share the myocardiotoxic potential of the phenothiazines.

Chlorpromazine and the other phenothiazines also lower the convulsive seizure threshold. Thus in theory their use with enflurane and ketamine, which can cause seizures during anesthesia, presents a potential problem. No reports of this interaction have appeared.[30]

On the other hand, antipsychotic agents prevent postoperative vomiting, presumably by blocking the medullary chemoreceptor trigger zone.[9] However, early studies on their use as antiemetics show that their advantages in this area are outweighed by their disadvantages, which include hypotension and delayed emergence from anesthesia.[4,20]

Interactions with conduction anesthesia

Serious hypotensive episodes have been reported when a patient taking chlorpromazine receives spinal or epidural anesthesia or celiac plexus block.[31] Apparently, the effects of sympathetic blockade following spinal, epidural, or celiac plexus block are additive with the hypotensive effects of chlorpromazine. As with inhalation anesthetics, the infusion of phenylephrine or norepinephrine may be indicated. However, two of the three patients described had conditions associated with deranged intravascular volume (intestinal obstruction, carcinomatosis); nor was mention made of evaluating and restoring circulating volume, an important procedure prior to any technique that causes major sympathectomy. The role of chlorpromazine under these circumstances is unclear.

Finally, one retrospective report has indicated an increased postoperative mortality rate in patients receiving long-term phenothiazine therapy.[37] In this report, 12 patients generally received ether or halothane anesthesia in combination with muscle relaxants and nitrous oxide. The eleven deaths that occurred within the first 12 postoperative days were due to several causes, including cardiac problems, respiratory arrest, and complications following adynamic ileus, a condition to which, apparently, patients receiving long-term phenothiazine therapy seem particularly susceptible.[24] Adrenocorticotropic hormone (ACTH) and "steroid hormones" have been recommended as a preventive measure during the pre- and intraoperative periods in such patients. Discontinuance of antipsychotic drugs has been recommended preoperatively and intensive monitoring has been recommended postoperatively to prevent postoperative mortality. The overall significance of the contribution of long-term phenothiazine therapy to perioperative morbidity and mortality is still undetermined. However, the autonomic imbalance created in these patients and the potential for toxic cardiomyopathy reinforce the need for careful preoperative evaluation—especially of the cardiovascular system—and the importance of intra- and postoperative monitoring.

RESERPINE (TABLE 13–2)

The rauwolfia alkaloids, including reserpine, continue to be used as effective antihypertensive agents.[2] During the 1950's, these drugs were widely used to treat mania and schizophrenia.[2,38] With the introduction of chlorpromazine as an antischizophrenic agent in the early 1950's, and with the subsequent development of related antipsychotic agents that presumably possessed fewer depressant, hypotensive, and cholinomimetic side effects, reserpine became clinically obsolete. At the height of its popularity as an antipsychotic agent, reserpine appeared to be successful in the treatment of manic and schizophrenic psychosis.[2,38]

During the past decade, psychiatrists and

Table 13–2

Some Interactions Between Reserpine and Drugs Used in Anesthesia

Reserpine	Interaction
Inhalation Drugs	↓ MAC (halothane)
Barbiturates	↑ sleep time
Sympathomimetics	↓ effect of indirect-acting agents ↑ effect of direct-acting agents
Muscle Relaxants	↑ duration of block with d-tubocurarine (animals)

psychopharmacologists have become aware that the more recent antipsychotic agents (the phenothiazines, butyrophenones, and thioxanthenes) also have serious drawbacks. Predominant among these drawbacks is that it has been discovered that long-term treatment with these agents often causes irreversible choreoathetoid tongue, body, and extremity movements, labeled "tardive dyskinesias." Considerable medicolegal and professional concern has centered on this problem.[39] Since reserpine does not cause tardive dyskinesias, it is possible that it will regain popularity and will be widely used as an alternative antipsychotic drug, especially in the treatment of chronically ill psychotic patients.

Mechanism of action

Reserpine depletes intraneuronally bound central and peripheral dopamine, norepinephrine, and serotonin, presumably by interfering with storage. Reserpine may also activate central and peripheral cholinoceptive sites. Catecholamine depletion is considered to underlie reserpine's antipsychotic and antihypertensive effects.[2,38]

Anesthetic implications

The anesthetic management of patients receiving reserpine deserves attention in several areas. These include: (1) anesthetic considerations in patients receiving electroconvulsive therapy, (2) anesthetic precautions in the administration of reserpine to patients receiving inhalation anesthetic agents, (3) anesthetic dose reduction in patients who were given reserpine and who were receiving barbiturates, and (4) analogous precautions in the administration of vasopressors.

Electroconvulsive therapy

In the 1950's, prolonged apnea and/or sudden death was reported in patients who had been given reserpine and who were receiving electroconvulsive therapy (ECT). In addition to apnea, patients developed profound hypotension and cardiac arrhythmias, leading to death in some cases. Details as to the type of anesthetics used for ECT, and, indeed, whether anesthetics were used at all, are not included in these early reports. Furthermore, the amount of reserpine administered to the patients preceding ECT was large, approximately 10 mg intramuscularly. The information on this interaction is incomplete, and, until more information is available, the use of reserpine probably should contraindicate ECT. A two-week reserpine-free period is suggested for patients who are recommended for ECT.[40,41] Alternative antihypertensive drugs should be used if possible for the patient who takes reserpine for blood pressure control and who requires ECT.

Inhalation anesthetic agents

Until the early 1960's, reserpine was incriminated in dangerous hypotensive reactions or in vascular instability when used in conjunction with such inhalation agents as cyclopropane, ether, halothane, methoxyflurane, and trichoroethylene. The literature recommended that any patient receiving general anesthesia, especially ether and halothane, be kept reserpine-free for a period of at least two weeks.[42-44] However, several well-controlled studies have demon-strated that reserpine treatment of hypertensive patients increases neither hypotensive reactions nor other adverse cardiovascular effects during general anesthesia. Currently, the consensus of opinion is that attention should be paid to the potential complications of reserpine therapy, and that its parasympathetic effects should be pretreated with an anticholinergic agent, such as atropine, in order to avoid discontinuing reserpine preoperatively.[45,46]

Reserpine decreased the minimum alveolar concentration (MAC) of halothane in an animal study; the effect appeared to be dose-dependent.[47] Speculation as to the mechanism of this interaction focused on the relationship between central catecholamine levels and anesthetic requirements. Interestingly, no comments were made as to the presence or absence of cardiovascular instability in these animals pretreated with reserpine and anesthetized with halothane.

Barbiturate-reserpine interactions

Several animal studies have demonstrated that reserpine increases barbiturate-induced sleeping time in small rodents and that the drug may increase sleeping time and sedation in man.[17,48-51] The mechanism for this effect is unknown, although it could be due to the depletion of central catecholamines and/or the augmentation of barbiturate-induced central nervous system depression. Since reserpine increases the effectiveness of a given dose of barbiturate, a lower dose of barbiturates in the patient who is given reserpine is suggested. However, few human experiments have demonstrated this interaction.[50]

Similarly, it has also been noted in rodents that reserpine decreases the ability of phenobarbital and diazepam to raise seizure thresholds, an observation that might be significant to the seizure-prone patient who receives anesthetics such as ketamine and enflurane, which are associated with the increased incidence of convulsive episodes.[52]

Interactions between reserpine and sympathomimetic drugs

Reserpine may affect exogenously administered sympathomimetic drugs. Since reserpine releases stored catecholamines, indirect-acting pressor amines, such as metaraminol, ephedrine, amphetamine, tyramine, mephentermine, phenylpropanolamine, and methylphenidate are less effective in animals that are given reserpine, and theoretically may decrease response in the patient who receives reserpine.[2,53] Conversely, probably because of the phenomenon of denervation hypersensitivity, an augmentation of the patient response to direct-acting sympathetic pressors, such as dopamine, phenylephrine, norepinephrine, and epinephrine, may occur if these agents are administered after reserpine pretreatment. Thus, in the reserpinized patient, conservative infusion of direct-acting sympathomimetic agents, rather than indirect-acting agents, is preferred for treating hypotension, should pressor agents be necessary.

Reserpine-narcotic analgesic interactions

The data on reserpine-morphine interactions in animals are difficult to evaluate. Potentiation of analgesia is apparent in some species, such as rats and rabbits. In mice, depending on the test system employed, reserpine may either potentiate or antagonize morphine analgesia.[54-56] The ability of reserpine to alter the effects of narcotic analgesics has not been well studied in man. Hence the importance of a narcotic analgesic-reserpine interaction is uncertain.

Additional reserpine-anesthetic interactions

In rabbits, the neuromuscular blocking effect of d-tubocurarine is antagonized by reserpine.[57] This is consistent with reserpine's cholinomimetic activity. Similarly, in rats,

reserpine pretreatment increases the lethality of sublethal doses of physostigmine and of neostigmine. This effect is prevented by prior administration of anticholinergic drugs.[58] No information on the significance of these interactions in human beings is available at present.

Digitalis glycosides may cause interactions when administered in patients who have received reserpine. These interactions include cardiac arrhythmias, bradycardia, and decreased ionotropic effect.[32,59] Reserpine may heighten the patient's responsiveness to thiazide diuretics. This interaction may require a readjustment of the dose of the diuretic.[59]

ANTICHOLINERGIC AGENTS

Anticholinergic agents are routinely used in the practice of psychiatry. These drugs, which include trihexyphenidyl and benztropine mesylate, are employed as antidotes to the frequent dystonias and parkinsonian side effects caused by the neuroleptic blockade of dopamine receptors. These agents treat related symptoms such as tremor, rigidity, shuffling gait, and drooling.[2]

Mechanism of action

Anticholinergic agents used in psychiatry generally exert their effects through their central and peripheral antimuscarinic actions. Thus, in addition to alleviating parkinsonian symptoms, anticholinergic drugs can cause hyperpyrexia, constipation, mydriasis, adynamic ileus, urinary retention, and other signs of heightened anticholinergic activity.[2]

Anesthetic implications

Patients who receive anticholinergic agents for the management of drug-induced parkinsonism, or who take anticholinergic drugs, such as tricyclic antidepressants, chlorpromazine, or thioridazine, are at greater risk of developing a central anticholinergic syndrome, consisting of disorientation, hallucinations, and memory loss, if centrally acting anticholinergic agents are added preoperatively.[25] Similarly, in the intraoperative and postoperative period, peripheral anticholinergic side effects are increased in patients who receive anticholinergic drugs.[24] The anticholinergic effects of various agents are additive; thus the effects of atropine or scopolamine, used preoperatively, may be augmented by the prior administration of other anticholinergics.[25] In addition, central and peripheral anticholinergic effects appear to be increased by methylphenidate, barbiturates, and procainamide. Anticholinergic agents and sympathomimetic drugs also may interact to enhance sympathetic effects caused by a shift in autonomic control (adrenergic-cholinergic imbalance).[24-60] Furthermore, meperidine has anticholinergic effects that may be additive to those of other anticholinergic agents.[61] To prevent a central anticholinergic syndrome, it may be appropriate either to eliminate completely or to reduce doses of atropine or scopolamine preoperatively, or to use a noncentrally acting anticholinergic drug, such as homatropine, glycopyrrolate, or methscopolamine as a preoperative medication.[27]

TRICYCLIC ANTIDEPRESSANTS (TABLE 13–3)

The tricyclic antidepressants are used to treat various psychiatric symptoms. These compounds, which include imipramine, amitriptyline, desipramine, nortriptyline, doxepin, and protriptyline, are related in structure to the phenothiazines; and indeed tricyclic antidepressants were originally developed as antipsychotic drugs, but were unsuccessful as such. Tricyclic antidepressants are used effectively in the treatment of severe depression. They may also be used in the treatment of chronic pain, phobic anxiety, and other psychosomatic disorders.

Table 13–3

Some Interactions Between Tricyclic Antidepressants and Drugs Used in Anesthesia

Tricyclic Antidepressants	Interaction
Narcotics	↑ analgesia ↑ respiratory depression
Barbiturates	↑ sleep time
Anticholinergics	↑ central activity ↑ peripheral activity
Sympathomimetics	↑ effect of direct-acting agents

Tricyclic antidepressants block the uptake of norepinephrine and/or of serotonin or dopamine into the presynaptic nerve ending, thereby increasing central and peripheral adrenergic tone. This effect has been linked to their antidepressant activity. The majority of tricyclic antidepressants also possess moderate anticholinergic effects, which may also alleviate depression. The anticholinergic and catecholamine uptake-blocking properties of the tricyclic antidepressants seem to cause their most significant clinical interactions with anesthetic agents.[2]

Vasopressor interactions

The tricyclic antidepressants, imipramine and desipramine, increase two- to tenfold the pressor response to injected, direct-acting sympathetic amines including norepinephrine, epinephrine, and phenylephrine. This response has resulted in hyperthermia, sweating, hypertensive crises, severe headache, rupture of cerebral blood vessels, and death. Indeed, these effects, elicited under controlled conditions, are more dramatic than the effects of a combination of direct-acting sympathetic amines and a monoamine oxidase inhibitor, a more widely feared drug-drug interaction.[62-65] Furthermore, tricyclic antidepressant-sympathetic amine interaction has occurred clinically in dental patients in Great Britain following the administration of local anesthetics to which norepinephrine was added as a vasoconstrictor.[66–68] The potentiation of the pressor action of epinephrine is not as pronounced as that of norepinephrine. However, epinephrine-induced changes in heart rate and rhythm may be dangerously potentiated by a tricyclic antidepressant.[64] Whether the same potential for hypertension and/or for disturbances in cardiac rate and rhythm exists with other drugs used during anesthesia that have sympathomimetic and/or anticholinergic effects, such as ketamine, pancuronium, gallamine, and fluroxene, is not known. However, in a recent study, pancuronium caused ventricular tachycardia and fibrillation in 40% of dogs anesthetized with halothane after two weeks of imipramine pretreatment.[62a] The mechanism of action by which these hypertensive crises occur has been tentatively linked to the amine reuptake-blocking properties of tricyclic antidepressants.[63] This ability to block amine reuptake is shared with several other drugs, including cocaine. Alternatively, it is possible that the induction of receptor hypersensitivity by the tricyclic antidepressant affects this drug interaction.[64]

In view of this possibility, it is advisable to stop all tricyclic antidepressants two weeks prior to an operation. If this is not possible because of the patient's psychiatric condition, and if a surgical procedure must be performed while tricyclic antidepressants are present, avoidance of direct-acting sympathetic pressor amines is suggested. Treatment of hypertensive crises, if they develop, consists in the administration of chlorpromazine or of an *alpha*-adrenergic blocking agent, such as phentolamine, or of the vasodilator, sodium nitroprusside. Cooling measures should be instituted if the patient is hyperpyrexic.

The synthetic vasoconstrictor felypressin (2-phenylalanine, 8-lysine vasopressin) does not interact adversely with tricyclic antidepressants. It has been recommended as a vasoconstrictor in a concentration of 0.03 IU/ml not to exceed a total of 8 ml, for use in conjunction with local anesthetics in patients receiving tricyclic antidepressants.[64,66] Currently, felypressin is not available in the United States.

Anticholinergic drug interactions

As mentioned previously, tricyclic antidepressants possess central and peripheral anticholinergic activity. Since the anticholinergic side effects of various drugs are additive, preoperative treatment with centrally active anticholinergic drugs may interact with tricyclic antidepressants and cause confusion and delirium (a central anticholinergic syndrome) during the postoperative period.[25,69] Preoperative use of noncentrally acting anticholinergic agents is suggested in the presence of tricyclic antidepressants, especially in elderly patients.[27]

Narcotic analgesic interactions

Although little data exist to support the contention that tricyclic antidepressants augment the analgesic and other effects of narcotic analgesics in human beings, imipramine and amitriptyline potentiate morphine analgesia in mice, and increase meperidine-induced respiratory depression.[70] These effects are theoretically important to the anesthesiologist and suggest lower doses of narcotics in patients taking tricyclic antidepressants.

Barbiturate-sedative hypnotic interactions

Some animal experiments suggest that tricyclic antidepressants increase the sedative and hypnotic effects of barbiturates. Increased tricyclic antidepressant lethality occurs in the presence of a barbiturate and vice versa. Imipramine has been known to prolong hexobarbital narcosis, possibly by means of enzyme inhibition, and to prolong apnea following thiopental administration in man. Thus tricyclic antidepressants probably enhance the CNS-depressant effects of barbiturates and related sedative hypnotics.[18] Awareness of this potential interaction suggests lower doses of barbiturates in patients receiving tricyclic antidepressants.

Other interactions

In addition to the interactions discussed, several other tricyclic antidepressant-anesthetic interactions have been described. In rabbits, the tricyclic antidepressants imipramine, amitriptyline, and protriptyline have increased the local anesthetic effect of lidocaine and procaine on the cornea.[71] This is probably related to the sedating effect of the tricyclic antidepressants, although other mechanisms may be implicated.

In animal experiments, tricyclic antidepressants antagonize the cardiovascular effects of propranolol. The mechanism of this interaction is probably related to the anticholinergic activity of antidepressants. The significance of this interaction in human beings is not known, although propranolol has successfully treated the cardiotoxicity associated with tricyclic antidepressant toxicity in man.[72,73]

MONOAMINE OXIDASE INHIBITORS (TABLE 13–4)

Prior to the development and popularization of tricyclic antidepressants, a variety of monoamine oxidase inhibitors (MAOI) were developed and were found to be effective as antidepressant agents. Although they have been superseded by the tricyclic antidepressants, MAOI are still used in psychiatry. At a time when the medicolegal sanctions against ECT are increasing, MAOI are not infrequently used as a "second line" of drugs to treat depression. Indeed, recent reviews suggest that these drugs may be used safely in combination with tricyclic antidepressants in the refractory-depressed patient. Currently, in the United States, only one MAOI, tranylcypromine, is approved for the treatment of depression. Another,

Table 13–4

Some Interactions Between Monoamine Oxidase Inhibitors (MAOI) and Drugs Used in Anesthesia

MAOI	Interaction
Inhalation Drugs	muscle stiffness, hyperpyrexia, (halothane in animals)
Narcotics	meperidine → excitatory syndrome → ↑ narcotic effect and coma
Barbiturates	↑ sleep time
Anticholinergics	↑ central activity
Sympathomimetics	↑ ↑ effects of indirect-acting agents ↑ effects of direct-acting agents ↑ dopamine effects
Muscle Relaxants	↑ duration of block with succinylcholine (phenelzine decreases plasma cholinesterase)

pargyline, is approved as an antihypertensive agent. However, other MAOI are used outside the United States.

Mechanism of action

MAOI are considered to be effective in the treatment of depression because they inhibit monoamine oxidase. These drugs also inhibit other enzymes, particularly hepatic microsomal enzymes involved in the metabolism of many drugs. Monoamine oxidase enzymes are ubiquitous in the body, with high concentrations in liver and intestine.[74] Monoamine oxidase is a major intraneuronal enzyme necessary for the oxidative deamination of serotonin, norepinephrine, and dopamine. The norepinephrine (catecholamine) hypothesis of depression asserts that MAOI are effective because they allow the repletion of monoamine stores in the brain. This ability to inhibit the metabolism of sympathetic amines and of other monoamines underlies the majority of their interactions with anesthetics and contributes to the inherent dangers of MAOI.[2,75]

Sympathetic amine interactions

Monoamine oxidase inhibitors are infamous for their ability to interact with some sympathetic compounds to cause the dangerous and often lethal hypertensive crisis. The hypertensive crisis may consist of precipitous hypertension, hyperpyrexia, sweating, tachycardia, throbbing occipital headache, and intracranial bleeding. It appears to be caused by a "sympathetic storm," and is similar to the effects of an overdose of amphetamines.[74,76–84]

Since MAOI act primarily intraneuronally in the central and peripheral nervous system, indirect-acting sympathetic amines are more likely to interact with them to cause hypertensive crises, because these compounds release intraneuronal monoamines. Thus amphetamine-like psychostimulants, including amphetamine, methamphetamine, methylphenidate, and other related drugs are likely to interact with MAOI in this connection. Similarly, indirect-acting vasopressors, including tyramine, mephentermine, metaraminol, ephedrine, and phenylpropanolamine, all of which release norepinephrine and dopamine from bound intracellular neuronal stores, can interact with MAOI and cause hypertensive crises.[64,65,77–79,85,86] Acute administration of reserpine to MAOI-pretreated patients may also lead to a hypertensive crisis, since reserpine depletes intracellular catecholamines by causing their release from bound stores.[87] The same phenomenon occurs with guanethidine and, similarly, with L-DOPA, a dopamine precursor, which may interact with MAOI to cause reactions that closely resemble a hypertensive crisis.[88,89] The MAOI augment and prolong the pressor effects and enhance the action of dopamine, but not of norepinephrine, on the contractile force of the heart.[81]

Interestingly, direct-acting sympathetic amines, including norepinephrine and epinephrine, interact less with MAOI.[64,65] Although some anecdotal reports indicate that these agents cause hypertension, controlled studies show only mild hypertensive effects when direct-acting sympathetic amines and MAOI are used concurrently.[64,90] Pharmacologically, the reason for this lack of reaction may be that exogenous, direct-acting sympathetic amines do not flood the intracellular site of action of the MAOI with monoamines, and are in part degraded in an alternative route by the extracellular enzyme, catechol-o-methyl transferase (COMT). The hypertensive response has been proposed because of the "denervation hypersensitivity" caused by the MAOI. This hypertension has been noted primarily during repeated MAOI administration, usually after orthostatic hypotension has developed. Oral, but not intravenous, phenylephrine (a sympathetic amine with more direct than indirect action) has been reported to cause hypertensive crisis in combination with MAOI. This interaction is believed to occur because of the inhibition of gastrointestinal monoamine oxidase, which usually degrades orally administered phenylephrine before its systemic absorption.

Investigators suggest that hypertensive crises can be avoided by the discontinuance of monoamine oxidase inhibitors two to three weeks prior to anesthetic administration. If pressor amines must be used during anesthesia in patients who are receiving MAOI, it is suggested that low doses of direct-acting amines, such as norepinephrine, be used, rather than indirect-acting amines. If a hypertensive crisis occurs, it is best treated with *alpha*-adrenergic blocking agents, such as phentolamine and/or chlorpromazine, or with the vasodilator, sodium nitroprusside, in addition to cooling the patient to alleviate hyperpyrexia.[64,83,91] Cardiac arrhythmias may be controlled by a *beta*-adrenergic blocking drug.[81] However, one must institute an *alpha*-blockade prior to the administration of *beta*-adrenergic blocking agents in order to prevent further hypertension from unopposed *alpha* activity.

Narcotic analgesic interactions

In addition to interactions with sympathetic amines, MAOI have been found to interact with the narcotic analgesic, meperidine[92-97] (see Chapter 16, second case report). In this case, a syndrome manifested by agitation, excitement, restlessness, hypertension, headache, rigidity, convulsions, and hyperpyrexia (all symptoms similar to the hypertensive crisis caused by MAOI-sympathetic amine interaction) occurs. A similar reaction has been observed between phenelzine and dextromethorphan.[98] Morphine has not been implicated as a cause of this effect clinically.[99] However, a study in mice did show that pretreatment with MAOI increased the mortality not only from meperidine, but from morphine, pentazocine, and phenazocine.[100] The mechanism by which this drug interaction occurs is uncertain. However, based on animal experiments, several authors postulate that the response is caused by the elevation of serotonin levels in the brain following monoamine oxidase inhibition in the presence of meperidine.[94,100,101]

Although prevention is the best treatment of a narcotic-MAOI interaction of this type, various authors recommend the administration of prednisolone hemisuccinate, 25 mg intravenously, as well as other supportive measures as indicated, and the control of the patient blood pressure if arterial blood pressure reaches excessive levels.[92,93]

Alternatively, narcotic analgesics, especially meperidine, have been reported to interact with MAOI to cause coma, depressed respiration, and hypotension, responses apparently caused by the potentiation of primary narcotic effects. The mechanism by which this interaction occurs has been attributed to the inhibition of narcotic metabolism in the liver by an action of MAOI on enzymes other than monoamine oxidase that increase free narcotic.[96,97] Treatment, which is primarily supportive, may include the narcotic antagonist, naloxone.[102,103]

In addition, prompt acidification of the urine, using lysine or arginine hydrochloride or sodium biphosphate intravenously, and the production of a large volume of urine have been used to hasten meperidine excretion.[84]

One-quarter to one-fifth of the usual narcotic amount should be given to the patient taking MAOI who, for whatever reason, must receive a narcotic; careful observation of the patient over the next 15 to 20 minutes for any changes in vital signs or level of consciousness is important. Churchill-Davidson described a "sensitivity test," using small incremental hourly injections of morphine (or meperidine), with careful observation of the patient for signs of adverse reaction.[104] However, the unpredictability of the response to meperidine of the patient receiving MAOI therapy probably warrants the avoidance of this drug altogether, with the use of morphine in reduced doses if a narcotic is necessary.

Sedative hypnotic and barbiturate interactions

MAOI have been reported to augment barbiturate and sedative hypnotic effects in animals and in man.[105] The mechanism by which this occurs is probably due to MAOI inhibition of liver microsomal enzymes necessary for barbiturate detoxification. Experimentally, a combination of an MAOI and a barbiturate increases sleep time, duration of anesthesia, and lethality in animals. Similar effects have been noted in man.[105] Thus, in a patient pretreated with MAOI, lower doses of barbiturates should be used.

Muscle relaxant interactions

One case of prolonged apnea following succinylcholine administration for ECT has been reported in a patient receiving the

MAOI phenelzine. This response was attributed to a decrease in plasma cholinesterase. Investigation of plasma cholinesterase levels in an additional series of 22 patients taking phenelzine and other MAOI revealed depressed enzyme activity in 40% of the patients taking phenelzine and normal levels in patients receiving the other MAOI.[106]

To date, no MAOI except phenelzine has been reported to exert this effect on plasma cholinesterase. After the discontinuance of phenelzine, plasma cholinesterase levels return to normal.[106]

One animal study has investigated the effect of d-tubocurarine on long-term MAOI therapy and found that the relaxant effect is not prolonged.[107] In the absence of clinical reports on this interaction, it is probably safe to use this nondepolarizing relaxant in patients. There are no studies available on gallamine or pancuronium in this context.

Miscellaneous MAOI-anesthetic interactions

Several other interactions between MAOI and agents used in anesthesia have been observed. In cats, MAOI in conjunction with halothane cause muscle stiffness.[108] In addition, pheniprazine and nialamide are reported to cause hyperpyrexia during halothane inhalation. Propranolol, given in association with an MAOI, has caused a hypertensive crisis, presumably by the blockade of *beta*-adrenergic receptors and the imbalanced activation of *alpha*-adrenergic receptors.[109] Hypotension has occurred when MAOI and thiazide diuretics are given concurrently.[110] Furthermore, MAOI have increased anticholinergic effects when given together with atropine.[81] Finally, one patient, receiving a large dose of droperidol in addition to a monoamine oxidase inhibitor, developed cardiovascular depression that lasted 36 hours.[111]

CASE REPORT

A 45-year-old 90-kg man required emergency repair of right wrist lacerations. He was moderately obese but was otherwise in good health. He was being treated for depression with tranylcypromine, 30 mg q.d. After premedication with diazepam, 10 mg p.o., he arrived in the operating room.

This patient presents several anesthetic problems: obesity, an emergency operation, and MAOI therapy. Detailed discussion of the patient's management as related to his obesity is omitted. Airway problems are anticipated, as well as possible intraoperative and postoperative problems with ventilation. A patient who requires an emergency operation may have a full stomach, and may also have an unknown intravascular volume status. Clinical tests of volume, such as tilting, may be misleading because of the MAOI therapy, which in itself can cause orthostatic hypotension. Because the operation is an emergency, a two-week MAOI-free period is not possible. The anesthetic technique and agents chosen must minimize the likelihood of an adverse drug interaction between anesthetic drugs and the MAOI.

Regional techniques may be considered. A brachial plexus block through the axillary route might be selected. A local anesthetic, such as bupivacaine, could offer a long-acting block, without concomitant vasoconstrictors such as epinephrine. Blood pressure change, due to sympathectomy, is not likely with this technique, although there is the possibility of inadvertent intravascular injection and subsequent hyper- and/or hypotension that might require treatment. In the event of hypotension, a direct-acting vasopressor, such as phenylephrine, in titrated amounts is preferred to indirect-acting vasopressors, such as ephedrine or mephentermine, because phenylephrine is less likely to cause extreme hypertension. Intravenous analgesic supplementation of the block with meperidine could be hazardous. Morpine should be selected if a narcotic is necessary, using small amounts of drug and watching for adverse effects such as a decreased level of consciousness or hypotension.

Alternatively, general anesthetic techniques may be considered. Balanced techniques, involving narcotics, are probably not advisable. Inhalation techniques with agents such as halothane or enflurane could be used with appropriate precautions, involving vasopressors as noted above. A rapid induction-intubation sequence is needed because of the "full stomach." Caution is indicated in the use of narcotics in the recovery room; to avoid meperidine and to use small increments of morphine is suggested. Constant temperature monitoring is important. Equipment for direct arterial pressure monitoring should be immediately available, as should agents for the rapid control of hypertension, such as sodium nitroprusside. Awareness of the patient's drug history and of the possible adverse drug interactions are crucial for the effective management of this patient.

LITHIUM CARBONATE (TABLE 13–5)

In 1949, Cade noted the effectiveness of lithium in the treatment of mania, and the drug has been used for this indication in the United States since the early 1960's.[112] More recently, lithium has proved useful in the prevention of recurrent depression.[113] In addition, lithium therapy has been tried in over 30 other disorders, psychiatric and nonpsychiatric, ranging from alcoholism and thyrotoxicosis to Huntington's chorea.[114]

Lithium is a monovalent cation, the lightest of the alkali metals, and in the same group of elements on the Periodic Table as sodium and potassium. It generally occurs in nature as a salt (lithium carbonate, lithium chloride), rather than as a free element, and is ubiquitous. The ion has no known physiologic role.[113] Approximately 95% of ingested lithium is excreted by the kidneys, complete excretion requiring 10 to 14 days in both short- and long-term therapy.[115]

At the cellular level, lithium acts as an imperfect substitute for Na^+. It moves intracellularly during depolarization, but is extruded from the cell at a rate only 10% of that of Na^+. Lithium, therefore, accumulates within the cell and is in a position to affect processes that depend on movement of monovalent cations.[115] Many studies have dealt with the effects of lithium on brain amine metabolism. Lithium inhibits the release of norepinephrine and serotonin, increases the reuptake of norepinephrine, and possibly increases the synthesis and the turnover rate of serotonin. This agent has little effect on dopaminergic systems. Lithium inhibits activation of adenylate cyclase in the CNS of experimental animals. It is not yet certain which, if any, of these actions are important for therapy.[112,113]

The anesthetic implications of lithium therapy have become a concern with the appearance of several case reports in the recent literature that describe probable anesthetic drug interactions with lithium.[116–118]

Lithium-muscle relaxant interaction

The first problem noted was prolonged neuromuscular blockade following pancuronium bromide and succinylcholine hydrochloride in patients receiving lithium carbonate.[116,118] Hill and colleagues subsequently investigated the effect of lithium treatment on the neuromuscular blockade in dogs following the administration of succinylcholine, decamethonium, d-tubocurarine, gallamine, or pancuronium.[119] They found that lithium prolonged the blockade of succinylcholine, decamethonium, and pancuronium, but that it had no effect on the

Table 13–5

Some Interactions between Lithium Carbonate and Drugs Used in Anesthesia

Lithium Carbonate	Interaction
Barbiturates	↑ sleep time
Muscle Relaxants	↑ duration of block with pancuronium, succinylcholine, decamethonium

blockade produced by gallamine or d-tubo-curarine. Lithium also prolonged the reversal time of pancuronium by neostigmine. There was no effect on plasma cholinesterase activity in 66 manic-depressive patients receiving chronic lithium therapy.[119] The effect of lithium on the neuromuscular blockade of succinylcholine and of decamethonium, as well as the prolonged reversal of pancuronium, are compatible with the findings of Vizi et al., who reported that lithium inhibited acetylcholine synthesis and release in animal preparations.[120] The effect on pancuronium blockade is more difficult to explain and implies differences in the mechanism of action between pancuronium and the two other nondepolarizing drugs—d-tubocurarine and gallamine. Pancuronium may have depolarizing as well as nondepolarizing activity at the neuromuscular junction. Another possibility is that, by virtue of the steroid moiety in its structure, pancuronium may have a more profound effect on the cellular distribution of sodium and potassium than either d-tubocurarine or gallamine, particularly if pancuronium possesses mineralocorticoid activity.

Lithium-barbiturate interaction

Jephcott and Kerry reported a case of prolonged recovery from barbiturate anesthesia following electroconvulsive therapy in a patient taking lithium carbonate.[117] The patient's serum lithium level was 3.4 meq/L (therapeutic range 0.9 to 1.5 meq/L), but preanesthetic evaluation had revealed no evidence of lithium toxicity. Mannisto and Saarnivaara studied the effects of short- and long-term lithium chloride treatment on sleeping time following the administration of intravenous thiopental, methohexital, ketamine, propanidid, alphaxalone-alphadolone acetate, and diazepam in white mice.[121] They found prolonged sleep time following thiopental, methohexital, and diazepam after short-term treatment with lithium chloride, but no significant effects after prolonged treatment (21 days). How-ever, serum lithium levels in the short-term experiments were much higher (2.3 ± 0.2 meq/L) than in the long-term experiments (0.6 ± 0.1 meq/L), which might account for some of the difference in results.

There have been no reports to date of interactions between lithium and either inhalation anesthetics or local anesthetics.

The therapeutic range for serum lithium concentration is narrow, with levels below 0.8 meq/L generally ineffective and levels above 1.5 meq/L toxic. Toxic symptoms are manifested primarily in the gastrointestinal, muscular, and central nervous systems, and range from very mild, such as nausea or fine tremor of the hands, to severe, including convulsions and death. It is not uncommon for patients to become intoxicated and to develop a confusional state with blood levels in the "therapeutic" range, particularly in elderly patients, who excrete lithium more slowly than do the young.[113,122,123]

Lithium crosses the placental barrier rapidly; concentrations of the ion at the time of delivery are similar in maternal, umbilical, and neonatal serum.[124] Severe maternal and neonatal lithium toxicity developed in a patient who took lithium during the last month of pregnancy. The patient received thiazide diuretics simultaneously, and in addition was on a sodium-restricted diet. Maternal serum lithium concentration immediately after delivery was 3.4 meq/L, whereas that of the newborn was 2.4 meq/L.[125]

Administration of diuretics or restriction of sodium is an added hazard to patients receiving lithium. Sodium loading promotes the excretion of lithium, and sodium depletion causes retention of the ion through renal mechanisms at the proximal tubule.[115] Short-term diuretic therapy can cause toxicity quickly.[126] Diuretics that deplete both sodium and potassium, such as thiazides, ethacrynic acid, and furosemide, are more hazardous in this regard than are the potassium-sparing agents, namely spironolactone and triamterene.[127] Treatment of lithium toxicity includes support of vital functions. Osmotic diuresis, alkalinization of the urine, and administration of aminophylline are important therapeutic modalities. Dialysis may be used in severe cases.[113]

Several side effects of lithium therapy may interest the anesthesiologist. Repeated lithium therapy causes a benign and reversible depression of electrocardiogram T-waves. In addition, some patients may develop a nephrogenic diabetes insipidus that is resistant to antidiuretic hormone. This syndrome resolves when lithium therapy is stopped. A few patients may develop goiter. These patients generally remain euthyroid, and the gland shrinks when lithium treatment is discontinued.[115]

CASE REPORT

A 64-year-old 70-kg man was scheduled for cataract extraction under general anesthesia. Preoperative evaluation revealed a long history of manic-depressive psychosis that had been successfully treated with lithium carbonate, 300 mg q.i.d., for the past two years. The remainder of his examination was unremarkable and preoperative laboratory studies including electrolytes were normal: The patient's lithium level was 1.2 meq/L.

In considering the anesthetic management of this patient, several points are important. First, from his preoperative evaluation, he seems to be in optimal condition for an elective operation. His lithium level is in the "therapeutic" range, and he manifests no signs of lithium toxicity. Second, the operation necessitates endotracheal anesthesia, which should be accomplished by maintaining the patient's intraocular pressure at or below preinduction levels. One could proceed with an inhalation induction using halothane and endotracheal intubation at the appropriate depth of anesthesia, thereby avoiding those muscle relaxants and barbiturates whose actions might be prolonged by lithium. If a muscle relaxant is deemed necessary, a nondepolarizing drug not known to interact with lithium (gallamine or d-tubocurarine) would be the best choice. Gallamine is preferable if used with

halothane because of its vagolytic effect, unless one seeks to obtain some degree of hypotension. The effect of barbiturates in man with nontoxic serum lithium levels is not known. However, in view of the animal data, low doses of barbiturate in the presence of "therapeutic" serum lithium levels are probably safe. Thus either an inhalation technique or a balanced anesthetic technique can be used in this patient, depending on the circumstances.

In conclusion, it is clear that psychotropic drugs frequently interact with drugs used in anesthesia. Psychotropic medications are widely used in the practice both of psychiatry and of general medicine. Thus it is important for an anesthesiologist to elicit a complete preoperative drug history for all patients. A close working relationship between the psychiatrist and the anesthesiologist is important for the anesthetic management of the patient who is treated with psychotropic medications.

REFERENCES

1. Snyder, S. H.: The dopamine hypothesis of schizophrenia. Am. J. Psychiatry, *133*:197, 1976.
2. Goodman, L. S., and Gilman, A. (Eds.): The Pharmacological Basis of Therapeutics. 5th Edition. New York, Macmillan, 1975.
3. Laborit, H., Huguenard, P., and Allaume, R.: Un nouveau stabilisateur végétatif (le 4460 RP). Presse Méd., *60*:206, 1952.
4. Inglis, J. M., and Barrow, M. E. H.: Premedication—a reassessment. Proc. R. Soc. Med., *58*:29, 1965.
5. Holderness, M. C., Chase, P. E., and Dripps, R.D.: A narcotic analgesic and a butyrophenone with nitrous oxide for general anesthesia. Anesthesiology, *24*:336, 1963.
6. Kreuscher, H.: Modifications of the classic neuroleptoanalgesic technique. Int. Anesthesiol. Clin., *11*:71, 1973.
7. Corssen, G.: Neuroleptanalgesia and anesthesia in obstetrics. Clin. Obstet. Gynecol., *17*:241, 1974.
8. Sadove, M.S., et al.: Clinical study of droperidol in the prevention of the side effects of ketamine anesthesia. Anesth. Analg., (Cleve.), *50*:526, 1971.
9. Foldes, F.F.: The prevention of psychotomimetic side effects of ketamine. Proceedings of the second ketamine symposium, Mainze, 1972. *In* Ketamine: New Information in Research and Clinical Practice. Edited by N. Gemperle, H.

Kreuscherz and D. Langrehr. Anesthesiology and Resuscitation Series, Vol. 69. Berlin and Heidelberg, and New York, Springer-Verlag, 1973.

10. Keats, A.S., Telford, J., and Kurosu, Y.: "Potentiation" of meperidine by promethazine. Anesthesiology, 22:34, 1961.

11. Jackson, C. L., and Smith, D.: Analgesic properties of mixtures of chlorpromazine with morphine and meperidine. Ann. Intern. Med., 45:640, 1956.

12. Lambertson, C. J., Wendel, H., and Longenhagen, J. B.: The separate and combined respiratory effects of chlorpromazine and meperidine in normal men controlled at 46 mm Hg alveolar P_{CO_2}. J. Pharmacol. Exp. Ther., 131:381, 1961.

13. Dundee, J. W., Nicholl, R. M., and Moore, J.: Clinical studies of induction agents. X: The effect of phenothiazine premedication on thiopentone anaesthesia. Br. J. Anaesth., 36:106, 1964.

14. Prasad, C. R., and Kar, K.: Effect of atropine alone and in combination with tranquilizers on morphine-induced analgesia. Curr. Sci., 35:308, 1966.

15. Morris, R. W.: Effects of phenothiazines on pentobarbital-induced sleep in mice. Arch. Int. Pharmacodyn Ther., 161:380, 1966.

16. Kissil, D., and Yelnosky, J.: A comparison of the effects of chlorpromazine and droperidol on the respiratory response to CO_2. Arch. Int. Pharmacodyn. Ther., 172:73, 1968.

17. Brodie, B. B.: Potentiating action of chlorpromazine and reserpine. Nature, 175:1133, 1955.

18. Dobkin, A. B.: Potentiation of thiopental anaesthesia by derivatives and analogues of phenothiazine. Anesthesiology, 21:292, 1960.

19. Dobkin, A. B.: Potentiation of thiopental anaesthesia with Tigan, Panectyl, Benadryl, Gravol, Marzine, Histadyl, Librium and Haloperidol. Can. Anaesth. Soc. J., 8:265, 1961.

20. Dripps, R.D., et al.: The use of chlorpromazine in anesthesia and surgery. Ann. Surg., 142:775, 1955.

21. Wallis, R.: Potentiation of hypnotics and analgesics: clinical experience with chlorpromazine. N. Y. State J. Med., 55:243, 1955.

22. Eggers, G. N., Corssen, G., and Allen, C.: Comparison of vasopressor responses in the presence of phenothiazine derivatives. Anesthesiology, 20:261, 1959.

23. Campbell, J. B.: Long-term treatment of Parkinson's disease with levodopa. Neurology, 20:18, 1970.

24. Warnes, H., Lehman, H. E., and Ban, T. A.: Adynamic ileus during psychoactive medication: a report of three fatal and five severe cases. Can. Med. Assoc. J., 96:1112, 1967.

25. El-Yousef, M. K., et al.: Reversal of antiparkinsonian drug toxicity by physostigmine: a controlled study. Am. J. Psychiatry, 130:141, 1973.

26. Grant, W. M.: Ocular complications of drugs. Glaucoma. J.A.M.A., 207:2089, 1969.

27. Janowsky, D. S., and Janowsky, E. C.: Methscopolamine as a preanesthetic medication (Letter to the Editor). Can. Anaesth. Soc. J., 23:334, 1976.

28. Gold, M. I.: Tranquilizers in the surgical patient. Surgery, 56:1027, 1964.

29. Gold, M. I.: Profound hypotension associated with preoperative use of phenothiazines. Anesth. Analg. (Cleve.), 53:844, 1974.

30. Hatch, R. C.: Ketamine catalepsy and anesthesia in dogs pretreated with antiserotonergic or antidopaminergic neuroleptics or with anticholinergic agents. Pharmacol. Res. Commun., 6:289, 1974.

31. Moore, D.C., and Bridenbaugh, L. D.: Chlorpromazine: a report of one death and eight near fatalities following its use in conjunction with spinal, epidural and celiac plexus block. Surgery, 40:543, 1956.

32. Swidler, G.: Handbook of Drug Interactions. New York, Wiley-Interscience, 1971.

33. Regan, A. G., and Aldrete, J. A.: Prolonged apnea after administration of promazine hydrochloride following succinylcholine infusion. Anesth. Analg. (Cleve.), 46:315, 1967.

34. Alexander, C. S., and Nino, A.: Cardiovascular complications in young patients taking psychotropic drugs. Am. Heart J., 78:757, 1969.

35. Fletcher, G. F., Kazamias, T. M., and Wenger, N. K.: Cardiotoxic effects of Mellaril: conduction disturbances and supraventricular arrhythmias. Am. Heart J., 78:135, 1969.

36. Editorial: Cardiovascular complications from psychotropic drugs. Br. Med. J., 1:3, 1971.

37. Matsuki, A., et al.: Excessive mortality in schizophrenic patients on chronic phenothiazine treatment. Agressologie, 13:407, 1972.

38. Alper, M. H., Flacke, W., and Krager, O.: Pharmacology of reserpine and its implications for anesthesia. Anesthesiology, 24:524, 1963.

39. Fann, W. E., Davis, J. M., and Janowsky, D. S.: The prevalence of tardive dyskinesias in mental hospital patients. Dis. Nerv. Sys., 33:182, 1972.

40. Foster, M. W., Jr., and Gayle, R. F., Jr.: Dangers in combining reserpine with electroconvulsive therapy. J.A.M.A., 154:1520, 1955.

41. Bracha, S., and Hes, J. P.: Death occurring during combined reserpine-electroshock therapy. Am. J. Psychiatry, 133:257, 1956.

42. Coakley, C. S., Alpert, S., and Boling, J. S.: Circulatory responses during anesthesia of patients on rauwolfia therapy. J.A.M.A., 161:1143, 1956.

43. Ziegler, C. H., and Lovette, J. B.: Operative complications after therapy with reserpine and reserpine compounds. J.A.M.A., 176:916, 1961.

44. Smessaert, A. A., and Hicks, R. G.: Problems caused by rauwolfia drugs during anesthesia and surgery. New York State J. Med., 61:2399, 1961.

45. Munson, W. M., and Jenicek, J. A.: Effect of anesthetic agents on patients receiving reserpine therapy. Anesthesiology, 23:741, 1962.

46. Katz, R. L., Weintraub, H. D., and Papper, E. M.: Anesthesia, surgery and rauwolfia. Anesthesiology, 25:142, 1964.

47. Miller, R. D., Way, W. L., and Eger, E. T.: The effects of *alpha*-methyldopa, reserpine, guanethidine, and iproniazid on minimum alveolar anesthetic requirement (MAC). Anesthesiology, 29:1153, 1968.

48. Child, K. J., Sutherland, P., and Tomich, E. G.: Some effects of reserpine on barbitone anesthesia in mice. Biochem. Pharmacol., *6*:252, 1961.
49. Lessin, A. W., and Parkes, M. W.: The relationship between sedation and body temperature in the mouse. Br. J. Pharmacol., *12*:245, 1957.
50. Ominsky, A. J., and Wollman, H.: Hazards of general anesthesia in the reserpinized patient. Anesthesiology, *30*:443, 1969.
51. Tammisto, T., et al.: The effect of reserpine, chlordiazepoxide and imipramine treatment on the potency of thiopental in man. Ann. Chir. Gynaecol. *356*:323, 1967.
52. Gray, W. D., and Rauh, C. E.: The anticonvulsant action of inhibitors of carbonic anhydrase: relation to endogenous amines in the brain. J. Pharmacol. Exp. Ther., *115*:127, 1967.
53. Gelder, M. G., and Vane, J. R.: Interaction of the effects of tyramine, amphetamine, and reserpine in man. Psychopharmacologia, *3*:231, 1962.
54. Matilla, M. J., and Saarnivaara, L.: Potentiation with indomethacin of the morphine analgesia in mice and rabbits. Ann. Med. Exp. Biol. Fenn., *45*:360, 1967.
55. Ross, J. W., and Ashford, A.: The effect of reserpine and *alpha* methyldopa on the analgesic action of morphine in the mouse. J. Pharm. Pharmacol., *19*:709, 1967.
56. Tabojnikova, M., and Kovalcik, V.: On the mechanism of the inhibiting effect of reserpine on morphine. Act. Nerv. Super., *9*:317, 1967.
57. Carrier, G. O., Pegram, B. L., and Carrier, O.: Antagonistic effects of reserpine on d-tubocurarine action on motor function of rabbits. Eur. J. Pharmacol., *6*:125, 1969.
58. Janowsky, D. S., Pechnick, R., and Janowsky, E. C.: Lethal effects of reserpine plus physostigmine and neostigmine in mice. Clin. Exp. Pharmacol. Physiol., *3*:483, 1976.
59. Therapeutic Drug Interactions. Edited by M. S. Cohen. Madison, Wisconsin, Drug Information Center, University of Wisconsin Medical Center, 1970.
60. Meyler, L., and Herxheimer, A. (Eds.): Side Effects of Drugs. Baltimore, Williams & Wilkins, 1968, Vol. VI.
61. Hartshorn, E. A.: Handbook of Drug Interactions. 2nd Edition. Hamilton, Illinois, Drug Intelligence Publications, 1973.
62. Vapaatalo, H. I., and Torofi, P.: Effect of some antidepressive drugs on the blood pressure responses to the sympathomimetic amines. Ann. Med. Exp. Biol. Fenn., *45*:399, 1967.
62a. Edwards, R. P., et al.: Cardiac responses to imipramine and pancuronium during anesthesia with halothane or enflurane. Anesthesiology, *50*:421, 1979.
63. Svedmyr, N.: The influence of a tricyclic antidepressive agent (protriptyline) on some of the circulatory effects of noradrenaline and adrenaline in man. Life Sci., *7*:77, 1968.
64. Boakes, A. J., et al.: Interactions between sympathomimetic amines and antidepressant agents in man. Br. Med. J., *1*:311, 1973.
65. Boakes, A. J.: Vasoconstrictors in Local Anaesthetics and Tricyclic Antidepressants. *In* Drug Interactions. Edited by D. G. Grahame-Smith. Baltimore, University Park Press, 1977.
66. Verrill, P. J.: Adverse reactions to local anaesthetics and vasoconstrictor drugs. Practitioner, *218*:380, 1975.
67. Goldman, V.: Local anaesthetics containing vasoconstrictors. Br. Med. J., *1*:175, 1971.
68. Jori, A.: Potentiation of noradrenaline toxicity by drug antihistaminic activity. J. Pharm. Pharmacol., *18*:824, 1966.
69. Milner, G., and Hills, N.: Adynamic ileus and nortriptyline. Br. Med. J., *1*:841, 1966.
70. Griffin, J. P., and D'Arcy, P. F.: A Manual of Adverse Drug Interactions. Bristol, John Wright and Sons, 1975.
71. Lechat, P., Fontagne, J., and Giroud, J. P.: Influence of previously given tricyclic antidepressants on the activity of local anesthetics. Therapie, *24*:393, 1969.
72. Marshall, L. J., and Green, V. A.: Propranolol and diazepam for imipramine poisoning. Lancet, 2:1249, 1968.
73. Vohra, J.: Cardiovascular abnormalities following tricyclic antidepressant drug overdosage. Drugs, *7*:323, 1974.
74. Goldberg, L. I.: Monoamine oxidase inhibitors, adverse reactions and possible mechanisms. J.A.M.A., *190*:456, 1964.
75. Jenkins, L. C., and Graves, H. B.: Potential hazards of psychoactive drugs in association with anesthesia. Can. Anaesth. Soc. J., *23*:334, 1976.
76. Hunter, K. R., et al.: Monoamine oxidase inhibitors and L-dopa. Br. Med. J., *3*:388, 1970.
77. Lewis, E.: Hyperpyrexia with antidepressant drugs. Br. Med. J., *2*:1671, 1965.
78. Krisko, I., Lewis, E., and Johnson, J.: Severe hyperpyrexia due to tranylcypromine-amphetamine toxicity. Ann. Intern. Med., *70*:559, 1969.
79. Hirsh, M.S., Walter, R.M., and Hasterlik, R. J.: Subarachnoid hemorrhage following ephedrine and MAO inhibitor. J.A.M.A., *194*:1259, 1965.
80. Blackwell, B., et al.: Hypertensive interactions between monoamine oxidase inhibitors and foodstuffs. Br. J. Psychiatry, *113*:349, 1967.
81. Sjoquist, F.: Psychotropic drugs. (2) Interaction between monoamine oxidase (MAOI) inhibitors and other substances. Proc. R. Soc. Med., *58*:967, 1965.
82. Elis, J., et al.: Modification by monoamine oxidase inhibitors of the effect of some sympathomimetics on blood pressure. Br. Med. J., *2*:75, 1967.
83. Raskin, A.: Adverse reactions to phenelzine, results of a nine hospital depression study. J. Clin. Pharmacol., *12*:22, 1972.
84. Editorial: Analgesics and monoamine-oxidase inhibitor. Br. Med. J., *4*:284, 1967.
85. Horler, A. R., and Wynne, N. A.: Hypertensive crisis due to pargyline and metaraminol. Br. Med. J., *2*:460, 1965.
86. Mason, A.: Fatal reaction associated with tranylcypromine and methylamphetamine. Lancet, *1*:173, 1962.

87. Davies, T. S.: Monoamine oxidase inhibitors and rauwolfia compounds. Br. Med. J. , *2*:739, 1960.
88. Hunter, K. R., Stern, G. M., and Laurence, D. R.: Use of levodopa with other drugs. Lancet *2*:1283, 1970.
89. Teychenne, P. F., et al.: Interactions of levodopa with inhibitors of monoamine oxidase and L-aromatic amino acid decarboxylase. Clin. Pharmacol. Ther., *18*:273, 1975.
90. Horwitz, D., Goldberg, L. I., and Sjoerdsma, A.: Increased blood pressure responses to dopamine and norepinephrine produced by monoamine oxidase inhibitors in man. J. Lab. Clin. Med., *56*:747, 1960.
91. Shepherd, M.: Psychotropic drugs. (1) Interaction between centrally acting drugs in man. Proc. R. Soc. Med., *58*:964, 1965.
92. Palmer, H.: Potentiation of pethidine. Br. Med. J., *2*:944, 1960.
93. Shee, J. C.: Dangerous potentiation of pethidine by iproniazid and its treatment. Br. Med. J., *2*:507, 1960.
94. Rogers, K. J.: Role of brain monoamines in the interaction between pethidine and tranylcypromine. Eur. J. Pharmacol., *14*:86, 1971.
95. Brownlee, G., and Williams, G. W.: Potentiation of amphetamine and pethidine by monoamine oxidase inhibitors. Lancet, *1*:699, 1963.
96. Eade, N. R., and Renton, K. W.: Effect of monoamine oxidase inhibitors on the n-demethylation and hydrolysis of meperidine. Biochem. Pharmacol., *19*:2243, 1970.
97. Eade, N. R., and Renton, K. W.: The effect of phenelzine and tranylcypromine on the degradation of meperidine. J. Pharmcol. Exp. Ther., *173*:31, 1970.
98. Rivers, N., and Horner, B.: Possible lethal reaction between Nardil and dextromethorphan. Can. Med. Assoc. J., *103*:85, 1970.
99. Jounela, A. J., and Mattila, M. J.: Modification by phenelzine of morphine and pethidine analgesia in mice. Ann. Med. Exp. Biol. Fenn., *46*:66, 1968.
100. Rogers, K. J., and Thornton, J. A.: The interaction between monoamine oxidase inhibitors and narcotic analgesics in mice. Br. J. Pharmacol., *36*:470, 1969.
101. Jounela, A. J.: Effect of phenelzine on the rate of metabolism of pethidine. Ann. Med. Exp. Biol. Fenn., *46*:531, 1968.
102. Vigran, I. M.: Dangerous potentiation of meperidine hydrochloride by pargyline hydrochloride. J.A.M.A., *187*:954, 1964.
103. Cocks, D. P., and Passmore-Rowe, A.: Dangers of monoamine oxidase inhibitors. Br. Med. J., *2*:1545, 1962.
104. Churchill-Davidson, H. C.: Anaesthesia and monoamine-oxidase inhibitors. Br. Med. J., *1*:520, 1965.
105. Domino, E., Sullivan, T. S., and Luby, E. D.: Barbiturate intoxication in a patient treated with a MAO inhibitor. Am. J. Psychiatry, *118*:941, 1962.
106. Bodley, P. O., Halwax, K., and Potts, L.: Low pseudocholinesterase levels complicating treatment with phenelzine. Br. Med. J., *3*:510, 1969.
107. Cheymol, J., et al.: Influence of chronic MAOI inhibitor administration on curarization. Therapie, *21*:355, 1966.
108. Summers, R. J.: Effects of monoamine oxidase inhibitors on the hypothermia produced in cats by halothane. Br. J. Pharmacol., *37*:400, 1969.
109. Frieden, J.: Propranolol as an anti-arrhythmic agent. Am. Heart J., *75*:283, 1967.
110. Moser, M.: Experience with isocarboxazid. J.A.M.A., *176*:276, 1961.
111. Penlington, G. N.: Droperidol and monoamine oxidase inhibitors. Br. Med. J., *1*:483, 1966.
112. Byck, R.: Drugs and the treatment of psychiatric disorders. *In* The Pharmacological Basis of Therapeutics. Edited by L. S. Goodman and A. Gilman, New York, Macmillan, 1975.
113. Davis, J. M., Janowsky, D. S., and El-Yousef, M. K.: The use of lithium in clinical psychiatry. Psychiatric Annals, *3*:78, 1973.
114. Greist, J. H., et al.: The lithium librarian. Arch. Gen. Psychiatry, *34*:456, 1977.
115. Peach, M. J.: Cations: calcium, magnesium, barium, lithium, and ammonium. *In* The Pharmacological Basis of Therapeutics. Edited by L. S. Goodman and A. Gilman. New York, Macmillan, 1975.
116. Borden, H., Clarke, M., and Katz, H.: The use of pancuronium bromide in patients receiving lithium carbonate. Can. Anaesth. Soc. J., *21*:79, 1974.
117. Jephcott, G., and Kerry, R. J.: Lithium: an anesthetic risk. Br. J. Anaesth. *46*:389, 1974.
118. Hill, G. E., Wong, K. C., and Hodges, M. R.: Potentiation of succinylcholine neuromuscular blockade by lithium carbonate. Anesthesiology, *44*:439, 1976.
119. Hill, G. E., Wong, K. C., and Hodges, M. R.: Lithium carbonate and neuromuscular blocking agents. Anesthesiology, *46*:122, 1977.
120. Vizi, E., et al.: The effect of lithium on acetylcholine release and synthesis. Neuropharmacology, *11*:521, 1972.
121. Mannisto, P. T., and Saarnivaara, L.: Effect of lithium and rubidium on the sleeping time caused by various intravenous anaesthetics in the mouse. Br. J. Anaesth., *48*:185, 1976.
122. Solomon, R., and Vickers, R.: Dysarthria resulting from lithium carbonate, a case report. J.A.M.A., *231*:280, 1975.
123. Wharton, R.: Geriatric Doses (Letter to the Editor). J.A.M.A., *233*:22, 1975.
124. Mackay, A.V.P., Loose, R., and Glen, A.I.M.: Labour on lithium. Br. Med. J., *1*:878, 1976.
125. Wilbanks, G. D., et al.: Toxic effects of lithium carbonate in a mother and newborn infant. J.A.M.A., *213*:865, 1970.
126. Macfie, A. C.: Lithium poisoning precipitated by diuretics. Br. Med. J., *1*:516, 1975.
127. Ascione, F. J.: Lithium with Diuretics. Drug Ther. (Hosp.), *7*:125, 1977.

14

Sedatives and Hypnotics

N. TY SMITH

The designation "sedative-hypnotic" may be one of the most confusing misnomers in modern therapeutics. It does not denote a specific drug action, but rather implies a spectrum of activity from sedative through hypnotic to general anesthesia and finally to coma.[1] We shall include under this heading a large group of chemically unrelated drugs that are, after aspirin, among the most used, as well as abused. The habitual intake of these drugs to relieve insomnia or to achieve tranquillity is a common preanesthetic finding. Thus the anesthesiologist should specifically inquire about the use of these agents, and should be aware of other drugs that might interact with them.

Although these agents are administered by several routes for several purposes, we shall consider mainly their long-term oral use and their short-term use as preanesthetic medication.

CASE REPORT

A 58-year-old man was admitted to the hospital for an acute myocardial infarction. In the hospital, he received digoxin, lidocaine, phenobarbital, and dicumarol. The latter agent was titrated according to the patient's prothrombin time, which, at the end of the stabilization period, was 18.4 sec, with a control of 12.1 sec. After two weeks, his barbiturate therapy was discontinued, but his anticoagulant therapy was maintained, without a readjustment in dosage. Two weeks later the patient was brought to the operating room with gastric bleeding. The anesthesiologist requested a prothrombin time before he would proceed with the anesthetic. The prothrombin time was 34 seconds, with a control of 11.8 seconds. Vitamin K was administered to the patient, with a subsequent lowering of prothrombin times to the therapeutic range of dicumarol—and with the cessation of the gastric bleeding.

This case occurred long before the barbiturate/dicumarol interaction was suspected. The mechanism for the interaction responsible for this patient's problems is covered in detail in this chapter. The case report brings up several important points. It demonstrates that one drug can alter the rate of metabolism, and hence the action, of another drug. It emphasizes a less well-appreciated fact: that discontinuing an interacting drug, in this case phenobarbital, can also have an impact. Finally, it points out that the anesthesiologist should be alert for *every* drug interaction, whether or not it may directly affect the course of the anesthetic management.

In the following paragraphs we describe the basic mechanism of the sedative-hypnotics, some of the more common agents, their mechanisms of action and uses, the more common drug interactions in which these agents are involved and a commentary on the clinical importance of these interactions. The drugs include the barbiturates, alcohol, diazepam, chlordiazepoxide, flurazepam, chloral hydrate, paraldehyde, antihistaminics, meprobamate, ethchlorvynol, and marijuana.

PHARMACOLOGIC MECHANISMS

The purpose of sedative therapy is to reduce anxiety or tension without interfering with the normal activities of the patient. The sedation produced can alleviate anxiety associated either with neurosis or with somatic disease. Sedatives are generally more useful in emotionally upset or neurotic persons than in psychotic patients. Drugs intended for the latter group of patients are discussed extensively in Chapter 13.

Although the sedative-hypnotic agents act at all levels in the central nervous system (CNS), the reticular-activating system is especially sensitive to their depressant effects. This action appears to be responsible for the sleep-inducing properties of these drugs.[2] The clinical effects of sedative-hypnotics are typified by the barbiturates, which are rapidly absorbed after oral administration and distributed throughout the body. Normal hypnotic doses can impair motor performance, judgment, and the performance of simple intellectual tasks.[3-6] It is unclear whether their action is at the cellular or synaptic level, and many theories have been advanced to explain their effects.[2] The barbiturates have an anticonvulsant activity, a property that may be shared by other sedative-hypnotic drugs. It should be noted, however, that the sedative and anticonvulsant activities of barbiturates have recently been recognized as being separate.[7]

The CNS depression that the sedative and hypnotic agents produce accounts for a substantial number of potentially serious interactions with other CNS-depressant drugs. Alcohol is a primary culprit in this regard. Although the classic "Micky Finn," a mixture of chloral hydrate and alcohol, has not been documented, the interaction of alcohol with CNS-depressant drugs can be serious.

Probably most of the interactions of sedative-hypnotics as preanesthetic medication have to do with additive central nervous system effects. Certainly most of us intuitively decrease the dosage of one preanesthetic medication when we add another. For example, we do not give as much pentobarbital in the presence of hydroxyzine as we would by itself. However, these interactions have not been well documented.

Even less clear is the effect of preanesthetic medication on anesthetic agents themselves. Preanesthetic agents certainly seem to alter anesthetic management. They facilitate the approach to the patient, and they may make the induction of anesthesia smoother. Whether these effects can be called true drug interactions is questionable. Similarly, a poorly timed or excessive dose of preanesthetic medication can prolong a patient's recovery time. How much of this phenomenon is due to interactions among the central nervous system effects of the agents and how much is due simply to the much longer action of the premedicant has not been determined.

Little information is available on the ability of the sedative-hypnotics to alter anesthetic depth when given as preanesthetic medication. A major problem is that the standard measurement of anesthetic depth (MAC) is related to pain, and most sedative-hypnotics have no analgesic action. To my knowledge, other, more appropriate, types of MAC, such as MAC awake, have not been used to study the effects of the sedative-hypnotics on anesthetic depth or duration.

When given in ordinary doses as preanesthetic medication, the sedative-hypnotics probably have little impact on the potency of inhalation anesthetics. Even morphine, with its known analgesic properties, changes the MAC of halothane by only 0.05 vol %.[8] If 0.2 mg/kg of diazepam are given intravenously 30 minutes before a surgical incision, halothane MAC is decreased from 0.73 to 0.48, a decrease of 34%.[9] One can assume that if given in smaller doses, intramuscularly or by mouth, two to three hours before an incision, the impact of diazepam would be considerably less. That, however, has not been examined.

Many hypnotic drugs stimulate hepatic microsomal enzyme production, which is the basis of the other common set of drug interactions of this class. Microsomal enzyme induction appears between two and seven days after administration of such a drug.[10-13] After the discontinuance of the drug, enzyme induction may persist for up to one month.[14] Phenobarbital, the best known of the enzyme-inducing drugs, increases the rate of synthesis and decreases the breakdown of mouse microsomal protein and rat microsomal phospholipid.[15,16] Thus phenobarbital increases liver microsomal protein by 20 to 40%.[17-19] The physiologic significance of enhanced liver growth and the function produced by microsomal enzyme-inducing drugs is not known.[10] However, many drug interactions occur because of the unsuspected and rapid metabolism of drugs given concurrently with microsomal enzyme-inducing agents. The case report is but one example of such an interaction.

SPECIFIC AGENTS

Barbiturates

The barbiturates are often implicated in drug interactions. They are used by all segments of the population for many indications, legal and illegal. Overdosage and physical and psychologic dependence are common medical and social problems.

Absorption of barbiturates is generally good. They are effective orally, parenterally, and rectally. All of these routes of administration are used clinically.

The duration of activity of a barbiturate is related to redistribution from the brain and plasma to other body tissues, to metabolic degradation in the liver, and to renal excretion of unchanged drug.[2] Biotransformation by the liver is apparently clinically less important in determining the duration of the drug's effect. Although it has been recommended that barbiturates be given cautiously to patients with liver disease, hepatic dysfunction must be severe to decrease appreciably the rate of barbiturate metabolism to a clinically significant degree.[2,20,21]

The distribution of the barbiturates is determined by their lipid solubility, protein binding, and degree of ionization.[2] The more lipid-soluble barbiturates act rapidly and for a short time. Albumin and other plasma proteins reversibly bind a portion of the barbiturate. The type and degree of binding vary greatly with the physicochemical characteristics of the barbiturate.[2] Barbiturates bound by proteins are unavailable for drug action. Thus anything that decreases protein binding by competing for binding sites (for example, aspirin and sulfonamides) increases the pharmacologic effects of the barbiturates, and vice versa. The degree of ionization affects the distribution across membranes such as the "blood-brain barrier'' and, therefore, the intracerebral concentration of barbiturates. Lower plasma pH increases brain tissue concentrations. The opposite is also true. Metabolic rather than respiratory acid-base alterations have a greater effect on barbiturate distribution and thus on central nervous system depression.[2]

Barbiturates alter the biotransformation and hence the action of a number of other drugs. The interaction is usually a biphasic enhancement followed by a reduction. If a barbiturate and another drug similarly metabolized are given for the first time together, the enzyme system is saturated and the effects of both drugs are enhanced.[20,22] The initially augmented effect takes place because barbiturates such as phenobarbital, by combining with cytochrome P-450, competitively inhibit the biotransformation of a number of drugs.

Probably the best-documented anesthetically related example of this acute inhibition phenomenon is the interaction between sedative premedications and ketamine in patients.[23] Secobarbital, diazepam, and hydroxyzine all prolong ketamine-induced sleep time in patients. These agents seem to work by inhibiting the metabolism of ketamine, as shown by an increase in the plasma half-life of the agent.

After prolonged use of a barbiturate, however, the subsequent administration of a drug similarly metabolized reduces the latter's effect because of the increase in the enzymes involved in its biotransformation.[24] (See Chap. 3 for further discussion.) The tolerance seen with the long-term use of barbiturates is due at least in part to this increased activity in the hepatic microsomal enzyme system.[24,25] One would expect an increased tolerance to most preanesthetic medications in patients taking long-term barbiturate therapy, but this has not been documented.

Central nervous system (CNS) depression by the barbiturates is well documented. A real danger of their abuse is seen with the additive effects of other CNS depressants (for example, ethanol, opiates).[26] Barbiturates, together with CNS stimulants such as amphetamines, can, conversely, result in agitation, although the clinical significance of this interaction is in doubt.[27]

Anticoagulants. The case report illustrates possibly the most common and certainly the best documented drug interaction. (Enzyme induction from barbiturates has also been incriminated in oral contraceptive failure.[28] Increasing the metabolism of some estrogen-like drugs renders these agents ineffective. This interaction does not directly affect the anesthesiologist—until the patient is in the labor/delivery room.) Enzyme induction secondary to the long-term use of barbiturates increases the metabolism of anticoagulants of the coumarin type. The result is a decreased coumarin effect, and the concomitant use of a barbiturate may create difficulties in the control of the coumarin dose and of the prothrombin time. Perhaps even more hazardous is the decrease in coagulability that follows cessation of the barbiturate if the dose of the anticoagulant is not decreased. Thus, in our case report, no problems occurred during barbiturate therapy, even though phenobarbital and dicumarol were started at the same time. The physicians were able to titrate the dose of dicumarol to compensate for the effects of phenobarbital. By the time the latter was discontinued, however, the prothrombin-time determinations were being made less frequently. Thus no one detected that a given dosage of dicumarol became more potent as its rate of metabolism decreased.

Considering all potential problems, it is preferable to use hypnotic drugs that do not appear to interact with anticoagulants, such as flurazepam or diazepam.

Digitoxin. A decreased therapeutic effect of digitoxin has also been ascribed to a similar metabolic mechanism. Barbiturates increase metabolism of digitoxin to digoxin, which has a shorter half life, and this may decrease the therapeutic effect.[29] (See Chap. 10.)

Miscellaneous Drugs. One cannot always depend on increased metabolism to protect against increased toxicity with long-term barbiturate therapy, however. For example, therapeutic levels of tricyclic antidepressants may be metabolized faster in patients who take barbiturates regularly. But high levels of tricyclic antidepressants may potentiate the respiratory depression produced by barbiturates.[30] As another example, the anticonvulsant phenytoin (diphenylhydantoin) is metabolized more rapidly in patients who have received moderate doses of barbiturates on a long-term basis, although higher doses of barbiturates can competitively inhibit the metabolism of this agent.[31]

Alkalinizers. Alkalinization of the urine could shorten the biological half-life of a weakly acidic barbiturate by rendering a greater proportion of it ionized and hence less readily absorbed from the tubular urine. This interaction, of modest significance except for slowly metabolized barbiturates such as phenobarbital, is covered in detail in Chapter 5.

CNS Depressants. It is well known that the CNS depressants interact with one another to produce at least additive effects. The combinations of barbiturates and other sedatives are no exception. Thus it behooves the anesthesiologist not only to examine the present therapy of any patient, but also to be careful in prescribing combinations for preanesthetic medication. A general rule is that most central nervous system depressants may have an additive or more than additive effect when used in combination with barbiturates. This is true with the phenothiazines, which can enhance not only sedation but also hypotension when used in combination with barbiturates. The combination of alcohol and barbiturates is particularly vicious and is discussed in the following section.

Ethyl alcohol

Alcohol is rapidly absorbed from the gastrointestinal tract, but only in limited amounts from subcutaneous tissue. Intravenous alcohol therapy is used for medicinal purposes, such as to arrest uterine contractions in premature labor. About 90 to 98% of alcohol is oxidized by the liver. The rest is excreted by the lungs and kidneys.

The majority of patients who undergo operations have a history of ethyl alcohol intake. Acute intoxication is a serious problem in an emergency operation, and its implications in anesthesia are well known. Ethyl alcohol is above all a CNS depressant and has additive effects when taken with any other CNS depressant. Long-term excessive ethyl alcohol intake is a different sort of problem, primarily because of hepatic enzyme induction. Ethanol ingestion initially decreases hepatic enzyme metabolism and then increases the enzyme activity.

Anticoagulants. The occasional use of small to moderate amounts of alcohol by patients who take oral anticoagulants is not contraindicated. However, if alcohol intake is prolonged and heavy enough to produce liver dysfunction, anticoagulant therapy may be affected.[32] In these patients, frequent determinations of prothrombin time are necessary, and the anesthetist should inquire about any sudden changes in alcohol consumption.

Barbiturates. The combined actions of barbiturates and alcohol have been described as antagonistic,[33] additive,[34] potentiating,[35] and synergistic.[36] The studies are difficult to compare, since they use different species, dose levels, and experimental designs.

Although the mechanism of the intensification of effect at the CNS level is not well understood, several theories have been proposed. One theory concerns the hepatic microsomal enzyme system, which not only is involved in metabolic transformations of numerous drugs, but also acts as an ethanol-oxidizing system and is responsible for adaptive increases of the rate of alcohol metabolism in alcoholics.[37] When the enzyme system is induced by phenobarbital, alcohol metabolism accelerates, and a greater tolerance to alcohol develops. When it is induced by long-term consumption of alcohol, phenobarbital is metabolized more quickly, and the patient becomes more tolerant to barbiturates. Thus phenobarbital appears to enhance the disappearance of ethanol from the blood, resulting in somewhat decreased blood ethanol concentrations.[38,39] The complete mechanism for this effect is not known, however. It may involve additional factors to a direct increase in hepatic metabolism of ethanol. When barbiturates and alcohol are ingested concurrently, competition for the enzyme system leads to the inhibition of oxidation and to the enhancement of CNS depressant effects.[40,41] However, this theory has been disputed,[42,43] because the physiologic significance of the microsomal ethanol-oxidizing system has been questioned.[44,45]

The clinical results of the additive interaction in the central nervous system are similar to the effects of either agent given alone, except more intense. Motor impairment and drowsiness are the most common symptoms.[46-50] Respiratory depression is mild at low doses of either drug,[49-51] but it can become serious at higher doses and may cause death.[46,49]

It is clear from the mechanisms just described (and probably from others as yet undiscovered) that the interrelationships between ethanol and the barbiturates are quite complex. Clinically the most important considerations are that they are both central nervous system depressants and that acute ethanol intoxication may impair barbiturate metabolism. Also, the enhanced drug metabolism with long-term ethanol intake may partially explain the tolerance to barbiturates seen in chronic alcoholics.

Although the precautions of combined ethanol-barbiturate use are well known, it bears repeating that the combination should be used cautiously with due attention to excessive central nervous system depression. Anesthesia should be administered with extreme care in patients who are already depressed by this combination.

Other Sedative-Hypnotic Agents. Alcohol given with any other sedative-hypnotic can result in a greater central nervous system depression than when either agent is taken alone. The mechanism varies slightly among agents, although in general it is the same as with barbiturates. An exception is glutethimide. The combined use of ethanol and glutethimide has *increased* blood ethanol concentration and has decreased plasma glutethimide concentration.[38] Although these effects may be clinically significant, it is probably more important to remember that both drugs are CNS depressants.

Guanethidine. Alcohol may enhance the antihypertensive effects of guanethidine. Guanethidine interferes with storage and release of catecholamines from postganglionic sympathetic nerve fibers and thereby causes adrenergic neuron blockade.[52] The reduction of vasomotor tone and the impairment of reflex adaptation to postural changes or to muscular exercise can lead to hypotension and syncope. Alcohol exerts profound vasodilator effects primarily on cutaneous vessels, whereas blood flow through skeletal muscle is either unchanged or decreased.[53-56] In addition, alcohol may directly depress the myocardium.[57,58] As little as 60 ml of whiskey can effect a statistically significant decrease in stroke volume, and thereby in cardiac output, in chronic alcoholics and in patients with cardiac disease of varying cause.[59]

No specific studies have been conducted concerning the guanethidine-alcohol interaction. However, the occurrence of hypotensive episodes induced by alcohol in patients treated with guanethidine has been frequent enough to warrant numerous comments and the inclusion of a warning in the manufacturer's drug package.[52,60,61] It seems that another stimulus is required to produce hypotension. This stimulus could include physical exercise, showers or baths, or rising quickly from a sitting or prone position.[52] Thus it is possible, although it is not documented, that general or spinal anesthesia in these patients could produce profound hypotension.

Hypoglycemic Agents. Diabetic patients treated with phenformin should avoid the ingestion of alcoholic beverages because concurrent use may cause hypoglycemic reactions or life-threatening lactic acidosis with shock. Some patients who take phenformin also experience pronounced anorexia and intolerance to alcohol. Insulin-dependent diabetic patients have been known to suffer dangerous hypoglycemic episodes after excessive alcohol intake. The concurrent use of insulin and alcohol by alcoholic patients has led to at least two deaths and three cases of permanent mental impairment.[62] In each case, patients stabilized with insulin were found comatose or semiconscious from hypoglycemia caused by the consumption of excessive amounts of alcohol. The anesthesiologist should be aware of this severe reaction in patients who ingest these combined agents; this applies not only in the operating room, but also when the anesthesiologist is confronted with a comatose patient in the emergency room or intensive care unit.

Sulfonylureas and alcohol interact by multiple mechanisms and cause unpredictable fluctuations in serum glucose levels. Alcohol ingestion may also precipitate a disulfiram-like reaction (for example, flushing, headache, palpitations, and a feeling of breathlessness) in patients stabilized with a sulfonylurea, particularly chlorpropamide.[63]

General Anesthetics. Clinical experience suggests that the induction of anesthesia in a long-term abuser of alcohol is prolonged, and is often seen in conjunction with marked excitement. Maintenance of anesthesia in these patients is characterized by the need for high anesthetic concentrations. These impressions are corroborated in part by Han, who showed an increase in the MAC of halothane in chronic alcoholics.[64] On the other hand, Munson could detect no motor response to a surgical incision at MAC concentrations.[65] One might expect lessened anesthetic requirements with the acutely intoxicated patient. Although this has not been documented in human beings, the interaction between alcohol and other CNS depressants is striking enough to warrant caution when anesthetizing the acute alcoholic.[66]

The interaction between ethanol and any of the general anesthetic agents can be delayed, so that ethanol consumed too soon after an anesthetic can be disastrous. Hugin has suggested handing a form to all patients who receive anesthetics on an outpatient basis. On the form they should acknowledge that they are not to drink alcohol or to drive a vehicle until the next day.[67]

Diazepam

Diazepam is a long-acting agent and is demethylated into active metabolites. One must certainly use less of other induction agents with this drug, particularly if the total dose is 20 mg or more.

The lack of interaction with the oral anticoagulants has been mentioned previously. I have also stated that diazepam, given as a preanesthetic medication, prolongs ketamine-induced sleep time.[23] Interestingly enough, patients premedicated with diazepam had higher plasma ketamine levels on awaking than did patients in any other group.

Lidocaine-Induced Seizures. Diazepam participates in other interactions. One of the most notable of these is its ability to protect against lidocaine-induced seizures. There is good evidence in several species of animals that diazepam, administered intramuscularly in doses in the range of those safe for premedication, can specifically antagonize the convulsant effect of lidocaine.[68–76] Thus a larger dose and a higher plasma concentration of lidocaine are required to produce seizures. Although this antagonism has not been shown in man, an anesthetist may wish to administer diazepam before performing a regional block that may require a large amount of lidocaine. Something could be gained and little should be lost. The use of diazepam should not create a false sense of security, however. Seizures can occur. And if they do develop, they seem to be more difficult to control, in that they require doses of an anticonvulsant drug that are larger than normally needed.

The *therapy* of lidocaine-induced seizures is another matter, since controversy exists over the desirability of diazepam as opposed to an ultrashort-acting barbiturate. Several points should be examined before treating an individual patient. Equiprophylactic doses of pentobarbital potentiate the cardiorespiratory depressant effects of local anesthetics more than does diazepam.[69,72,73,75] This property, combined with the lesser central nervous system effects of diazepam under the same conditions, would seem to give this drug the advantage over oxybarbiturates. Certainly, diazepam can prevent local anesthetic-induced convulsions with increasing lidocaine cardiovascular toxicity.[77] I prefer, however, to use a thiobarbiturate such as thiopental, for several reasons. First, the onset of action of the barbiturate is more rapid than that of diazepam, and allows quick titration of anticonvulsant effects. Second, since small amounts of thiopental (25 to 50 mg) can abort a lidocaine-induced seizure, the chances of producing respiratory or cardiovascular depression are minimal. Third, its duration of action is less than that of diazepam. Thus if small amounts of the barbiturate have been given and the patient has a prolonged awakening, one can probably attribute it to a postictal phenomenon, rather than to a pharmacologic effect.

Since diazepam antagonizes the central nervous system toxicity of lidocaine, it was feared that the antiarrhythmic action of lidocaine might also be antagonized by diazepam. However, studies in dogs have indicated that diazepam actually enhances the antiarrhythmic effect of lidocaine.[78]

Physostigmine. Physostigmine is unique among commonly used anticholinergic agents in that it has a tertiary rather than a quaternary nitrogen. Therefore, it can rapidly cross the blood-brain barrier to exert its effect in the central nervous system. There have been several reports that physostigmine can reverse the sedative or respiratory depressant effects of diazepam or lorazepam.[79-83] Although physostigmine has reversed the effects of anticholinergic agents, such as atropine, scopolamine, the phenothiazines, or the tricyclic antidepressants, it is surprising that it could have such an action with the benzodiazepines.

There are, of course, many problems with the case reports described. It is possible that physostigmine is acting as a nonspecific analeptic. It causes an arousal response in the electroencephalogram of cats, presumably by acting on the reticular activating system.[84] In many reports, other agents were given, some of these capable of being reversed by physostigmine. Thus it is impossible to separate simple two-drug interactions. More important, none of the reports attempted to use a placebo in a double-blind fashion. This may be significant in light of an unfortunately uncompleted study.[85] When diazepam was the only agent administered during spinal anesthesia, there was no difference between saline and physostigmine in producing arousal. There was, however, a suggestion of a greater incidence of side effects in the physostigmine group. Although only 12 patients were studied, *if* physostigmine had produced arousal in every patient and *if* saline had had no effect, 23 additional patients would have had to be studied before a significant difference would have been obtained.

On the other hand, preliminary evidence indicates that physostigmine does shorten the duration of somnolence induced by diazepam in rats[86] and rapidly reverses that induced in healthy volunteer subjects.[87] The latter group involved a randomized, double-blind, cross-over study. Accompanying the arousal in these latter studies were definite signs of electroencephalographic arousal.

Physostigmine is not a benign drug, however. During the investigations by Karen[85] and by Avant, two of the 20 patients experienced atrial dysrhythmia—one atrial flutter and one atrial fibrillation. These did convert to normal after one to two hours.

Neuromuscular Blocking Agents. A preliminary clinical study indicated that diazepam increased the duration of action of gallamine, and decreased the duration of succinylcholine activity.[88] However, subsequent work[89,90] has not substantiated these findings, and it appears likely that diazepam itself does not significantly affect the response to numerous neuromuscular blocking agents.

Chlordiazepoxide

Since several studies have demonstrated a lack of interaction between chlordiazepoxide and oral anticoagulants, no special precautions appear necessary when administering this agent to patients who are taking oral anticoagulants.[91-93]

Flurazepam

Flurazepam has become a popular nighttime hypnotic in recent years. Because it is a benzodiazepine compound, it might be expected to share the same interactions as diazepam. However, to date, no clinically significant interaction has been documented with flurazepam.[94-98] As with diazepam, this agent does not seem to change the activity of any anticoagulants and thus can be used safely with them.[97]

Chloral hydrate

Chloral hydrate is still a popular oral hypnotic. It is rapidly metabolized in the liver and in other tissues to trichloroethanol, which is responsible for its CNS depressant effects. Excretion of its metabolites is through the urine and the bile.

Some disagreement exists as to the ability of chloral hydrate or of trichloroethanol to induce the microsomal enzyme system.[99-100] Although one report has suggested such

an induction and has been cited, most studies, both laboratory and clinical, have not demonstrated this phenomenon.[12,14,99,101-107] This is not surprising, since neither agent is metabolized by the hepatic microsomal enzyme system.[99]

However, chloral hydrate can affect the action of the anticoagulants, probably by another mechanism. A major metabolite, trichloroacetic acid, can displace acidic drugs from plasma proteins, resulting in a shortened half-life but in increased blood levels. Thus, trichloroacetic acid appears to displace warfarin from plasma-protein binding. This causes a transient increase in the amount of free (active) plasma warfarin and also increases its rate of metabolism. Bishydroxycoumarin is probably affected similarly, but almost all available data deal with warfarin. Results from several clinical studies indicate that chloral hydrate temporarily increases the hypoprothrombinemic effect of warfarin in some patients.[101,103,104,108] Reports to the contrary have dealt with longer-range effects, thus demonstrating that continued administration of the two drugs probably normalizes the hypoprothrombinemic effect of warfarin.[96,109] The interaction resulting from the administration of chloral hydrate to patients already receiving long-term warfarin therapy is likely to be adverse.

Paraldehyde

Paraldehyde is a hypnotic drug used in the management of convulsions, tetanus, eclampsia, and status epilepticus. It is effective orally, but is a local irritant when given parenterally. After administration, 70 to 80% is metabolized by the liver, 11 to 28% is exhaled, and 0.1 to 2.5% is excreted in the urine.

Paraldehyde is metabolized to acetaldehyde by the liver. Thus disulfiram may impair the metabolism of acetaldehyde by decreasing acetaldehyde dehydrogenase, so that paraldehyde is not advised in patients receiving disulfiram.

Antihistaminics

Concurrent administration of an antihistaminic and a barbiturate may enhance the central nervous system depression caused by either drug. There is no clinical documentation, however, that this enhanced effect occurs.[110] However, one should still be cautious when concomitantly administering agents from these two classes.

Although frequently discussed in the scientific literature, no clinically significant interactions between warfarin and the antihistamines have been reported. Therefore, no additional precautions are necessary when these drugs are given concurrently.[111] This also means that sedative antihistaminics, such as diphenhydramine, would be satisfactory for preanesthetic medication in a patient who is receiving an oral anticoagulant.

Meprobamate

Meprobamate is a tranquilizer with central nervous system depressant actions similar to those of the barbiturates. It is well absorbed from the gastrointestinal tract and, like the barbiturates, can induce hepatic microsomal enzymes.[10] It interacts with ethanol in that short-term ethanol ingestion may decrease meprobamate metabolism, whereas the long-term use of ethanol and the resultant enzyme induction hastens the metabolism of meprobamate.[10,112] The suspicion that meprobamate may interfere with coumarin-type anticoagulants has not been sufficiently documented.

Ethchlorvynol

Ethchlorvynol is an alcohol used as a nighttime sedative. It is effective orally and metabolized by the liver, although up to 10% may be excreted unchanged. This drug has been reported to increase the metabolism of coumarin-type anticoagulants, in a fashion similar to the barbiturates. However, the clinical significance of this interaction has not been established.[113]

Δ-9-Tetrahydrocannabinol (THC) ("Marijuana")

Although one could argue that marijuana is not a sedative-hypnotic agent, it does produce sedation, and a significant fraction of the American population has been exposed to this plant.[114-115] The question must arise, then, whether this drug alters the response to anesthetic agents. In independent studies, Stoelting et al. and Vitez et al. observed a decrease in anesthetic requirement for halothane (dogs) and for cyclopropane (rats) after the short-term administration of Δ-9-tetrahydrocannabinol (THC), an active, purified component of marijuana.[116,117] Long-term administration, on the other hand, did not alter the MAC of either agent. Marijuana is often consumed together with alcohol, and the acute additive effects of this combination might decrease anesthetic requirements.[118] Enzyme induction[119,120] after long-term marijuana smoking might alter biotransformation and potential toxicity of certain agents.

The purified agent THC had interesting effects when administered *after* either oxymorphone or pentobarbital.[121] The administration of THC further increased the sedation and the respiratory depression caused by oxymorphone. Although oxymorphone alone caused no significant cardiovascular changes, the addition of THC increased the cardiac index and heart rate and decreased systemic vascular resistance. When added to pentobarbital, THC induced hallucinations and anxiety in five of seven volunteers. The cardiovascular effects of the addition of THC were the same as with oxymorphone. Again, the experimental protocol did not imitate the clinical situation, but these studies must give us pause.

That THC must be administered within a few hours before the administration of the anesthetic or during it to affect anesthetic requirements might seem to minimize the clinical significance of these observations; presumably few patients smoke marijuana the morning of an operation.[107,108] On the other hand, some patients admitted for an emergency operation may have been exposed to street drugs, and the possibility of altered anesthetic requirement must always be kept in mind. Perhaps more pertinent is that the experimental doses of THC were 10 to 20 times those needed to produce a satisfactory "high." However, one or more of the agents contained in marijuana may ultimately become a routine preanesthetic medication, and it is presently impossible to predict the dosage.

In summary, the anesthesiologist is probably more likely to encounter patients taking the sedative-hypnotic agents than any other type of agent, particularly if one includes ethanol. It would seem that the interaction between these agents and the oral anticoagulants represents the most commonly encountered of all interactions. This impression is partly due to the ease with which the interaction is detected; few agents are served by a laboratory test that defines their action so precisely as does the prothrombin time for the anticoagulant agents. Other common interactions involve those among the sedative-hypnotic agents themselves. In general, they produce additive CNS depression if given concomitantly. Awareness of the possibility of these interactions facilitates their detection and control. Because there is more awareness among physicians of these interactions than of many others, the incidence *seems* to be high. Actually, the number of serious interactions has been small, considering the enormous amount of these agents given and the theoretical potentials for interactions.

REFERENCES

1. Way, W. L., and Trevor, A. J.: Sedative-hypnotics. Anesthesiology, *34*:170, 1971.
2. Harvey, S. C.: Hypnotics and sedatives. The barbiturates. *In* The Pharmacological Basis of Therapeutics. 5th Edition. Edited by L. S. Goodman and A. Gilman. New York, Macmillan, 1975.
3. Kornetsky, C. O., et al.: Comparison of psychological effects of certain centrally acting drugs in man. Arch. Neurol. Psychiat., *77*:318, 1957.
4. Goldstone, S., et al.: Effect of quinalbarbitone, dextroamphetamine and placebo on apparent time. Br. J. Psychol., *49*:324, 1958.
5. Smith, G. M., and Beecher, H. K.: Amphetamine, secobarbital and athletic performance III: Quantitative effects on judgment. J.A.M.A., *172*:623, 1960.
6. Goldstein, A. B., et al.: Effects of secobarbital and of d-amphetamine on psychomotor performance of normal subjects. J. Pharmacol. Exp. Ther., *130*:55, 1960.
7. MacDonald, R. L., and Barker, J. L.: Different actions of anticonvulsant and anesthetic barbiturates revealed by use of cultured mammalian nerves. Science, *200*:775, 1978.
8. Saidman, L. J., and Eger, E. I.: Effect of nitrous oxide and of narcotic premedication on the alveolar concentration of halothane required for anesthesia. Anesthesiology, *25*:302, 1964.
9. Perisko, J. A., Buechel, D. R., and Miller, R. D.: The effect of diazepam (Valium) on minimum alveolar anesthetic requirement in man. Can. Anaesth. Soc. J., *18*:536, 1971.
10. Conney, A. H.: Pharmacological implications of microsomal enzyme induction. Pharmacol. Rev., *19*:317, 1967.
11. Corn, M.: Effect of phenobarbital and glutethimide on the biological half-life of warfarin. Thromb. Diath. Haemorrh., *16*:606, 1966.
12. Cucinell, S. A., et al.: The effect of chloral hydrate on bishydroxycoumarin metabolism. J.A.M.A., *197*:366, 1968.
13. Robinson, D. S., and MacDonald, M. G.: The effect of phenobarbital administration on the control of coagulation achieved during warfarin therapy in man. J. Pharmacol. Exp. Ther., *153*:250, 1966.
14. MacDonald, M. G., et al.: The effects of phenobarbital, chloral betaine, and glutethimide administration on warfarin plasma levels and hypoprothrombinemic response in man. Clin. Pharmacol. Ther., *10*:80, 1969.
15. Shuster, L., and Jick, H.: The turnover of microsomol protein in the livers of phenobarbital-treated mice. J. Biol. Chem., *241*:5361, 1966.
16. Holtzman, J. L., and Gillette, J. R.: The effect of phenobarbital on the synthesis of microsomal phospholipid in female and male rats. Biochem. Biophys. Res. Commun., *24*:639, 1966.
17. Conney, A. H., et al.: Adaptive increases in drug-metabolizing enzymes induced by phenobarbital and other drugs. J. Pharmacol. Exp. Ther., *130*:1, 1960.
18. Conney, A. N., and Gilman, A. G.: Puromycin inhibition of enzyme induction by 3-methylcholanthrene and phenobarbital. J. Biol. Chem., *238*:3682, 1963.
19. Remmer, H., and Merker, H. J.: Drug-induced changes in the liver endoplasmic reticulum: Association with drug metabolizing enzymes. Science (N.Y.), *142*:1657, 1963.
20. Brodie, B. B., Burns, J. J., and Weiner, M.: Metabolism of drugs in subjects with Laennec's cirrhosis. Med. Exp., *1*:290, 1959.
21. Sessions, J. T., Jr., et al.: The effect of barbitu-

rates in patients with liver disease. J. Clin. Invest., *33*:1116, 1954.

22. Rubin, A., Tephly, T. R., and Mannering, G. J.: Kinetics of drug metabolism by hepatic microsomes. Biochem. Pharmacol., *13*:1007, 1964.
23. Lo, J. N., and Cumming, J. F.: Interaction between sedative premedicants and ketamine in man and in isolated perfused rat livers. Anesthesiology, *43*:307, 1975.
24. Fingl, E., and Woodbury, D. M.: General principles. *In* The Pharmacological Basis of Therapeutics. 5th Edition. Edited by L. S. Goodman and A. Gilman. New York, Macmillan, 1975.
25. Ascione, F. J.: Sedative and hypnotic therapy. *In* Evaluations of Drug Interactions. 2nd Edition. Washington, D. C., American Pharmaceutical Association, 1976.
26. Hansten, P. D.: Drug Interactions. 3rd Edition. Philadelphia, Lea & Febiger, 1975, p. 201.
27. Hansten, P. D.: Drug Interactions. 3rd Edition. Philadelphia, Lea & Febiger, 1975, p. 198.
28. Janz, D., and Schmidt, D.: Anti-epileptic drugs and failure of oral contraceptives (Letter). Lancet, *1*:1113, 1974.
29. Hansten, P. D.: Drug Interactions. 3rd Edition. Philadelphia, Lea & Febiger, 1975, p. 129.
30. Hansten, P. D.: Drug Interactions. 3rd Edition. Philadelphia, Lea & Febiger, 1975, p. 191.
31. Hansten, P. D.: Interaction between anticonvulsant drugs: primidone, diphenylhydantoin and phenobarbital. Northwest Med. J., *1*:17, 1974.
32. Ascione, F. J.: Warfarin-alcohol. *In* Evaluations of Drug Interactions. 2nd Edition. Washington, D.C., American Pharmaceutical Association, 1976.
33. Carriere, G., et al.: Etude experimental des injections intraveineuses d'alcool au cours d'intoxications par le gardenal. C. R. Soc. Biol. (Paris), *116*:188, 1934.
34. Gruber, C. M., Jr.: A theoretical consideration of additive and potentiated effects between drugs with a practical example using alcohol and barbiturates. Arch. Int. Pharmacodyn. Ther., *102*:17, 1955.
35. Morselli, P. L., et al.: Further observations on the interaction between ethanol and psychotrophic drugs. Arzneim. Forsch., *21*:20, 1971.
36. Jetter, W. W., and McLean, R.: Poisoning by the synergistic effect of phenobarbital and ethyl alcohol. An experimental study. Arch. Pathol., *36*:112, 1943.
37. Ascione, F. J.: Phenobarbital-alcohol. *In* Evaluations of Drug Interactions. 2nd Edition. Washington, D.C., American Pharmaceutical Association, 1976.
38. Mould, G. P., et al.: Interaction of glutethimide and phenobarbitone with ethanol in man. J.Pharm. Pharmacol., *24*:894, 1972.
39. Mezey, F., and Robles, E. A.: Effects of phenobarbital administration on rates of ethanol clearance and on ethanol-oxidizing enzymes in man. Gastroenterology, *66*:248, 1974.
40. Lieber, C. S., and DeCarli, L. M.: Effect of drug administration on the activity of the hepatic mi-

crosomal ethanol oxidizing system. Life Sci., *9*:267, 1970.
41. Lieber, C. S., and DeCarli, L. M.: The role of the hepatic microsomal ethanol oxidizing system (MEOS) for ethanol metabolism *in vivo*. J. Pharmacol. Exp. Ther., *181*:279, 1972.
42. Khanna, J. M., et al.: Significance *in vivo* of the increase in microsomal ethanol-oxidizing system after chronic administration of ethanol, phenobarbital and chlorcyclizine. Biochem. Pharmacol., *21*:2215, 1972.
43. Roach, M. K., et al.: Ethanol metabolism *in vivo* and the role of hepatic microsomal ethanol oxidation. Quart. J. Stud. Alc., *33*:751, 1972.
44. Khanna, J. M., and Kalant, H.: Effect of inhibitors and inducers of drug metabolism on ethanol metabolism *in vivo*. Biochem. Pharmacol., *19*:2033, 1970.
45. Carter, E. A., and Isselbacher, K. J.: Hepatic microsomal ethanol oxidation. Mechanism and physiologic significance. Lab. Invest., *27*:283, 1972.
46. Forney, R. F., and Hughes, F.: Combined Effects of Alcohol and Other Drugs. Springfield, Ill., Charles C Thomas, 1968.
47. Kielholz, P., et al.: Fahrversuche zur frage der beeintrachtigung der verkehrstuchtigkeit durch alkohol, tranquilizer und hypnotika. Dtsch. Med. Wochenschr., *94*:301, 1969.
48. Joyce, C. R. B., et al.: Potentiation by phenobarbitone of effects of ethyl alcohol on human behavior. J. Ment. Dis., *105*:51, 1959.
49. Mathew, H.: Acute Barbiturate Poisoning. Amsterdam, Excerpta Medica Foundation, 1971.
50. Evans, M. A., et al.: Quantitative relationship between blood alcohol concentration and psychomotor performance. Clin. Pharmacol. Ther., *15*:253, 1974.
51. Johnstone, R. E., and Reier, C. E.: Acute respiratory effects of ethanol in man. Clin. Pharmacol. Ther., *14*:501, 1973.
52. Nickerson, M., and Collier, B.: Drugs inhibiting adrenergic nerves and structures innervated by them. *In* The Pharmacological Basis of Therapeutics. 5th Edition. Edited by L. S. Goodman and A. Gilman. New York, Macmillan, 1975.
53. Cook, E., and Grown, G.: The vasodilating effects of ethyl alcohol on the peripheral arteries. Proc. Mayo Clin., *7*:449, 1932.
54. Docter, R., and Perkins, R.: The effects of ethyl alcohol on autonomic and muscular responses in humans. Quart. J. Stud. Alc., *22*:374, 1960.
55. Fewings, E., et al.: The effects of ethyl alcohol on the blood vessels of the hand and forearm in man. Br. J. Pharmacol. Chemother., *27*:93, 1966.
56. Gillespie, J.: Vasodilator properties of alcohol. Br. Med. J., *2*:274, 1967.
57. Gimena, A., et al.: Effects of ethanol on cellular membrane potentials and contractility of isolated rat atrium. Am. J. Physiol., *203*:194, 1962.
58. Regan, T., et al.: The acute metabolic and hemodynamic responses of the left ventricle to ethanol. J. Clin. Invest., *45*:270, 1966.
59. Gould, L., et al.: Cardiac effects of a cocktail. J.A.M.A., *218*:1799, 1971.

60. Bienvenu, O.: Essential hypertension. Med. Clin. North Am., *51*:967, 1967.
61. Meyer, F. H., et al.: Review of Medical Pharmacology. Los Altos, Calif., Lange Medical Publications, 1968.
62. Arky, R. A., et al.: Irreversible hypoglycemia, A complication of alcohol and insulin. J.A.M.A., *206*:575, 1968.
63. Ascione, F. J.: Tolbutamide-alcohol. *In* Evaluations of Drug Interactions. 2nd Edition. Washington, D.C., American Pharmaceutical Association, 1976.
64. Han, Y. H.: Why do chronic alcoholics require more anesthesia? Anesthesiology, *30*:341, 1969.
65. Munson, E. A.: Unpublished data.
66. Fitzgerald, M. G., et. al.: Alcohol sensitivity in diabetics receiving chlorpropamide. Diabetes, *11*:40, 1962.
67. Hugin, W.: Intentional beneficial and accidental or undesirable drug interactions in anesthesia. *In* Drug Interactions. Edited by P. L. Morselli, S. Garattini, and S. N. Cohen. New York, Raven Press, 1974.
68. De Jong, R. H., and Heavner, J. E.: Diazepam prevents and aborts lidocaine convulsions in monkeys. Anesthesiology, *41*:226, 1974.
69. Feinstein, M. B., Lenard, W., and Mathias, J.: The antagonism of local anesthetic induced convulsions by the benzodiazepine derivative diazepam. Arch. Int. Pharmacodyn. Ther., *187*:144, 1970.
70. Wale, N., and Jenkins, L. C.: Site of action of diazepam in the prevention of lidocaine induced seizure activity in cats. Can. Anaesth. Soc. J., *20*:146, 1973.
71. De Jong, R. H., and Heavner, J. E.: Diazepam prevents local anesthetic seizures. Anesthesiology, *34*:523, 1971.
72. Aldrete, J. A., and Daniel, W.: Evaluation of premedicants as protective agents against convulsive (LD_{50}) doses of local anesthetic agents in rats. Anesth. Analg. (Cleve.), *50*:127, 1971.
73. Wesseling, H., Bovenhorst, G. H., and Wiers, J. W.: Effects of diazepam and pentobarbitone on convulsions induced by local anesthetics in mice. Eur. J. Pharmacol., *13*:150, 1971.
74. Munson, E. S., and Wagman, I. H.: Diazepam treatment of local anesthetic-induced seizures. Anesthesiology, *37*:523, 1972.
75. De Jong, R. H., and Heavner, J. E.: Local anesthetic seizure prevention: Diazepam versus pentobarbital. Anesthesiology, *36*:449, 1972.
76. Munson, E. S., Gutnick, M. J., and Wagman, I. H.: Local anesthetic drug-induced seizures in rhesus monkeys. Anesth. Analg. (Cleve.), *49*:986, 1970.
77. De Jong, R. H., and Heavner, J. E.: Diazepam and lidocaine-induced cardiovascular changes. Anesthesiology, *39*:633, 1973.
78. Dunbar, R. W., et al.: The effect of diazepam on the antiarrhythmic response to lidocaine. Anesth. Analg. (Cleve.), *50*:685, 1971.
79. Larson, G. F., Hurlbert, B. J., and Wingard, D. W.: Physostigmine reversal of diazepam-induced arousal. Anesth. Anesth. Analg. (Cleve.), *56*:348, 1977.
80. Bernards, W.: Case history number 74: Reversal of phenothiazine-induced coma with physostigmine. Anesth. Analg. (Cleve.), *52*:938, 1973.
81. DiLiberti, J., O'Brien, M. L., and Turner, T.: The use of physostigmine as an antidote in accidental diazepam intoxication. J. Pediatr., *86*:106, 1975.
82. Rosenberg, H.: Physostigmine reversal of sedative drugs (letter). J.A.M.A., *229*:1168, 1974.
83. Blitt, C. D., and Petty, W. C.: Reversal of lorazepam delirium by physostigmine. Anesth. Analg. (Cleve.), *54*:607, 1975.
84. Bradley, P. B. and Elkes, J.: The effect of atropine, hyoscyamine, physostigmine, and neostigmine on electrical activity of the conscious cat. J. Physiol., *120*:14, 1953.
85. Karen, D.: Unpublished observations.
86. Berman, M. L., and Harbison, R. D.: Induction of consciousness by physostigmine. Pharmacologist, *18*: Abstract 406, 1976.
87. Avant, G. R., et al.: Physostigmine reversal of diazepam-induced hypnosis in human volunteers. *In* Abstracts of Scientific Papers. Park Ridge, Ill., American Society of Anesthesiologists, 1978.
88. Feldman, S. A., and Crawley, B. E.: Interaction of diazepam with the muscle-relaxant drugs. Br. Med. J., *2*:336, 1970.
89. Dretchen, K., et. al.: The interaction of diazepam with myoneural blocking agents. Anesthesiology, *34*:463, 1971.
90. Webb, S. N., and Bradshaw, E. G.: Diazepam and neuromuscular blocking drugs (Letter). Br. Med. J., *3*:640, 1971.
91. Whitfield, J. B., et al.: Changes in plasma α-glutamyl transpeptidase activity associated with alterations in drug metabolism in man. Br. Med. J., *1*:316, 1973.
92. Robinson, D. S., and Sylwester, D.: Interaction of commonly prescribed drugs and warfarin. Ann. Intern. Med., *72*:853, 1970.
93. Lackner, H., and Hunt, V. E.: The effect of Librium on hemostasis. Am. J. Med. Sci., *256*:368, 1968.
94. Ascione, F. J.: Amitriptyline-chlordiazepoxide. *In* Evaluations of Drug Interactions. 2nd Edition. Washington, D.C., American Pharmaceutical Association, 1976.
95. Ascione, F. J.: Diazepam-alcohol. *In* Evaluations of Drug Interactions. 2nd Edition. Washington, D.C., American Pharmaceutical Association, 1976.
96. Ascione, F. J.: Gallamine triethiode-diazepam. *In* Evaluations of Drug Interactions. 2nd Edition, Washington, D.C., American Pharmaceutical Association, 1976.
97. Ascione, F. J.: Levodopa-diazepam. *In* Evaluations of Drug Interactions. 2nd Edition, Washington, D.C., American Pharmaceutical Association, 1976.
98. Ascione, F. J.: Warfarin-chlordiazepoxide. *In* Evaluations of Drug Interactions. 2nd Edition. Washington, D. C., American Pharmaceutical Association, 1976.

99. Harvey, S. C.: Hypnotics and sedatives. Miscellaneous Agents. *In* The Pharmacological Basis of Therapeutics. 5th Edition. Edited by L. S. Goodman and A. Gilman. New York, Macmillan, 1975.

100. Ascione, F. J.: Warfarin-chloral hydrate. *In* Evaluations of Drug Interactions. 2nd Edition. Washington, D.C., American Pharmaceutical Association, 1976.

101. Weiner, M.: Species differences in the effect of chloral hydrate on coumarin anticoagulants. Ann. N. Y. Acad. Sci., *179*:226, 1971.

102. Griner, P. F., et al.: Chloral hydrate and warfarin interaction: Clinical significance. Ann. Intern. Med., *74*:540, 1971.

103. Sellers, E. M., and Koch-Weser, J.: Kinetics and clinical importance of displacement of warfarin from albumin by acidic drugs. Ann. N.Y. Acad. Sci., *179*:213, 1971.

104. Sellers, E. M., and Koch-Weser, J.: Potentiation of warfarin-induced hypoprothrombinemia by chloral hydrate. N. Engl. J. Med., *283*:827, 1970.

105. Van Dam, I. E., and Gribnau-Overkamp, M. J. H.: The effect of some sedatives (phenobarbital, glutethimide, chlordiazepoxide, chloral hydrate) on the rate of disappearance of ethyl biscoumacetate from the plasma. Folia Med. Neerl., *10*:141, 1967.

106. Breckeneridge, A., et al.: Drug interactions with warfarin: Studies with dichloralphenazone, chloral hydrate and phenazone (Antipyrine). Clin. Sci., *40*:351, 1971.

107. Breckenridge, A., and Orme, M.: Clinical implications of enzyme induction. Ann. N. Y. Acad. Sci., *179*:421, 1971.

108. Boston Collaborative Drug Surveillance Program: Interaction between chloral hydrate and warfarin. N. Engl. J. Med., *286*:53, 1972.

109. Udall, J. A.: Chloral hydrate and warfarin therapy (Letter). Ann. Intern. Med., *75*:141, 1971.

110. Ascione, F. J.: Chlorcyclizine-phenobarbital. *In* Evaluations of Drug Interactions. 2nd Edition. Washington, D.C., American Pharmaceutical Association, 1976.

111. Ascione, F. J.: Warfarin-diphenylhydramine. *In* Evaluations of Drug Interactions. 2nd Edition. Washington, D.C., American Pharmaceutical Association, 1976.

112. Hunninghake, D. B., and Azarnoff, D. L.: Drug interactions with warfarin. Arch. Intern. Med., *121*:349, 1968.

113. Ascione, F. J.: Anticoagulant therapy. *In* Evaluations of Drug Interactions. 2nd Edition. Washington, D.C., American Pharmaceutical Association, 1976.

114. Hollister, L. E., Richard, R. K., and Gillespie, H. K.: Comparison of tetrahydrocannabinol and synhexyl in man. Clin. Pharmacol. Ther., *9*: 783, 1968.

115. Brill, N. Q.: The marihuana problems. Ann. Intern. Med., *73*:449, 1970.

116. Stoelting, R. K., et al.: Effects of delta-9-tetrahydrocannabinol on halothane MAC in dogs. Anesthesiology, *38*:521, 1973.

117. Vitez, T. S., et al.: Effects of delta-9-tetrahydrocannabinol on cyclopropane MAC in the rat. Anesthesiology, *38*:525, 1973.

118. Beaconsfield, P., Ginsburg, J., and Rainsbury, R.: Marihuana smoking. Cardiovascular effects in man and possible mechanisms. N. Engl. J. Med., *287*:209, 1972.

119. Berman, M. L.: "Pot" and anesthetics—how do they mix. J.A.M.A., *220*:914, 1972.

120. Lemberger, L., Axelrod, J., and Kopin, I.: Metabolism and disposition of delta-9-tetrahydrocannabinol in man. Pharmacol. Rev., *23*:371, 1971.

121. Johnstone, R. E., et al.: Combination of Δ-9-Tetrahydrocannabinol with oxymorphone or pentobarbital: Effects on ventilatory control and cardiovascular dynamics. Anesthesiology, *42*:674, 1975.

Intravenous Agents

RONALD D. MILLER
and
LEO D.H.J. BOOIJ

Many types of drugs are injected intravenously either to produce anesthesia or to be adjuncts to it. Thus the potential for drug interactions is enormous. Interactions with psychotropic drugs are covered in Chapter 13; with sedative-hypnotics in Chapter 14; and with narcotics in Chapter 16. This chapter describes those interactions involving ketamine and several new intravenous anesthetics that have been used extensively in other countries and to a limited extent in the United States.

KETAMINE (Ketalar, Ketaject)

Ketamine, a phencyclidine derivative, produces a state called "dissociative anesthesia" characterized by what appears to be catatonia. It also renders the patient amnesic and analgesic. Although it is desirable in many respects, ketamine has been associated with disorientation, sensory and perceptual illusions, and vivid dreams following anesthesia that are termed "emergence phenomena." Garfield et al.[1] performed one of the most objective studies in this regard and concluded that ketamine produces visual, auditory, proprioceptive and/or confusional illusions at much higher incidence than do other general anesthetics. Diazepam, 0.2 to 0.3 mg/kg, given intravenously five minutes prior to the administration of ketamine, reduces the incidence of all dreams and illusions.[2] No doubt drugs other than diazepam will be tried in an effort to eliminate the "emergence phenomena." For example, fewer dreams occur when thiopental is also used for induction of anesthesia.[3]

Other than possibly attenuating the incidence of illusions and dreams, diazepam, hydroxyzine, and secobarbital will alter the sleeping time of the patient and the metabolism of ketamine.[4] Ketamine, a lipophilic drug, is rapidly distributed into highly vascular organs and subsequently redistributed to less well-perfused tissues, with concurrent hepatic metabolism and urinary and biliary excretion. Pretreatment with phenobarbital, a well-known enzyme-inducer, accelerates the rate at which ketamine is metabolized and reduces plasma half-life.[5] However, because sleeping times were not prolonged, Cohen and Trevor concluded that the metabolic inactivation of ketamine was not responsible for the termination of the drug's hypnotic effects.[5] The researchers assumed that the redistribution of ketamine from brain to other tissues helps to eliminate ketamine's hypnotic effect. However, phenobarbital pretreatment did decrease the duration of posthypnotic ataxia and agitation.

Although phenobarbital did not alter the hypnotic effects of ketamine in the study discussed, premedication with diazepam increases sleeping time (Fig. 15–1A) probably because of delayed plasma clearance (Fig. 15–1B) and decreased metabolism.[4] Lo and Cumming suggest that diazepam and ketamine are biotransformed by the hepatic microsomal system in such a way that diazepam inhibits the metabolism of ketamine.[4] In conclusion, although premedication with diazepam attenuates "emergence phenomena," clinicians should be aware that sleeping time is prolonged and that plasma clearance of ketamine is delayed. Tolerance to ketamine could counteract diazepam's effect. However, since tolerance to ketamine does not develop until six hours after the initial dose, this interaction usually would not be of clinical relevance.[6]

When ketamine is given during halothane anesthesia several interactions occur, some of which are clinically important (Table 15–1). Ketamine reduces the minimum alveolar anesthetic concentration (MAC) of

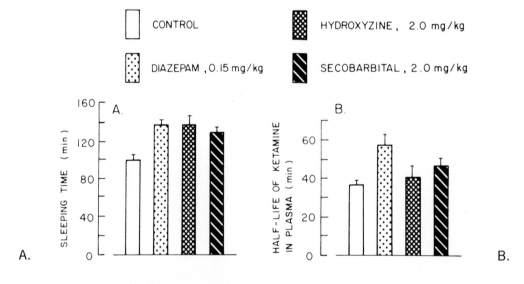

Fig. 15–1A, & B: Sleeping times of patients given ketamine, 10 mg/kg, intramuscularly. Premedications above were given 30 minutes prior to induction of anesthesia with ketamine (Fig. 15–1A). To the right, plasma half-lives of ketamine in patients receiving atropine, 0.02 mg/kg intramuscularly, 30 minutes prior to induction of anesthesia (control) and those receiving the same dose of atropine plus the sedative indicated (Fig. 15–1B). (From Lo, J. N., and Cumming, J. F.: Interaction between sedative premedicants and ketamine in men and in isolated perfused rat livers. Anesthesiology, *43*:307, 1975.)

Table 15–1

Summary of Interaction Between Ketamine and Halothane

1. Ketamine reduces the MAC of halotheane[7]
2. Halothane prolongs the pharmacologic effects of ketamine[8]
3. Halothane decreases plasma clearance, redistribution and metabolism of ketamine[8]
4. Ketamine causes hypotension when given during halothane anesthesia[9,11]
5. Ketamine and halothane both enhance the arrhythmogenicity of epinephrine[15]
6. Ketamine and halothane both enhance a nondepolarizing neuromuscular blockade.[9]

halothane.[7] Furthermore, White et al. suggest that ketamine is not a short-acting drug.[7] The MAC of halothane was reduced for several hours (Fig. 15–2). Also, doses of ketamine that produced less than ten minutes of hypnosis resulted in analgesia and ataxia lasting an hour or longer. The researchers estimate that the prolonged effect of ketamine on halothane MAC is due to ketamine's high lipid solubility and the conversion of ketamine to metabolite I, which itself possesses weak anesthetic properties. White et al. estimated that approximately 75% of the prolonged depression of anesthetic requirement following ketamine administration is attributable to ketamine itself and that the remaining 25% is related to the formation of metabolite I, which has an anesthetic potency one-third that of ketamine.[7]

The emphasis of this study has been on what ketamine does to halothane. However, halothane has profound effects on ketamine. Although only halothane was studied, these conclusions probably also apply to other inhalation anesthetics. Halothane prolongs the sleeping time and ataxia induced by ketamine. This can partly be explained by the influence of halothane on the pharmacokinetics of ketamine : (1) halothane delays the attainment of peak plasma levels and rate at which ketamine leaves the plasma (Fig. 15–3); (2) time to achievement of peak levels and plasma clearance of metabolite I are also delayed by halothane

(Fig. 15–3); and (3) levels of metabolite I are lower in plasma when halothane is given.

Thus halothane prolongs the pharmacologic effect of ketamine by decreasing its uptake, distribution, redistribution, and metabolism.[8]

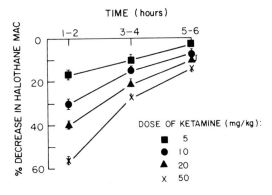

Fig. 15–2. Changes in halothane MAC (minimum alveolar anesthetic concentration) at various times after the intramuscular injection of ketamine. (From Winter, P. F., Johnston, R. R., and Pudwill, C. R.: Interaction of ketamine and halothane in rats. Anesthesiology, *42*:179, 1975.)

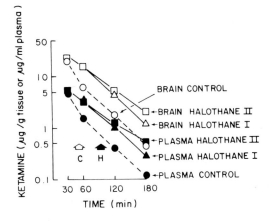

Fig. 15–3. Plasma and brain levels of ketamine on a logarithmic scale as a function of time after ketamine administration (50 mg/kg intramuscularly) in unanesthetized animals (control), in rats exposed to anesthesia during the first 60 minutes only (halothane I) and in animals continuously anesthetized (halothane II). Time to the termination of ataxia for control (C) and halothane I (H) are indicated by arrowheads. (From White, P. F., et al.: Effects of halothane anesthesia on the biodisposition of ketamine in rats. J. Pharmacol. Exp. Ther., *196*:545, 1976.)

CASE REPORT

A 35-year-old woman was scheduled for a vaginal hysterectomy. She had a negative medical history. Anesthesia was induced and maintained with halothane. Neuromuscular function was quantitated for measuring force of thumb adduction in response to stimulation of the ulnar nerve. This anesthetic was part of a clinical study to evaluate the effect of ketamine on neuromuscular blockades produced by muscle relaxants. Ketamine, 75 mg/m^2 was given intravenously. The patient's systolic blood pressure decreased from 105 to 74 torr and her pulse rate fell from 76 to 60/min. Administration of atropine, 0.4 mg intravenously, resulted in a prompt increase in blood pressure and pulse rate to the preketamine values. No further problems occurred.[9]

The cardiovascular effects of ketamine include increases in heart rate, blood pressure, and cardiac output. The mechanism of these effects is reviewed elsewhere.[10] However, we found that ketamine caused hypotension when given during halothane anesthesia in 38 patients, including the patient in our case report. Bidwai et al. later confirmed our original observation that ketamine causes hypotension when given during halothane anesthesia.[11] Although ketamine still caused an increase in arteriolar peripheral resistance, the marked decrease in cardiac output and stroke volume resulted in arterial hypotension. We speculated that halothane, which obtunds baroreceptor activity and ganglionic transmission, might have prevented the usual increase in blood pressure and pulse rate following ketamine administration.[9,12,13] Ketamine alone produces cardiac depression in denervated isolated hearts.[14] We then might have added to the cardiac depression produced by halothane, which resulted in hypotension. This explanation was extended by Koehntop et al., who suggested that ketamine owes part of its cardiovascular effect to blockade of the intraneuronal uptake of catecholamines.[15] During halothane anesthesia, the release of catecholamines is depressed and the quantity of catecholamines that could be prevented

from being taken up into the adrenergic nerve endings by ketamine is correspondingly decreased. As a result, less than the usual amount of catecholamines is diverted back to, or is prevented from leaving, the area of the receptor, thereby allowing the direct depressant effects of ketamine on the heart to predominate. In addition, Koehntop et al. found that ketamine enhances the arrhythmogenicity of epinephrine, an effect augmented by halothane.[15] Caution should be exercised in the administration of ketamine during halothane anesthesia.

Finally, ketamine enhances a d-tubocurarine neuromuscular blockade during halothane anesthesia. The ED$_{50}$ of d-tubocurarine (dose that caused a 50% depression of twitch tension) was 4.9 mg/m^2 with halothane alone and 2.8 mg/m^2 with halothane plus ketamine, 75 mg/m^2.[9]

This section illustrates only a few interactions involving ketamine and other drugs during anesthesia.

FLUNITRAZEPAM (Rohypnol)

Flunitrazepam, a benzodiazepine and a homologue of diazepam, represents continued efforts to develop a sedative-hypnotic superior to the popular and successful diazepam. In initial reports, flunitrazepam appeared to have all the advantages of diazepam, namely minimal cardiovascular effects and a faster onset of sedation (<1 min).[16] With more detailed investigations, Dundee et al. found that the maximum sedative effect occurred in about the same time required for diazepam.[17] Using approximately equipotent doses, Clarke and Lyons found the drug's depression of arterial blood pressure similar to that following the administration of diazepam or of thiopental (Fig. 15–4).[18] Thus flunitrazepam appears to have no advantage over more commonly used drugs such as diazepam or thiopental. Flunitrazepam has been used in combination with diazepam and procaine to produce general anesthesia.[19,20] Although these

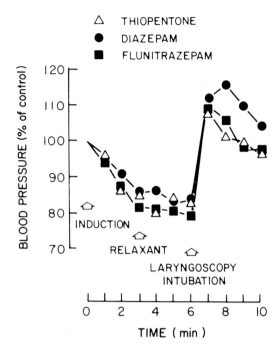

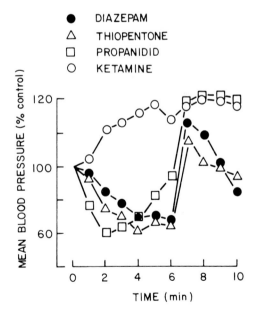

Because of the dependence of cholinesterase activity for the drug's degradation, a prediction was made that propanidid may interfere with the biotransformation of succinylcholine. This prediction was confirmed. Propanidid prolongs succinylcholine-induced apnea.[23,24] However, the prolongation is insufficient (<4 min) to be of clinical significance.

Propanidid causes hypotension primarily due to peripheral vasodilation and secondarily due to a slight negative inotropic effect.[25] At the same time, filling pressures of the heart are increased. However, the hypotension induced by propanidid is transient and is no greater than that induced by diazepam or by thiopental (Fig. 15–5). Propanidid produces a biphasic ventilatory effect. As unconsciousness ensues, a short period (~30 sec) of hyperventilation develops, fol-

Fig. 15–4. The mean arterial blood pressure (% of control) during induction with flunitrazepam, 0.036 mg/kg, diazepam, 0.32 mg/kg, and thiopentone (thiopental), 4 mg/kg. (From Clarke, R. S. J., and Lyons, S. M.: Diazepam and flunitrazepam as induction agents for cardiac surgical operations. Acta Anaesthesiol. Scand., *21*:282, 1977.)

drugs clearly interact with one another, the interaction has not been quantitated.

PROPANIDID

Propanidid (3-methoxy-4-(N,N-diethylcarbamoylmethoxy) phenylacetic acid-n-propylester) produces anesthesia with about the same rapidity as thiopental. However, some authors claim that recovery is more complete and that cumulation is less likely to occur with propanidid than with thiopental.[21] This is because propanidid is rapidly degraded by cholinesterase into inactive metabolites.[22] Predictably, when cholinesterase activity is low, the rate of degradation of propanidid is slower. Also, protein binding appears to be important. With low levels of plasma protein, higher levels of propanidid activity are observed, and greater cholinesterase inhibition occurs.

Fig. 15–5. The mean arterial blood pressure (% of control) during induction with diazepam, 0.46 mg/kg, ketamine, 2.0 mg/kg, propanidid, 4.0 mg/kg, and thiopentone (thiopental), 4.3 mg/kg, followed by pancuronium, 0.1 mg/kg, and endotracheal intubation three and six minutes later respectively. (From Lyons, S. M., Clarke, R. S. J., and Dundee, J. W.: Some cardiovascular and respiratory effects of four nonbarbiturate anesthetic induction agents. Eur. J. Clin. Pharmacol., *1*:275, 1974.)

lowed by hypoventilation and sometimes by apnea.[27] Usually the duration of apnea is only about 30 seconds from a dose of 10 mg/kg.

Because of the patient's rapid recovery, the apparent lack of cumulative effect, and the minimal cardiorespiratory effects, propranidid is a promising anesthetic. However, numerous adverse reactions have been reported. Major epileptiform convulsions occasionally occur both in patients with and without epilepsy.[28] Thornton has summarized some of these reactions as "severe hypotension: cyanosis following flushing and hypotension: morbilliform rash with facial edema 15 to 20 minutes after injection: glottic spasm before loss of consciousness and an anesthesiologist who developed edema and itching of the fingers on skin contact with propanidid."[29] In more severe reactions, cardiac arrest has occurred.[30] Although the cause is often not apparent, these reactions appear to limit the usefulness of propanidid.

ALPHADIONE (Althesin)

The considerable interest in using steroids as an anesthetic that has been generated has been reviewed by Gyermek and Soyka.[31] As a result of this interest, a mixture of two steroids has been found to be effective. Alphadione, a combination of alphaxalone and its 21 acetoxy ester, induces sleep in less than 60 seconds with a duration ranging from two to 13 minutes. Although not well studied, it appears to have no cumulative effect. The potency and duration of hypnosis probably depend, in part, on the rapidity with which the drug is infused (Fig. 15–6).[32] Alphadione rapidly disappears from plasma and appears in bile within ten minutes after injection.[33] The drug can be detected in urine within 30 minutes after injection. After five days, about 80% of the drug is excreted in the urine. Strunin et al. speculate that alphadione is rapidly taken up by the liver, metabolized to a more polar compound possibly by conjugation, and then ex-

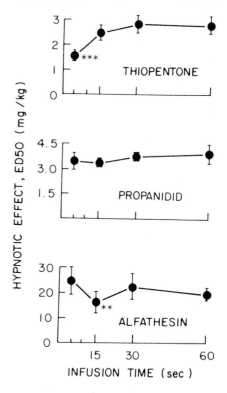

Fig. 15–6. The effect of intravenous infusion times (sec) on the ED_{50} values for the hypnotic effect of thiopentone (thiopental), alfathesin, and propanidid. (From Aveling, W., Bradshaw, A. D., and Crankshaw, D. P.: The effect of speed of injection on the potency of anaesthetic induction agents. Anaesth. Intensive Care, 6:116, 1978.)

creted in the urine.[33] Consistent with this, Novelli et al. found the effects of alphadione to depend on the functional state of the liver.[34] Alphadione is, indeed, rapidly broken down in the liver by microsomal enzymes and especially by glucuronyltransferase. Sleeping time is reduced with enzyme induction. Therefore, if a patient is receiving those drugs known to induce enzymes (for example, phenobarbital), the duration of hypnosis may be reduced. Conversely, depression of hepatic activity by cholestasis or by decreased microsomal enzyme activity increases sleeping time.

Alphadione causes hypotension to a degree similar to thiopental and either does not change or increases a patient's heart rate.[35]

Although the mechanism of alphadione's cardiovascular effects has not been elucidated, Broadley and Taylor concluded that "Althesin (alphadione) can be used satisfactorily as an induction agent for poorly compensated myocardial and valvular diseased patients when used in small increments slowly, but does produce a more pronounced fall in cardiac output than thiopental, over which it offers no special advantage."[36] However, alphadione appears to be useful for intracranial surgery, as does thiopental. Alphadione decreases intracranial pressure, cerebral blood flow, cerebral blood volume, and cerebral metabolic rate for oxygen and it increases cerebral vascular resistance.[37,38]

Adverse reactions to alphadione include skin changes, hypotension, bronchospasm, and abdominal symptoms, in order of frequency. Watkins has reviewed these reactions and has found that of 90 cases reported, only one resulted in death.[39] Alphadione reactions generally involve excessive activation of complement C_3, leading to histamine release, and are not reagin-antibody mediated. For further information, the review of Watkins is recommended.[39]

Although several drug interactions involving alphadione probably exist, we could only find two of interest to anesthesiologists. The claim has been made that benzodiazepines (for example, diazepam) and the steroid anesthetics act in a synergistic manner; however, support of this claim is not convincing.[40] Another interaction not unique with alphadione is an increased incidence of involuntary movements when patients are premedicated with hyoscine. Substitution with atropine attenuates the incidence of involuntary movement.[41] Perhaps neither hyoscine nor atropine is necessary for premedication.

ETOMIDATE

Etomidate, a carboxylated imidazole derivative, produces hypnosis rapidly (one circulation time) with a duration of action of four to ten minutes. The duration can be increased by augmenting the dose or by using a constant infusion. Distribution of etomidate is rapid, with early distribution half-lives of 2.6 and 28.7 min.[42] The drug is lipid-soluble and therefore has a large volume of distribution of about 4.5 times body weight. When distribution of etomidate is nearly complete, only 7% of the drug is in the central compartment, available for elimination at any time. Preliminary studies in man indicate that almost 90% of the label eventually appears in the urine, of which only 2% is unchanged etomidate. This suggests that total clearance of etomidate primarily represents clearance for metabolism, with the liver being the primary site of metabolism. Therefore, etomidate clearance is influenced by changes in hepatic blood flow and metabolism; such changes commonly occur intraoperatively. Whether this is clinically important has not been documented.

Initial reports were encouraging and stated that etomidate produces hypnosis within seconds with no effect on heart rate, slight hypotension, and a low frequency of apnea.[43] Unlike many other intravenous anesthetics, histamine is not released. However, Fragen et al. observed a 70% incidence of myoclonia (only 10% were severe cases) and a 50% incidence of pain during injection.[44] The speed of injection appeared not to affect the incidence of side effects. Ghoneim and Yamada found that myoclonic movements were not associated with epileptiform discharges on the electroencephalogram.[45] Prior administration of fentanyl or diazepam will reduce the incidence of myoclonic movements. They observed that patients who received both etomidate and thiopental for short operations reported quicker recovery with no hangover effect after etomidate. Ghoneim and Yamada then suggested that etomidate would constitute a significant advantage for outpatients and for minor operations.[45] Rapid, full recovery of mental and psychomotor function is uncommon with other intravenous anesthetics. However, we believe that until the problems of myoclonic movement and pain with injection are resolved, etomidate's value is limited.

GAMMA HYDROXYBUTYRIC ACID

Gamma hydroxybutyric acid (GHBA) is interesting because of its close association with normal chemicals in the brain. Gamma aminobutyric acid has been isolated from the brain and is a central and peripheral synaptic inhibitor. However, it does not cross the blood-brain barrier. In 1960 Laborit et al. developed a form of GHBA that crossed the blood-brain barrier and exerted the same neuroinhibitory action as the amino derivative.[46] Apparently GHBA has the advantage of being nontoxic with a wide safety margin. As an anesthetic, GHBA has a unique pathway of metabolism. GHBA is probably degraded to succinic semialdehyde, then to succinic acid, which then enters the Krebs cycle as a normal metabolite. This process forms carbon dioxide and water.[47] Less than 2% is excreted through the kidney, which makes GHBA ideal in the presence of impaired renal function.[48]

Because GHBA is principally a hypnotic with few hypnotic properties, it must be supplemented with narcotics or with nitrous oxide.[49] In our experience, administration of GHBA, 60/80 mg/kg, with thiopental, 1 mg/kg, intravenously, produces anesthesia in about five minutes that, with the addition of 50 to 70% nitrous oxide, lasts for about 60 minutes. Cardiorespiratory function is stable except for a tendency to develop bradycardia. This tendency can be corrected by the administration of atropine. A significant drawback of GHBA is that it occasionally causes extrapyramidal motor activity during the induction of anesthesia.[50] In our experience, this activity can be prevented by premedication either with droperidol or with the combination of diazepam and a narcotic. Alcohol enhances GHBA's hypnotic effect by interfering with its metabolism through the liver. Relative

contraindications are epilepsy (because of extrapyramidal activity) and alcoholism (because of decreased metabolism).

In addition to intraoperative anesthesia, one of us has found that GHBA can successfully provide a sedative effect that aids in a patient's acceptance of controlled ventilation. GHBA is no longer used in the United States, which we think is unfortunate.

In summary, with the exception of ketamine and possibly of GHBA, the intravenous anesthetics described probably have limited if any value. One major problem of comparing intravenous anesthetics is not knowing what constitutes an equipotent dose. For example, how can the cardiovascular effects of two drugs be compared if the equipotent dose is not known? How can one determine the equipotent dose of an intravenous anesthetic? Crankshaw and Allt-Graham have attempted to solve this problem.[51] They determined the ED_{50} for various intravenous anesthetics by a cumulative dose-response technique, using the inability of the patient to grasp a light object as the end point. With this method precise potency can be determined, and this will allow more accurate comparison of the various intravenous anesthetics.

REFERENCES

1. Garfield, J.M., et al.: A comparison of psychologic responses to ketamine and thiopental-nitrous oxide-halothane anesthesia. Anesthesiology, 36:329, 1972.
2. Kothary, S. P. and Zsigmond, E. K.: A double-blind study of the effective antihallucinatory doses of diazepam prior to ketamine anesthesia. J. Clin. Pharmacol. Ther., 21:108, 1977.
3. Liang, H. S., and Liang, H. G.: Minimizing emergence phenomena: subdissociative dosage of ketamine in balanced surgical anesthesia. Anesth. Analg. (Cleve.), 54:312, 1975.
4. Lo, J. N., and Cumming, J. F.: Interaction between sedative premedicants and ketamine in man and in isolated perfused rat livers. Anesthesiology, 43:307, 1975.
5. Cohen, M. L., and Trevor, A. J.: On the cerebral accumulation of ketamine and the relationship between metabolism of the drug and its pharmacological effects. J. Pharmacol. Exp. Ther., 189:351, 1974.
6. Cumming, J. E.: The development of an acute tol-

erance to ketamine. Anesth. Analg. (Cleve.), *55*:788, 1976.

7. White, P. F., Johnston, R. R., and Pudwill, C. R.: Interaction of ketamine and halothane in rats. Anesthesiology, *42*:179, 1975.

8. White, P. F., et al.: Effects of halothane anesthesia on the biodisposition of ketamine in rats. J. Pharmacol. Exp. Ther., *196*:545, 1976.

9. Johnston, R. R., Miller, R. D., and Way, W. L.: The interaction of ketamine with d-tubocurarine, pancuronium and succinylcholine in man. Anesth. Analg. (Cleve.), *53*:496, 1974.

10. Tweed, W. A., Minuck, M., and Mymin, D.: Circulatory responses to ketamine anesthesia. Anesthesiology, *37*:613, 1972.

11. Bidwai, A. V., et al.: The effects of ketamine on cardiovascular dynamics during halothane and enflurane anesthesia. Anesth. Analg. (Cleve.), *54*:588, 1975.

12. Bristow, J. P., et al.: Effects of anesthesia on baroreceptor control of heart rate in man. Anesthesiology, *31*:422, 1969.

13. Alper, M. H., Fleisch, T. H., and Flacke, W.: The effects of halothane on the response of cardiac ganglia to various stimulants. Anesthesiology, *31*:429, 1969.

14. Dowdy, E. G., and Kayo, K.: Studies of the mechanism of cardiovascular responses to CI-581. Anesthesiology, *29*:931, 1968.

15. Koehntop, D. E., Liao, J. C., and Van Bergen, F. H.: Effects of pharmacologic alterations of adrenergic mechanisms by cocaine, tropolone, aminophylline and ketamine on epinephrine-induced arrhythmias during halothane-nitrous oxide anesthesia. Anesthesiology, *46*:83, 1977.

16. Stover, J., Endresen, R., and Osterud, A.: Intravenous anaesthesia with a new benzodiazepine. Acta Anaesthesiol. Scand., *17*:163, 1973.

17. Dundee, J. W., et al.: Clinical studies of induction agents XLIII: flunitrazepam. Br. J. Anaesth., *48*:551, 1976.

18. Clarke, R. S. J., and Lyons, S. W.: Diazepam and flunitrazepam as induction agents for cardiac surgical operations. Acta Anaesthesiol. Scand., *21*:282, 1977.

19. de Castro, J.: Atar-analgesia with Ro 5-4200, pancuronium and ketamine. Symposium No. 4 Abstracts, 5th World Congress of Anesthesiology, Kyoto, 1972. Amsterdam, Excerpta Medica, North-Holland Publishing Co.

20. Vega, D.: Technique of intravenous general anesthesia utilizing a new benzodiazepine (Ro 5–4200), procaine and succinylcholine. *In* Abstracts 5th World Congress of Anesthesiology, Kyoto, 1972. Amsterdam, Excerpta Medica, North-Holland Publishing Co.

21. Conway, C. M., and Ellis, D. B.: Propanidid. Br. J. Anaesth., *42*:249, 1970.

22. Doenicke, A., et al.: Experimental studies of the breakdown of Epontol determinations of propanidid in human serum. Br. J. Anaesth., *40*:415, 1968.

23. Torda, T. A., Burkhart, J., and Toh, W.: The interaction of propanidid with suxamethonium and decamethonium. Anaesthesia, *27*:159, 1972.

24. Monks, P. S., and Norman, J.: Prolongation of suxamethonium-induced paralysis by propanidid. Br. J. Anaesth., *44*:1303, 1972.

25. Bernhoff, A., Eklund, B., and Kaijser, L.: Cardiovascular effects of short-term anaesthesia with methohexitone and propanidid in normal subjects. Br. J. Anaesth., *44*:2, 1972.

26. Lyons, S. M., Clarke, R. S. J., and Dundee, J. W.: Some cardiovascular and respiratory effects of four nonbarbiturate anaesthetic induction agents. Eur. J. Clin. Pharmacol., *7*:275, 1974.

27. Harnik, E.: A study of the biphasic ventilatory effects of propanidid. Br. J. Anaesth., *36*:655, 1964.

28. Barron, D. W.: Propanidid in epilepsy. Anaesthesia, *29*:445, 1974.

29. Thornton, H. L.: Apparent anaphylactic reaction to propanidid. Anaesthesia, *26*:490, 1971.

30. Johns, G.: Cardiac arrest following induction with propanidid. Br. J. Anaesth., *42*:74, 1970.

31. Gyermek, L., and Soyka, L. F.: Steroid anesthetics. Anesthesiology, *42*:331, 1975.

32. Aveling, W., Bradshaw, A. D., and Crankshaw, D. P.: The effect of speed of injection on the potency of anaesthetic induction agents. Anaesth. Intensive Care, *6*:116, 1978.

33. Strunin, L., et al.: Metabolism of ^{14}C-labelled alphaxalone in man. Br. J. Anaesth., *46*:319, 1974.

34. Novelli, G. P., Marsili, M., and Lorenzi, P.: Influence of liver metabolism on the actions of Althesin and thiopentone. Br. J. Anaesth., *47*:913, 1975.

35. Aronski, A., et al.: Cardiovascular effects of Althesin. Anaesthesia, *31*:195, 1976.

36. Broadley, J. N., and Taylor, P. A.: An assessment of Althesin for the induction of anaesthesia in cardiac surgical patients. Br. J. Anaesth., *46*:687, 1974.

37. Sari, A., et al.: Effects of Althesin on cerebral blood flow and oxygen consumption in man. Br. J. Anaesth., *48*:545, 1976.

38. Pickerodt, V. W. A., et al.: Effects of Althesin on cerebral perfusion, cerebral metabolism and intracranial pressure in the anaesthetized baboon. Br. J. Anaesth., *44*:751, 1972.

39. Watkins, J.: Anaphylactoid reactions to I.V. substances. Br. J. Anaesth., *51*:51, 1979.

40. Gyermek, L.: Benzodiazepines for supplementing steroid anesthesia. Life Sci., *14*:1433, 1974.

41. Clarke, R. S. J., et al.: Clinical studies of induction agents. XL: Althesin with various premedicants. Br. J. Anaesth., *44*:845, 1972.

42. Van Hamme, M. J., Ghoneim, M. M., and Ambre, J. J.: Pharmacokinetics of etomidate, a new intravenous anesthetic. Anesthesiology, *49*:274, 1978.

43. Morgan, M., Lumley, J., and Whitwam, J. G.: Etomidate, a new water-soluble nonbarbiturate intravenous induction agent. Lancet, *2*:955, 1975.

44. Fragen, R. J., Caldwell, N., and Brunner, E. A.: Clinical use of etomidate for anesthesia induction. Anesth. Analg. (Cleve.), *55*:730, 1976.

45. Ghoneim, M. M., and Yamada, T.: Etomidate: A clinical and electroencephalographic comparison with thiopental. Anesth. Analg. (Cleve.), *56*:479, 1977.

46. Laborit, H., et al.: First report on experimental and clinical studies of sodium gamma-4-hydroxy-

butyrate in anesthesiology and neuropsychiatry. Neuropsychopharmacology, *2*:490, 1961.

47. Nirenberg, M. W., and Jakoby, W. B.: Enzymatic utilization of gamma hydroxybutyric acid. J. Biol. Chem., *235*:954, 1960.

48. Helrich, M., et al.: Correlation of blood levels of 4 hydroxybutyrate with state of consciousness. Anesthesiology, *25*:771, 1964.

49. Appleton, P. J., and Burn, J. M. B.: Gamma hy-

droxybutyric acid. Anesth. Analg. (Cleve.), *47*:164, 1968.

50. Solway, J., and Sadove, M. S.: 4-hydroxybutyrate. Anesth. Analg. (Cleve.), *44*:532, 1965.

51. Crankshaw, D. P., and Allt-Graham, J.: The ED_{50} values for thiopentone, methohexital, propanidid and alfathesin: a clinical experiment. Anaesth. Intensive Care, *6*:36, 1978.

Chapter 16

Narcotics and Narcotic Antagonists

DAVID E. LONGNECKER

Narcotics are widely used in the practice of medicine, in anesthesia in particular, and in nonmedical circumstances (so-called ''street use''), where their abuse is frequent. There are two fundamental pharmacologic actions of narcotics that account for their widespread use: analgesia (without anesthesia) and euphoria. Perhaps the most striking examples of the use of opiates as analgesics are the high-dose narcotic techniques frequently employed in ''anesthesia'' for cardiovascular surgery. On the other end of the spectrum, the illicit user of narcotics consumes these drugs for their euphoric effect rather than for their analgesic properties. The most frequent medical applications for narcotics are in cases where both analgesia and euphoria are desirable. The alleviation of acute or chronic pain by narcotics results from both properties of these compounds and accounts for their prevalent use in medical practice.

Since opiates are used so commonly, the potential for significant interactions with other drugs is considerable. Although many interactions with opiates may occur, perhaps the most important involve their analogs, the narcotic antagonists. Narcotic antagonists minimize both the acute and chronic effects of narcotic overdosage. In persons who suffer from narcotic addiction, the antagonists are used to obtund the euphoria that the abuser craves and to antagonize toxic side effects as well. In anesthetic practice, the antagonists are used to treat either accidental or intentional (the inevitable respiratory depression that accompanies narcotic ''anesthesia'') overdoses of the opiates.

221

This chapter reviews briefly: the pharmacology of the narcotics and illustrates some drug-drug interactions that may occur with narcotic agents; the pharmacology of the narcotic antagonists, and describes their important interactions with the narcotics; and, finally, potential drug interactions between the narcotic antagonists and nonnarcotic drugs.

NARCOTICS

Pharmacology of narcotics

Central Nervous System. As noted above, narcotics are used and abused mainly because of their effects on the central nervous system (CNS). The major therapeutic indication for opiates is the alleviation of pain, and the analgesic qualities of these compounds are unsurpassed. Although new evidence suggests that narcotics may act peripherally, it is widely held that the primary site of action of the opiate is in the central nervous system. In addition to their intrinsic analgesic properties, opiates also modify the perception of pain. Not only is the pain threshold elevated by narcotics, but also the subjective perception of pain is alleviated by the administration of opiates. In the absence of pain, opiates frequently induce a state of euphoria (occasionally dysphoria) and apathy. As the dose of narcotic is increased, progressive drowsiness, difficulty in concentrating, mental clouding, and, finally, loss of consciousness occur.

Cardiovascular System. The widespread and growing use of narcotic anesthetic techniques in patients with impaired myocardial performance attests to their innocuous effects on the human cardiovascular system.[1,2] In general, arterial blood pressure, heart rate, heart rhythm, and cardiac output are not altered by opiates *providing* the recipient is supine. However, orthostatic hypotension frequently accompanies the administration of opiates to patients who are erect. Such hypotension results primarily from the peripheral vascular effects of opiates on the capacitance vessels, with pooling of blood in the dependent veins and a resultant decrease in venous return, cardiac output, and arterial blood pressure.

Respiratory System. Because of its potentially lethal consequences, respiratory depression is perhaps the most important side effect of the narcotics. Marked slowing of respiratory rate or even complete apnea may occur with large doses of opiates. Respiratory depression results from direct effects of the drugs on the respiratory control centers in the central nervous system. Ventilatory depression is rapid in onset and has been shown to persist for several hours when sensitive tests, such as the carbon dioxide challenge test, evaluate respiratory function. Death from narcotic overdose is almost invariably attributable to respiratory depression.

Miscellaneous Effects. Nausea and vomiting are common side effects of narcotic administration and result from the stimulation of the chemoreceptor trigger zone in the medulla oblongata. Bowel peristalsis is reduced, whereas sphincter tone is increased, leading to paralytic ileus in some patients. Narcotics may produce biliary spasm, with resultant biliary colic. Enhanced bladder sphincter tone occasionally produces urinary retention.

DRUG INTERACTIONS WITH NARCOTICS

Unfortunately, there are few clinical studies of drug interactions among the narcotics and other compounds. Although numerous single-case reports exist, the absence of both systematic investigation and controlled studies is striking. Much of what is known about drug interactions with narcotics has been derived from animal studies, and even these results are inconsistent and often confusing. In part, the lack of clinical studies and the conflicting laboratory data reflect the difficulties in the reliable documentation of the effects of these drugs. The intensity of analgesia is difficult to quantitate in human beings, and inconsistent data may result from placebo effects, suggestion, tolerance, and measurement errors. The subjective properties of these compounds are also difficult to quantitate in human beings, and almost impossible in animals. Perhaps the one property of opiates that can be assessed quantitatively is the respiratory depressant effect. It must be remembered, however, that respiratory depression is a side effect of these drugs, and is not the desired therapeutic effect. Although it is tempting to do so, one must not conclude that interactions in the respiratory system can be extrapolated either quantitatively or qualitatively to any other system. No doubt one could increase respiratory depression if d-tubocurarine were administered along with morphine, but it is difficult to imagine that either increased analgesia or enhanced euphoria would result from this combination.

Thus the literature on the subject is not illuminating. One finds reports that show both potentiation and inhibition of narcotic potency for each of the following drugs: dopamine, reserpine, phenoxybenzamine, MAO inhibitors, L-DOPA, dexamethasone, and chlorpromazine. In light of these problems, the following discussion focuses only on those interactions that appear to be well documented in either human beings or animals, or on those interactions founded in clinical experience despite the lack of firm laboratory confirmation.

CASE REPORT

A 27-year-old man with a suspected fracture of the right femur was brought to the emergency room following an automobile accident. There was a strong smell of alcohol in his expired breath. He was incoherent, frequently somnolent, and occasionally combative. There was no evidence of head trauma, and witnesses indicated that he never lost consciousness. The emergency room physician administered morphine sulfate, 15 mg IM (intramuscularly), and sent the patient for roentgenograms of the right lower extremity. Twenty minutes later the physician was urgently called to the radiology department. The technician reported that the patient became increasingly somnolent

until he was no longer responsive, and then he vomited. Examination revealed small pupils, vomitus in the pharynx, and a respiratory rate of six breaths per minute. There were coarse moist rhonchi in both upper lung fields. He was only slightly responsive to deep pain. After consultation with a colleague, a presumptive diagnosis of narcotic overdose and polydrug abuse, involving at least alcohol, was made and appropriate treatment for narcotic overdose and associated aspiration of gastric contents was instituted. Following recovery, the patient recalled that he had been at a party and had ingested approximately 500 ml of vodka and several "downers" (thought to be barbiturates) before the accident.

CNS Depressants. This case illustrates an important principle of narcotic interactions: in general, the CNS-depressant properties of narcotics add to the CNS-depressant effects of other drugs. Under ordinary circumstances, the prescription of morphine, 15 mg, would have been appropriate for this patient. However, in the presence of two other CNS-depressants (alcohol and barbiturates), this amount of narcotic was sufficient to induce a profound loss of consciousness and consequent regurgitation and pulmonary aspiration of gastric contents. Morphine has potentiated acute alcohol intoxication in mice.[3] In human beings, the incidence of mortality of former addicts in methadone maintenance programs is greater among alcohol abusers than among nonabusers.

Narcotics enhance the effects of other CNS-depressants as well, including the general anesthetics. In both man and animals the anesthetic requirements for several of the inhalation anesthetics are reduced by narcotic premedication.[4]

In general, narcotics act in consort with other CNS depressants to alter states of consciousness, although the exact type of interaction (simple additivity or true synergism) is generally not known.

Although the interactions between the opiates and other CNS depressants on the level of consciousness seem well established, the effect of the CNS depressants on analgesia produced by the narcotics is less clear. For example, barbiturates (including thiopental, pentobarbital, and phenobarbital) have antagonized the analgesic properties of narcotics in both human beings and animals.[5,6] Results obtained in mice suggest that the overall effect of diazepam is to antagonize morphine analgesia, although some enhancement of analgesia may occur briefly (less than 30 min) after both drugs are administered.[7]

Other Drugs. A great number of drugs have altered the analgesic properties of narcotics in animals, and a recent publication summarizes many of these interactions.[8] However, the mechanism of these interactions is poorly understood at best, and the clinical significance of most of them remains unknown. In general, it appears that drugs that deplete central nervous system stores of biogenic amines antagonize narcotic analgesics, whereas sympathomimetic agents appear to enhance narcotic analgesia in both human beings and animals. On the other hand, adrenergic blocking drugs (either *alpha* or *beta*) do not alter morphine analgesia. The cholinergic nervous system appears to be a positive modulator of narcotic analgesia. In animals, drugs that increase cholinergic activity, such as physostigmine, enhance morphine analgesia, whereas atropine antagonizes opiate analgesia.[9]

Occasionally narcotics are administered in combination with other drugs in order to produce a tranquil state for cardiac catheterization or radiologic procedures. Although it is often hoped that the combination will produce greater sedation without increasing toxic manifestations, this is rarely the case. In human beings, careful studies of the respiratory depressant properties of meperidine and chlorpromazine, alone or in combination, revealed that there was potentiation of respiratory depression when the drugs were combined, clearly indicating that the combination did not result in increased sedation without increased toxicity.[10]

CASE REPORT

A 43-year-old woman was scheduled for excision of a ganglion of the wrist. She had a long history of depression and anxiety for which she was taking phenelzine, 45 mg daily. She was anxious about the proposed operation and refused regional anesthesia. All medications were stopped 24 hours preoperatively. She was premedicated with meperidine, 75 mg IM, and with atropine, 0.4 mg IM, 60 minutes prior to the procedure. Shortly after premedication, she developed agitation, diaphoresis, stupor, and hypotension, followed by coma and marked cyanosis with slow respirations.

MAO Inhibitors. This case demonstrates an uncommon but severe drug interaction involving narcotics and monoamine oxidase (MAO) inhibitors (also known as MAOI) (pargyline, furazolidone, isocarboxazid, phenelzine, nialamide, and tranylcypromine).[11] These potent compounds are notorious for their toxicity and for their propensity to interact with other drugs, especially narcotics. Interaction with narcotics may produce hypertension or hypotension, tachycardia, coma, convulsions, diaphoresis, respiratory depression, and hyperpyrexia. Meperidine has been implicated most frequently but all narcotics should be considered to be potential sources for this severe interaction. The MAO inhibitors should be discontinued at least two weeks before any elective surgical procedure. When emergency circumstances demand narcotic treatment in patients who are receiving these drugs, therapy should be initiated very cautiously with morphine. Meperidine should not be used. Although this is an infrequent reaction, numerous deaths have been reported and it is essential that this interaction be avoided.

NARCOTIC ANTAGONISTS

CASE REPORT

A 73-year-old, 55-kg woman was scheduled for open reduction and internal fixation of a fractured hip. She had a long history of hypertension, angina, and occasional congestive heart failure. Physical examination revealed an elderly patient with bilateral ankle edema, dyspnea when supine, moderate jugular venous distension, and bilateral rales and rhonchi in the lung bases. The presumptive diagnosis was mild congestive heart failure, in addition to the hip fracture. The anesthesiologist selected a nitrous oxide-oxygen-narcotic anesthetic technique. She was anesthetized for 90 minutes, during which time she received 30 mg of morphine intravenously (IV) in addition to the 6 mg administered preoperatively. The narcotic was antagonized with naloxone, 0.3 mg intravenously, and she was taken to the recovery room in satisfactory condition. She was alert and comfortable during the first hour in the recovery room. Ninety minutes later the recovery room nurse reported that the patient had become cyanotic, lethargic, and was breathing only six times per minute. The presumptive diagnosis was recurrent narcotism. Naloxone, 0.3 mg, was administered again and promptly reversed both the mental clouding and the respiratory depression.

This case illustrates the principal drug interaction involving the narcotics: the antagonism of the opiates by narcotic antagonists. The following section reviews the principal features of narcotic antagonists and summarizes their interactions with the opiates. Other drugs that may interact with the antagonists are also discussed.

Pharmacology

History. The narcotic-antagonist properties of *N*-allylnorcodeine were first observed in 1914 and *N*-allylnormorphine (nalorphine) was synthesized and its narcotic antagonist properties were demonstrated in animals in 1940. Nevertheless, it was not until 1952 that nalorphine was introduced into clinical medicine. Naloxone was synthesized in 1966 and, because of the unique pharmacologic properties of this compound it has become the drug preferred for the antagonism of respiratory depression associated with narcotics.

Structure. Most opiates contain a methylated nitrogen atom, and nearly all narcotic antagonists are synthesized by replacing the methyl group with a longer side chain, usually an allyl group (Fig. 16–1). Although other substitutions are possible, the major narcotic antagonists currently available are *N*-allyl substitutions of an opiate. Nalorphine is the *N*-allyl derivative of morphine, levallorphan is the *N*-allyl substitution of

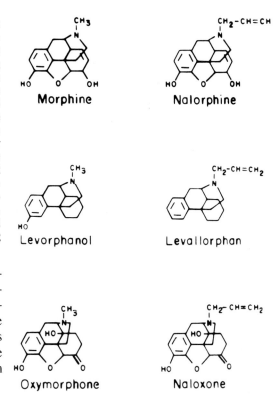

Fig. 16–1. Chemical structures of narcotics and of their related antagonists. Note that all three potent antagonists are allyl (C_3H_5) substitutions of the corresponding narcotic.

levorphanol, and naloxone is the *N*-allyl congener of oxymorphone.

Classification. Whereas there are other compounds with some opiate antagonist properties, the potent antagonists are basically three: nalorphine, levallorphan, and naloxone. Narcotic antagonists may be classified into two major groups based on their agonist potential: partial agonists and pure antagonists. Both nalorphine and levallorphan are partial agonists; that is, when these drugs are administered to a patient who has not received any narcotic, there will be evidence of mild to moderate agonist activity, including respiratory depression.[12] In essence, the therapeutic rationale for these drugs is the substitution of a weak agonist for a potent one. The problems associated with this form of therapy are obvious. If, for example, a comatose patient is incorrectly

diagnosed as suffering from narcotic overdose, when in fact the cause is some hypnotic or sedative agent, the administration of a
partial agonist will aggravate the problem
rather than correct it. Naloxone is the only
pure antagonist currently available. No evidence of narcotic activity is associated with
the administration of even large doses of this
drug to volunteer subjects.[12] (Naltrexone,
another pure antagonist, is not yet approved
for human use.)

Mechanism of Action. The action of narcotic antagonists can be explained in terms of
the agonist-antagonist-receptor theory of
drug interactions; that is, that narcotic antagonists bind to opiate receptors in the central nervous system and either displace or
prevent the narcotics from binding to these
receptors.

Recently, specific opiate receptors have
been identified and characterized within the
central nervous system.[13] These receptors
are more abundant in the amygdala,
hypothalamus, and thalamus of primates,
and a similar distribution pattern appears to
exist in man also. Opiate receptors can be
isolated from other areas of the gray matter,
but there is no evidence of receptor activity
in white matter. Structure-activity relationships are prominent, since nonopiates do not
bind to the receptor and only levorotatory
forms of the narcotics exhibit agonist properties. The binding of both agonists and antagonists depend on the sodium concentration in the area of the receptor. *In vitro*, the
binding of narcotic agonists is reduced by
increasing sodium concentration in brain
homogenates, whereas the opiate antagonists are more tightly bound to the receptor when the sodium concentration is increased. This "sodium effect" may be clinically important, since it may explain the
greater potency of antagonists as compared
to that of agonists (that is, small doses of
naloxone antagonize large doses of narcotics). At normal body sodium concentrations, the antagonists are 10 to 100 times
more tightly bound to the receptor than are
the agonists and, therefore, a one-to-one

antagonist/agonist ratio is not necessary to
displace the narcotic from the receptor site.

Actions of Antagonists. In general, antagonists counteract nearly all the properties
of the opiates. In the central nervous system, the drowsiness, apathy, lethargy,
euphoria, and loss of consciousness associated with narcotics are reversed. In the cardiovascular system, the orthostatic hypotension and peripheral vasodilation induced
by narcotics are abolished. By far the most
important application of the opiate antagonists in anesthesia is the reversal of the
respiratory depression associated with these
potent analgesics. The antagonists promptly
reverse the respiratory depression produced
by even large doses of narcotics. In patients
subjected to morphine-nitrous oxide anesthesia for approximately 2½ hours,
naloxone, 5 µg/kg/IV, provided rapid reversal of a total morphine dose that averaged
1.5 mg/kg.[14] These results indicate the potency of naloxone as a narcotic antagonist.
Others have reported similar results and
have successfully employed smaller doses
of naloxone (approximately 2 µg/kg) when
correspondingly smaller amounts of narcotic were used to supplement nitrous oxide
anesthesia.[15,16] All investigators noted the
brief duration of action of naloxone when
morphine or, in many cases, even when fentanyl was the agonist.

Duration of Action of Naloxone. The
short duration of action of naloxone is extremely important to the clinician. It has
been confirmed by clinical studies in human
beings and by laboratory studies. The kinetics of both morphine and naloxone have
been determined in animals.[17] After intravenous administration of naloxone, the brain
concentrations of the drug exceed the
plasma concentrations by a factor of three to
four. In contrast to naloxone, the initial
brain concentration of morphine is only
one-tenth that detected in the plasma. However, the brain concentration of naloxone
declines much more rapidly than that of
morphine, suggesting that the rapid loss of
naloxone from the CNS could explain its

short duration of action. The plasma half-life of naloxone was estimated to be 64 minutes in human beings, a value consistent with the clinical data, indicating that *supplemental naloxone is required to insure adequate antagonism of morphine (or large doses of fentanyl)*. Various protocols for supplementing intravenous naloxone have been described, but intramuscular supplements are consistently effective and the dosage schedule is much simpler than either a constant intravenous infusion or intermittent bolus injections of the drug.[14,15] In general, twice the successful intravenous dose may be given intramuscularly.

Side Effects of Antagonism by Naloxone. The antagonism of narcotics by naloxone is associated with three major problems: nausea and vomiting, cardiovascular stimulation, and reversal of analgesia.

Nausea and vomiting appear to be closely related to the speed of injection and to the total dose of naloxone. When the drug is injected rapidly into patients who have received narcotics, we have observed nausea and vomiting following 60% of the injections.[14] Others have reported no greater incidence of nausea and vomiting in postoperative patients who receive smaller doses of naloxone than in patients who do not receive the drug.[16] More recently, it is our impression that administering the drug slowly over two to three minutes reduces the incidence of nausea and vomiting in postoperative patients. Fortunately, arousal occurs either before or simultaneously with the vomiting, which means that the patient's protective reflexes are present and that aspiration has not been a problem. However, the potential does exist.

Cardiovascular stimulation following intravenous naloxone has been reported in both human beings and animals.[18-20] In general, the response is that of sympathetic nervous system stimulation manifested by hypertension and tachycardia. Others have reported ventricular irritability associated with the reversal by naloxone of morphine anesthesia, although these patients were in the early postcardiotomy period and were receiving other cardiovascular drugs as well.[21] Severe cardiovascular reactions to naloxone appear to be rare, although some increase in heart rate and blood pressure is not uncommon when postoperative patients receive narcotic antagonists.

Whereas it is inevitable that some loss of analgesia will accompany the administration of naloxone to postoperative patients, this problem is minimized by careful titration of the dose of antagonist.[15,16] After intravenous naloxone, there will be prompt arousal and some patients may complain briefly of pain. Within two to three minutes this effect is greatly reduced (again, consistent with the pharmacokinetics of the antagonist). It would be unwise to conclude that respiratory depression could be reversed without some loss of analgesia; nevertheless, data suggest that the problem of loss of analgesia is minimal and that narcotic antagonists should not be withheld in postoperative patients for this reason if they are warranted otherwise.[16] Certainly one can attempt to titrate naloxone so that most of the respiratory depression disappears without seriously affecting the analgesia.

OPIATE ANTAGONIST INTERACTIONS WITH NONNARCOTICS

Although there are isolated reports of the effectiveness of naloxone in reversing overdoses of nonnarcotics such as diazepam and propoxyphene, the efficacy of this drug in treating nonnarcotic overdoses must be questioned until convincing data are available. One study has suggested partial reversal of inhalation anesthesia (produced by halothane, enflurane, or cyclopropane) in rats, whereas other investigators have been unable to demonstrate such an action.[22] At present, it appears likely that naloxone is a *potent* antagonist of narcotics only. Although the drug may have general analeptic properties in other circumstances, these effects are not well documented in human beings. Naloxone therefore should not be considered appropriate to treat CNS depression produced by non-narcotics until more indicative data are available.

The interaction of opiate antagonists with non-narcotic drugs has received little attention. In animals, the following drugs have been reported to potentiate narcotic antagonists: cortisone, ACTH (adrencorticotropic hormone), L-DOPA, and propranolol, whereas atropine and physostigmine appear to inhibit narcotic antagonists.[8] The clinical significance of these observations is unknown at this time.

In summary, narcotics and narcotic antagonists are potent drugs that interact with one another as well as with other drugs. Narcotic antagonists can reverse nearly all the agonist properties of the opiates, but they are usually employed therapeutically to abolish the respiratory depression associated with morphine and related compounds. Naloxone is the only pure narcotic antagonist and is the drug preferred for opiate antagonism. However, naloxone has a brief duration of action, and narcotic depression may recur unless the drug is readministered intravenously or administered intramuscularly. Although cardiovascular stimulation may accompany narcotic reversal, these effects are generally mild and infrequent, if the antagonist is administered judiciously.

The most important of the interactions of narcotics with other drugs involves additive effects with other CNS depressants and the rare but dramatic interactions with MAO inhibitors. Narcotic antagonists are either potentiated or inhibited by several drugs in laboratory animals, but the clinical importance of these effects is uncertain.

REFERENCES

1. Lowenstein, E., et al.: Cardiovascular responses to large doses of intravenous morphine in man. N. Engl. J. Med., *281*:1389, 1969.
2. Stanley, T. H., and Webster, L. R.: Anesthetic requirements and cardiovascular effects of fentanyl-oxygen and fentanyl-diazepam-oxygen anesthesia in man. Anesth. Analg. (Cleve.), *57*:411, 1978.
3. Eerola, R., et al.: Acute alcohol poisoning and morphine. Ann. Med. Exp. Biol. Fenn., *33*:253, 1955.
4. Eger, E. I., II: Anesthetic Uptake and Action. Baltimore, Williams & Wilkins, 1974.
5. Dundee, J. W.: Alterations in response to somatic pain associated with anesthesia. II. The effects of thiopentone and pentobarbitone. Br. J. Anaesth., *32*:407, 1960.
6. Neal, M. J.: The hyperalgesic action of barbiturates in mice. Br. J. Pharmacol., *24*:170, 1965.
7. Fennessy, M. R., and Sawynok, J.: The effect of benzodiazepines on the analgesic effect of morphine and sodium salicylate. Arch. Int. Pharmacodyn. Ther., *204*:77, 1973.
8. Takemori, A. E.: Pharmacologic factors which alter the action of narcotic analgesics and antagonists. *In* Interactions of Drugs of Abuse. Edited by E.S. Vessell and M. C. Braude. Ann. N.Y. Acad. Sci., *281*:262, 1976.
9. Takemori, A. E., Tulunay, F. C., and Yano, I.: Differential effects on morphine analgesia and naloxone antagonism by biogenic amine modifiers. Life Sci., *17*:21, 1975.
10. Lambertsen, C. J., Wendel, H., and Longenhagen, J. B.: The separate and combined respiratory effects of chlorpromazine and meperidine in normal men controlled at 46 mmHg alveolar P_{CO_2}. J. Pharmacol. Exp. Ther., *131*:381, 1961.
11. Goldberg, L. I.: Monoamine oxidase inhibitors. Adverse reactions and possible mechanisms. J.A.M.A., *190*:456, 1964.
12. Foldes, F. F., and Torda, T. A. G.: Comparative studies with narcotics and narcotic antagonists in man. Acta Anaesthesiol. Scand., *9*:121, 1965.
13. Snyder, S. H.: Opiate receptors and internal opiates. Sci. Am., *236*:44, 1977.
14. Longnecker, D. E., Grazis, P. A., and Eggers, G. W. N., Jr.: Naloxone for antagonism of morphine-induced respiratory depression. Anesth. Analg. (Cleve.), *52*:447, 1973.
15. Heisterkamp, D. V., and Cohen, P. J.: The use of naloxone to antagonize large doses of opiates administered during nitrous oxide anesthesia. Anesth. Analg. (Cleve.), *53*:12, 1974.
16. Kripke, B. J., et al.: Naloxone antagonism after narcotic-supplemented anesthesia. Anesth. Analg. (Cleve.), *55*:800, 1976.
17. Ngai, S. H., et al.: Pharmacokinetics of naloxone in rats and in man. Basis for its potency and short duration of action. Anesthesiology, *44*:398, 1976.
18. Tanaka, G. Y.: Hypertensive reaction to naloxone. J.A.M.A., *228*:25, 1974.
19. Flacke, J. W., Flacke, W. E., and Williams, G. D.: Acute pulmonary edema following naloxone reversal of high-dose morphine anesthesia. Anesthesiology, *47*:376, 1977.
20. Patschke, D., et al.: Antagonism of morphine with naloxone in dogs: Cardiovascular effects with special reference to the coronary circulation. Br. J. Anaesth., *49*:525, 1977.
21. Michaelis, L. L., et al.: Ventricular irritability associated with the use of naloxone hydrochloride. Ann. Thorac. Surg., *18*:608, 1974.

22. Finck, A. D., Ngai, S. H., and Berkowitz, B. A.: Antagonism of general anesthesia by naloxone in the rat. Anesthesiology, *46*:241, 1977.
23. Harper, M. H., et al.: Naloxone does not antagonize general anesthesia in the rat. Anesthesiology, *49*:3, 1978.

This work was supported in part by Research Career Development Award HL 00037 from the National Institutes of Health, Bethesda, Maryland.

The author gratefully acknowledges the expert assistance of Mrs. Sherry Aldridge and of Mrs. Anne Lescanic in the preparation of this manuscript.

Chapter 17

Inhalation Agents

JOHN L. NEIGH

Multiple drug exposure prior to inhalation anesthesia is common today. Not only are anesthesiologists presented with patients who receive numerous medications, but also inhalation anesthesia is often induced and maintained by agents that produce unconsciousness, analgesia, abolition of noxious reflexes, and muscle relaxation. The following case report is a common example of a patient who undergoes anesthesia and operation and who is receiving multiple drug therapy.

CASE REPORT

A 54-year-old man was admitted to a hospital with a four-day history of abdominal pain and intermittent light stools. He had noted chills and icteric sclerae on the day prior to admission. The patient's past medical history included 13-year treatment of hypertension; several hospitalizations for substernal pain without electrocardiographic or enzyme evidence of acute myocardial infarction; syncope and seizures; alcoholic intake of up to a gallon of wine daily; and a 40-year smoking history. His current medications were *alpha*-methyldopa, 250 mg q.i.d.; hydralazine, 50 mg q.i.d.; propranolol, 40 mg q.i.d.; dyazide capsules, one daily; phenytoin (diphenylhydantoin), 100 mg t.i.d., and phenobarbital, 15 mg q.i.d.

On admission to the hospital, icteric sclerae, cardiomegaly with a grade 3 holosystolic murmur, and right upper quadrant tenderness were noted. The patient's blood pressure was 130/90, his pulse was 72, his respiratory rate was 18, and his oral temperature was 101²°F. Laboratory values were hemoglobin 13.1 g/100 ml, hematocrit 41%, white blood cell count 15,400 with a shift to the left, serum sodium 141 meq/L, serum potassium 4.2 meq/L, serum chloride 105 meq/L, serum bicarbonate 23 meq/L, blood urea nitrogen 16 mg/100 ml, creatinine 1.1 mg/100 ml, and total bilirubin 9 mg/100 ml. The chest roentgenogram was normal except for cardiomegaly, the ECG (electrocardiogram) indicated left ventricular hypertrophy with a strain pattern, and a percutaneous transhepatic cholangiogram demonstrated a common duct stone. He was scheduled for cholecystectomy and for common duct exploration the following day.

This chapter discusses the interaction of inhalation anesthetics with prior drug therapy as well as the interaction of agents administered during anesthesia. It demonstrates that under optimal conditions the patient may continue to benefit from prior drug therapy up to the time of anesthesia and an operation.

INFLUENCE OF PRIOR DRUG THERAPY

Antihypertensive drugs

Antihypertensives can be categorized by their mechanism of action. The majority of these agents inhibits the sympathetic nervous system centrally or peripherally.[1-3] The rauwolfia alkaloids, of which reserpine is the prototype, deplete norepinephrine stores in central and peripheral neurons. *Alpha*-methyldopa enters the norepinephrine biosynthetic pathway with the formation of methylnorepinephrine, a false neurotransmitter that produces hypotension owing to its lesser potency. Guanethidine both inhibits the release of norepinephrine and depletes it. Clonidine stimulates postsynaptic *alpha*-adrenergic receptors in the medulla, decreasing sympathetic tone. *Beta* receptor blockers lower blood pressure by several mechanisms such as the interference with cardiac inotropism, the inhibition of renin secretion, and the resetting of baroreceptors.

Sympathetic tone is also altered by *alpha*-adrenergic blocking drugs, although they are rarely used except in the management of pheochromocytoma. Ganglionic blocking agents reduce arterial pressure through venodilation, decreased venous return, and reduction of cardiac output. Other antihypertensives are those with direct-acting vasodilating actions (for example, hydralazine) and drugs that enhance the Bezold-Jarish reflex, thus reflexly inhibiting central sympathetic control (for example, veratrum alkaloids).

The thiazide diuretics reduce plasma fluid volume by means of a loss of sodium chloride and, to a lesser extent, potassium. They are the mainstay of antihypertensive treatment since they have few side effects.

Originally, it was feared that because antihypertensive agents alter sympathetic tone as well as fluid and electrolyte balance, changes in cardiovascular function, especially hypotension, should be expected during anesthesia. Cyclopropane, diethyl ether, and, to a lesser extent, fluroxene, agents that depend on sympathetic nervous system stimulation for cardiovascular support, may produce cardiovascular depression secondary to catecholamine depletion.[4] Halothane or enflurane, which cause myocardial depression or vasodilatation, may produce hypotension in conjunction with antihypertensives. Hypotension may be exacerbated by hypovolemia due to thiazide therapy.

The potential interaction of antihypertensive drugs with inhalation anesthetics has frequently been studied by the evaluation of side effects detected in patients who have received reserpine. Early reports of hypotension, bradycardia, and lack of response to vasopressors during general anesthesia in such patients led to the practice of discontinuing reserpine ten days to two weeks prior to anesthesia. Subsequently, the impression that hypotension could be due to other causes, such as hemorrhage or reflex responses to surgical manipulations, and the awareness that hypertensive patients are prone to greater oscillations in blood pressure, coupled with the necessity of an emergency operation in patients who had taken reserpine, led to the conclusion that these patients were similar to normotensive patients.[5] Evaluations of patients whose blood pressure is controlled by reserpine up to the time of operation compares well with patients in whom reserpine has been discontinued, and confirms the safety of antihypertensive treatment.[6-9]

The persistence of compensatory reflexes

caused by the incomplete depletion of the neurotransmitter applies also to patients pretreated with either *alpha*-methyldopa or guanethidine. Although these drugs produce more orthostatic hypotension, current opinion indicates that they should be administered up to the time of anesthesia.[2,3]

Another approach to the study of the interaction of antihypertensive medication and inhalation anesthetics is directed to the effects of a chosen anesthetic technique on the cardiovascular response of normal, treated, or untreated hypertensive patients. The most extensive evaluation has been with halothane, 1%, and with nitrous oxide and oxygen in patients receiving various antihypertensive medications.[10] Decreases in arterial pressure with ECG evidence of myocardial ischemia occur more frequently in patients with untreated or inadequately treated hypertension. The major alteration in cardiovascular function in the untreated patient is decreased peripheral vascular resistance. Patients with adequately controlled arterial pressure exhibit circulatory changes analogous to those that occur in normotensive patients who receive halothane.[10] Hypotension is most pronounced during the induction of anesthesia; endotracheal intubation is frequently marked by hypertension, tachycardia, and arrhythmias.[11] Responses to endotracheal intubation may be controlled by *beta* blockade.[12]

Drugs that deplete central nervous system catecholamines decrease anesthetic requirements. In the dog, treatment with either *alpha*-methyldopa or reserpine reduces the minimal alveolar concentration (MAC) for halothane, whereas guanethidine, which depletes only peripheral catecholamine stores, does not alter MAC.[13]

The management of hypotension in patients receiving antihypertensive therapy requires a reduction in anesthetic concentration, changes in position, modification of positive airway pressure, appropriate fluid therapy, atropine, and vasopressor therapy. Direct-acting vasopressors, such as methoxamine and phenylephrine, are preferable to indirect-acting ones. Since direct-acting pressors may induce excessive responses owing to receptor oversensitivity in the treated patient, the dose of the pressor drug should be reduced. Increased peripheral vascular resistance, which occurs with increased blood pressure, may be dangerous if myocardial contractility is depressed by an inhalation agent.

In summary, the evidence indicates the safety and the desirability of continuing antihypertensive medications up to the time of anesthesia. The value of controlling arterial pressure seems clearly established, and remains the most important consideration in the anesthetic management of the hypertensive patient.

Propranolol

The most important actions of *beta* receptor blockade are cardiac. The strength of myocardial contraction, the rate of shortening and tension development, heart rate, and blood pressure are invariably reduced. The total oxygen demand on the heart is decreased, and this increases myocardial oxygen consumption and exercise tolerance. Atrioventricular (AV) node refractory time and AV conduction are prolonged.[14,15] Propranolol is the only *beta* blocker presently available in the United States, although other selective and nonselective *beta* blockers (practolol, for example) are available in Europe. Practolol is more cardiospecific since it cannot block H_2 *beta* receptors in bronchial smooth muscle. Hence practolol is safer to use in asthmatic subjects.

Propranolol is an increasingly common treatment for angina pectoris, cardiac arrhythmias, hypertension—especially systolic hypertension concomitant to a hyperdynamic circulatory state—hypertrophic obstructive cardiomyopathy, and some forms of tremor. Abrupt discontinuance of propranolol may lead to an increase in arterial pressure, anginal symptoms, and a serious risk of myocardial infarction. Consequently, *beta* blocker therapy is usually continued until the time of anesthesia. At the same time, the anesthesiologist must understand the effects of *beta* blockade and of diminished cardiac reserve on a patient's tolerance to anesthesia and to the additional stresses of an operation.

Considerable data are available on the interaction of propranolol and inhalation anesthetics. A major consideration is the inherent ability of the anesthetic to induce *beta*-adrenergic stimulation. The problem has been studied by means of the intravenous or long-term oral administration of *beta* blockers in dogs, although intravenous administration may have an effect different from long-term oral administration. Intravenous propranolol reduces cardiac output 47%, and decreases stroke volume, myocardial contractility, and systolic blood pressure in dogs receiving cyclopropane.[16] Similar results are obtained with diethyl ether anesthesia.[17] Dogs anesthetized with trichloroethylene show a 25% reduction in cardiac output following oral propranolol therapy.[18] An additive myocardial-depressant action, in which cardiac output is reduced by 15%, can be shown in dogs receiving methoxyflurane and intravenous *beta* blockers.[19] Methoxyflurane is supposedly devoid of sympathetic nervous system stimulation.[20]

In the dog, halothane and prolonged large-dose propranolol slightly decrease cardiac output, stroke volume, myocardial contractility, and heart rate.[21,22] Increasing concentrations of halothane further decrease arterial pressure, cardiac output, and stroke volume without changing heart rate or peripheral resistance.[21] The added depression produced by propranolol is equivalent to an additional 0.5% halothane concentration. The administration of intravenous propranolol to dogs anesthetized with enflurane, which does not stimulate sympathetic function, causes deterioration in cardiovascular function, with large decreases in mean arterial pressure, cardiac output, and myocardial contractility.[23,24] In contrast, isoflurane, an isomer of enflurane, and intravenous propranolol produce only mild depression, comparable to halothane.[25]

The results of the retrospective analysis of patients and of prospective studies do not always confirm the animal data. Previous experience led to a recommendation, not currently accepted, of a two-week interval between anesthesia and the cessation of oral propranolol administration. This study involved a few cardiopulmonary bypass patients with severe cardiac lesions who were not able to recover cardiovascular stability following cardiopulmonary bypass and who subsequently died. Although they received methoxyflurane, the disease itself is now believed to have been a more likely cause of their deaths.[26] Recent results from a larger number of coronary artery bypass graft patients show no difference in arterial pressure, heart rate, or in the incidence of hypotension irrespective of whether propranolol had been discontinued 24 hours, between 24 and 48 hours, or over 48 hours before the induction of nitrous-oxide, enflurane, and oxygen anesthesia.[27] In another large group of patients who were not undergoing cardiac operations, a similar plan of propranolol administration associated with nitrous oxide-relaxant or nitrous oxide-halothane anesthesia did not change the incidence of hypotension or of bradycardia in any group irrespective of the anesthetic used.[28] In a group of cardiac patients given propranolol up to six hours before an operation and anesthetized with nitrous oxide-halothane, there was a decrease in heart rate, but no difference in cardiac output, mean arterial pressure, stroke volume, or peripheral resistance when compared to cardiac patients not receiving propranolol.[29] The stability afforded by halothane is also demonstrated in hypertensive patients who receive *beta* blockers and many conventional antihypertensives up to the morning of an operation. Following intravenous atropine, patients with *beta* blockade showed higher mean arterial pressure, higher cardiac output, and lower peripheral resistance than a group of hypertensive patients receiving only conventional antihypertensive medication.[12] Fewer arrhythmias and less ECG evidence of myocardial ischemia were observed in patients with *beta* blockade following endotracheal intubation.[11]

The addition of the stress imposed by hemorrhage has been evaluated in dogs by the acute reduction of 20 to 25% of their blood volume. *Beta*-blocked dogs anesthetized with halothane both with and without induced myocardial infarction tolerate hemorrhage well, as do dogs receiving isoflurane.[25,30,31] The imposition of both hemorrhage and *beta* blockade on trichloroethylene, methoxyflurane, and particularly enflurane anesthesia is poorly tolerated.[18,19,24]

This evidence indicates that oral propranolol can be given to within six to 12 hours of anesthesia with some inhalation anesthetics under some clinical circumstances. The depression produced in certain animal studies may be related to the use of intravenous *beta* blockers, but clinical reports indicate the safety of halothane, enflurane, and nitrous oxide. Therefore, initial intravenous doses of 0.25 mg to 0.5 mg are recommended.

Propranolol dosage may be modified over several days since its half-life is three to six hours and since the drug has been shown to disappear from plasma and myocardium in 24 to 48 hours.[32,33] The discontinuance or the lowering of a therapeutic dose is less common today because of the potential increase in symptoms for which propranolol was administered, because effective oral doses may need to be large owing to hepatic destruction of propranolol that occurs prior to distribution to cardiac muscle, and because of the documented safety of inhalation anesthetics with propranolol.

Hypotension associated with propranolol during anesthesia is treated by decreasing the inspired anesthetic concentration, by increasing fluid administration, with atropine, and with vasopressors. Calcium may improve myocardial performance. Since the *beta* block is competitive in nature, isoproterenol competes for the receptor. Increased doses of isoproterenol may be required and arrhythmias and tachycardia may precede inotropic effects. Glucagon and digitalis also bypass the *beta* blockade.

L-DOPA

Levodopa is the immediate precursor of dopamine. Unlike dopamine, it can cross the blood-brain barrier. Thus the rate-limiting step in catecholamine synthesis is bypassed and levodopa is rapidly converted to dopamine. Dopamine inhibits dopamine neurons in basal ganglia that control extrapyramidal function. Levodopa is also converted to dopamine in peripheral tissues, and increased amounts of dopamine are responsible for the cardiovascular side effects of levodopa therapy.[34,35,36] Postural hypotension is due to several mechanisms, such as a dopaminergic effect on the peripheral vasculature, the replacement of norepinephrine by dopamine, and a possible central action of levodopa itself. Arrhythmias and hypertension also occur, although less frequently than hypotension, and a decrease in intravascular volume is seen. Because of the effectiveness of levodopa in controlling the symptoms of Parkinson's disease, because of its short duration of action, and because of the chest rigidity and excessive salivation that occur shortly after discontinuance of the drug, levodopa should be administered up to the time of anesthesia.[37]

The interaction between levodopa and inhalation anesthetics is minor and is probably caused by rapidly diminishing peripheral dopamine concentrations. Hypotension is a potential problem owing to the effects of dopamine in combination with the vasodilatation and the cardiac depression produced by anesthetic agents. Arrhythmias may be precipitated by dopamine in conjunction with anesthetics that sensitize the heart to catecholamines, although dopamine is approximately one-seventy-fifth as arrhythmogenic as norepinephrine.[38] Butyrophenones block the dopaminergic activity of dopamine, and droperidol in neuroleptanesthesia produces muscle rigidity.[39]

Tricyclic antidepressants

Tricyclic antidepressants block the mechanism of reuptake of catecholamines from the synaptic cleft to intracellular storage areas, as well as the mechanism of catecholamine storage. The important side effects of these agents are cardiac and involve an atropine-like action, myocardial depression, and arrhythmias seen with high therapeutic doses or with overdosage. Therapeutic doses of tricyclic antidepressants usually produce no cardiovascular side effects.[40] Tricyclic antidepressants need not be discontinued prior to anesthesia. However, the cardiac depressant and arrhythmogenic potential associated with tricyclic antidepressant therapy should be considered when selecting anesthetic agents. Interaction with inhalation anesthetics is uncommon, although a delayed awakening of the patient and a decrease in MAC is reported.[41,42] Interactions between these antidepressants and antihypertensive agents may cause problems with preoperative blood pressure control, and an exacerbated pressor response may follow the administration of vasopressors.[3,43] The use of pancuronium in patients who are anesthetized with halothane and who are receiving chronic tricyclic antidepressant therapy is contraindicated. Pancuronium may cause ventricular arrhythmias in this situation.[42]

MAO inhibitors

At present, monoamine oxidase inhibitors (MAO inhibitors, or MAOI) are rarely administered as psychotherapeutic or antihypertensive agents. The inhibition of monoamine oxidase alters the catecholamine balance and, consequently, interferes with norepinephrine release and elevates the levels of other catecholamines, such as dopamine. The important drug interactions involving MAO inhibitors are severe hypertension following the administration of indirect-acting sympathomimetic amines, and hypertension, hypotension, tachycardia, convulsions, coma, and respiratory depression following the administration of meperidine. Other narcotic analgesics may produce similar actions and should be used

carefully.[44] Interactions with inhalation anesthetics are not clearly defined; it has been suggested that inhalation anesthetics should be avoided in patients receiving MAO inhibitors for several reasons. Certain anesthetics or techniques stimulate the sympathetic nervous system. There may be difficulty associated with narcotic and pressor therapy. Delayed awakening of the subject may follow barbiturate administration, perhaps owing to partial interference with barbiturate metabolism by MAO inhibition. Other sedatives and narcotics may similarly prolong the effects of MAO inhibitors. Delayed awakening in patients receiving MAO inhibitors following inhalation anesthetics may occur, although the halothane MAC in the dog is not increased by pretreatment with iproniazid, whereas iproniazid increases MAC in the rat.[13] Current opinion recommends that MAO inhibitors be discontinued two weeks prior to anesthesia because of the slow reversal of enzyme inhibition. Hypotensive responses should be treated with small doses of direct-acting vasopressors, whereas hypertension may be managed by adrenolytic or ganglionic blocking drugs or by direct-acting vasodilators.

Phenothiazines

Phenothiazines and their congeners and derivatives are especially effective in the treatment of schizophrenia. These drugs are usually administered in increasingly large doses until a therapeutic benefit or extrapyramidal side effects occur. The cardiovascular effects and sedation produced by phenothiazines may have important consequences when inhalation anesthetics are administered.

The interaction has two important clinical aspects. Although the phenothiazines are not good hypnotics, they have been used as premedicants, often in combination with narcotics. Hypotension and, less commonly, tachycardia may occur, which decreases the desirability of phenothiazines as medicants.[45–47] The administration of small doses of these agents prior to inhalation anesthesia does not cause major cardiovascular changes. In large doses, chlorpromazine, 400 mg or more daily, may increase hypotension during and may delay awakening after inhalation anesthesia.[48] The mechanism of the hypotension produced by phenothiazines is unclear. However, weak *alpha*-adrenergic blockade, peripheral vasodilatation, and central nervous system effects have been implicated. Current opinion suggests that if phenothiazine therapy is essential to the patient's emotional stability, the drug should be administered until the induction of anesthesia. If a modification of dosage is required, phenothiazine levels may be effectively altered within 48 hours. Maintenance of adequate blood volume and appreciation of the additional cardiovascular depression produced by certain inhalation anesthetics and by other adjunct drugs is important for the successful management of these patients. The effectiveness of vasopressor agents may be compromised by epinephrine reversal. It seems that norepinephrine, an *alpha* and *beta* receptor stimulator, is more effective in the treatment of hypotension than are pure *alpha* stimulants.[49]

Large-dose administration of butyrophenones may cause similar problems. Experience gained with the intravenous administration of smaller doses of droperidol in neuroleptanesthesia indicates that a brief decrease in blood pressure may occur secondary to peripheral vasodilatation and to weak *alpha*-adrenergic blockade.[50,51] There is little alteration in cardiovascular function following the addition of nitrous oxide except in the patient who is hypovolemic or who has significant myocardial pathology, in which cases arterial pressure may decrease.[50,51]

Ethanol

The induction of anesthesia in alcoholics is often prolonged and is characterized by excitement and an increased anesthetic requirement. These impressions are collaborated by studies showing that continuous ethanol ingestion for 10 to 20 days increases the required anesthetizing concentration (ED_{50}, or median effective dose) of isoflurane in rats.[52] Tolerance to anesthesia persists for more than two months following the discontinuance of ethanol. Chronic ethanol ingestion increases the minimal alveolar concentration of halothane in man.[53] Sudden ethanol intoxication reduces the ED_{50} for isoflurane in the rat.[52] One should expect lessened anesthetic requirements for the acutely intoxicated patient.

INFLUENCE OF DRUGS ADMINISTERED DURING ANESTHESIA

Premedication

Barbiturates, benzodiazepines, butyrophenones, and other sedatives used for premedication minimally depress the circulation and respiration, although phenothiazine premedication may cause hypotension.[47,51] These agents rarely produce a clinically significant increase in depression after the induction of inhalation anesthesia, although evaluations of MAC indicate that the amount of inhalation anesthetic required is less than otherwise needed.[54] The time for awakening after anesthesia is not prolonged. Narcotic analgesics used singly or in combination with other sedatives may increase cardiovascular or respiratory depression following inhalation anesthetics, reduce anesthetic requirements, and increase sleep time.[55,56]

Intravenous induction agents

The administration of thiopental decreases myocardial contractility, decreases arterial pressure slightly, and increases heart rate.[57] This agent decreases systemic vascular resistance in the patient with uncontrolled hypertension.[11] The cardiorespiratory-depressant effects of thiopental are so short in duration that they usually do not alter a patient's response to inhalation anesthesia; however, in the hypovolemic patient, cardiovascular depression may occur with anesthesia.

In spite of a longer duration of action, diazepam produces minimal cardiovascular alterations by decreasing arterial pressure and cardiac output without changing peripheral resistance. This response to diazepam is usually seen with intravenous doses in excess of 10 mg.[58-60] Respiratory depression is more common following intravenous diazepam.[58,59] Both the cardiovascular and the respiratory effects of this drug may interact with inhalation agents. Diazepam induction reduces anesthetic requirements.[54]

The interaction of ketamine and inhalation anesthetics is becoming an important clinical consideration with the increasing use of ketamine in a rapid-sequence induction in cases where the increase in blood pressure, heart rate, and cardiac output may be desirable in critically ill patients.[61] Hypertension predominates with the subsequent administration of nitrous oxide.[61] However, the cardiovascular-stimulating properties of ketamine are blocked when administered to patients receiving halothane and enflurane; a decrease in cardiac output and blood pressure are observed in those patients.[61a,61b] Ketamine reduces the minimal alveolar concentration of halothane, and a similar action with other inhalation agents would be expected.[61c]

Anesthesia may be induced slowly with high-dose morphine administration (1 mg/kg or greater), with meperidine, or with combinations of fentanyl and droperidol. Intravenous morphine rarely produces circulatory alterations in healthy persons;[62] the fentanyl-droperidol combination may decrease arterial pressure and systemic vascular resistance.[40,51,63] The addition of nitrous oxide, 70%, to a high dose of morphine in volunteers increases peripheral resistance and decreases heart rate and cardiac output without altering arterial pressure.[64] Similar changes are seen with morphine and nitrous

oxide in patients who have valvular or coronary artery disease; these changes include a decrease in arterial pressure, stroke volume, and cardiac output and an increase in peripheral resistance.[65]

Smaller concentrations of nitrous oxide (10% to 50%) in patients who receive morphine for valve replacement operations produce a reduction in cardiac output and in mean arterial pressure that is concentration-related.[66] When combined with morphine, low concentrations of halothane cause similar cardiovascular depression in patients with coronary artery disease.[67] Following fetanyl (10 μg/kg) and droperidol (100 μg/kg) induction, nitrous oxide, 60%, produces the same effect as that observed in patients with vascular heart disease who are anesthetized with morphine and nitrous oxide.[68]

Inhalation anesthetics

The most common interaction between inhalation anesthetics occurs during nitrous oxide anesthesia with other, more potent volatile agents. The results of this interaction can affect several organ systems.

The use of nitrous oxide reduces the minimum alveolar concentration of the volatile anesthetic. This interaction is additive. Assuming a MAC of nitrous oxide of 100%, the addition of 70% nitrous oxide should reduce the MAC of the other agent by 70%. If the halothane-oxygen MAC is 0.74%, the addition of 70% nitrous oxide reduces MAC to 0.29%.[69] If the fluroxene-oxygen MAC is 3.4%, the addition of 70% nitrous oxide reduces MAC to 0.8%.[70] If the methoxyflurane-oxygen MAC is 0.16%, the addition of 70% nitrous oxide reduces MAC to 0.07%.[71] With enflurane-oxygen, MAC is 1.68%, and the addition of 70% nitrous oxide reduces MAC to 0.7%.[72] With isoflurane-oxygen, MAC is 1.28%, and the addition of 70% nitrous oxide reduces MAC to 0.56%.[73]

Nitrous oxide increases the speed of induction when used simultaneously with another agent. This increase is due in part to the rapid equilibration of alveolar with inspired concentration of nitrous oxide. Owing to its rapid onset, nitrous oxide anesthesia minimizes the irritative properties of the other agent. The high initial uptake of nitrous oxide increases the uptake of the other anesthetic at a rate higher than if the second agent is administered either in oxygen or in air (second gas effect).[74] Both a concentrating effect of the second gas due to the high nitrous oxide uptake and an increase in ventilation replenishing the lung with the same initial concentration of the delivered anesthetic mixture increase the concentration of the other anesthetic.[75] Whereas the second gas effect is of some importance, rapid induction is usually accomplished by increasing either ventilation or the inspired concentration of the volatile agent.

The addition of nitrous oxide decreases the respiratory effects of volatile anesthetics. At equipotent anesthetic doses, the use of nitrous oxide may result in less respiratory depression than would occur with the use of the volatile agent alone. An increase in respiratory rate is responsible for the maintenance of minute ventilation. At MAC for halothane and nitrous oxide, 70%, resting ventilation and carbon dioxide retention are depressed less than at MAC for halothane-oxygen.[76] During equi-MAC isoflurane-nitrous oxide and isoflurane-oxygen anesthesia, the respiratory rate and minute ventilation are higher with nitrous oxide, although arterial carbon dioxide tension is similar.[77] The addition of nitrous oxide, 70%, to halothane, 0.8% or 1.5%, decreases tidal volume, and increases respiratory frequency with only minor increases in carbon dioxide tension.[76] The responsiveness of respiration to inhaled carbon dioxide is not altered by the addition of nitrous oxide to halothane, 0.8% or 1.5%, in volunteers.[76] This mild respiratory stimulation of nitrous oxide has also reduced the respiratory depression following thiopental provided that no narcotic has been administered before thiopental.[78] The use of nitrous oxide with volatile anesthetics coupled with the respiratory stimulation consequent to surgical incision decreases respiratory depression.[79]

Important advantages are derived by the interaction of nitrous oxide and volatile anesthetics in the presence of diminished cardiovascular depression. This depression is usually less marked than that accompanying the volatile anesthetic used with oxygen. Halothane, 0.3%, in nitrous oxide depresses arterial pressure and cardiac output less than does halothane, 0.8%, in oxygen in volunteers with spontaneous ventilation.[76] During controlled ventilation at 1.2 to 2.4 MAC equivalents, halothane-nitrous oxide depresses cardiac output, mean arterial pressure, and ventricular work less than does halothane oxygen.[80]

The addition of nitrous oxide to halothane, 0.8%, during spontaneous ventilation in volunteers increases cardiac output, heart rate, stroke volume, and mean arterial pressure with no alteration in peripheral resistance.[76] Conversely, the addition of nitrous oxide to halothane, 1.5%, in these volunteers resulted in cardiovascular depression.[76] In another study, the addition of nitrous oxide for 15 minutes to light halothane (0.8% to 1.2%) during controlled ventilation in volunteers increased arterial pressure and peripheral resistance without changing cardiac output, whereas the addition of nitrous oxide to deeper halothane (1.5 to 2.0%) produced a greater increase.[81] The administration of nitrous oxide for longer periods of time following several hours of halothane anesthesia in volunteers decreased peripheral resistance and increased stroke volume and cardiac output at halothane, 0.8%. With halothane, 1.2% and 1.6%, nitrous oxide neither changed these variables nor increased peripheral resistance with a decrease in cardiac output respectively. Cardiac output was determined by a method different from that of the previous study. Arterial pressure and heart rate are unchanged at any halothane concentration.[82] In patients with acquired valvular heart disease the addition of nitrous oxide to halothane, 0.55%, does not change arterial pressure, heart rate, stroke volume, cardiac index, or peripheral resistance.[83] Cardiovascular stimulation occurs at low concentrations of halothane; high halothane concentrations are invariably cardiodepressant.

Cardiovascular stimulation by nitrous oxide is seen during its addition to diethyl ether, where systemic vascular resistance and mean arterial pressure increase without changing cardiac output.[84] Similar stimulation is observed with equipotent anesthetic concentrations of fluroxene, 5%, in oxygen and fluroxene, 2.5%, with nitrous oxide, 70%. Arterial pressure increases, with less elevation in peripheral resistance and without the change in cardiac output that is associated with nitrous oxide and fluroxene. The addition of nitrous oxide to fluroxene, 5%, increases arterial pressure and peripheral resistance, but the addition of nitrous oxide to fluroxene, 9%, increases heart rate and cardiac output and lowers peripheral vascular resistance.[85]

At equi-MAC levels, enflurane-nitrous oxide depresses the cardiovascular system less than enflurane-oxygen; cardiovascular support is most pronounced at 1.5 MAC levels. In volunteers, the addition of nitrous oxide to steady state enflurane-oxygen anesthesia does not alter cardiovascular function.[86] This combination decreases arterial pressure and cardiac output and increases peripheral resistance in patients who are undergoing operations wherein several adjunct anesthesia drugs are also administered.[87]

Comparative studies of nitrous oxide-isoflurane and isoflurane-oxygen at equianesthetic concentrations show that there is less hypotension owing to higher peripheral resistance. Heart rate, stroke volume, and cardiac output are similarly affected by both combinations.[77]

Data concerning the interaction of nitrous oxide with other inhalation anesthetics vary because of differences between patients and volunteers, alterations in ventilation and arterial carbon dioxide tension, second gas effect, attempts at equipotent levels of anesthesia, and variations in the dose and sequence of administration of the two anesthetics as well as the duration of anesthetic administration. Alteration in arterial oxygen tension has been implicated when shifting from a high-oxygen concentration as carrier gas to oxygen, 30%, during the addition of nitrous oxide. However, studies with halothane, ether, fluroxene, and enflurane that use nitrogen to reduce oxygen tension demonstrate that there is no change when oxygen tension is decreased.

The addition of nitrous oxide to volatile anesthetics or to narcotic induction induces a combination of *alpha-* and *beta-*stimulating effects as well as myocardial depression. With volatile anesthetics, sympathetic activation prevails, as evidenced by pupillary dilatation and by increased plasma norepinephrine following nitrous oxide.[81] In the cat, the discharge from preganglionic cervical sympathetic nerves and the splanchnic nerve are increased.[88] The increase in sympathetic outflow depends on an action at the suprapontine level.[89] The direct action of nitrous oxide depresses vasomotor neurons at the brain stem and spinal level.[89]

The interaction of nitrous oxide with volatile anesthetics and narcotics can vary cardiovascular responses. Normally one can expect less cardiovascular depression when nitrous oxide is combined with volatile anesthetics. In other circumstances, the addition of nitrous oxide results in cardiovascular depression. Obviously, nitrous oxide should not be considered to be a benign carrier gas without important effects of its own or devoid of significant interactions with other agents.

Neuromuscular blocking drugs

The interaction between inhalation anesthetics and neuromuscular blocking agents is of major importance. Muscle relaxation sufficient to permit abdominal operations may be achieved with high concentrations of some inhalation anesthetics through their action on the central nervous system that depresses spinal cord reflexes.[90] Inhalation anesthetics produce a small degree of blockade at the nerve-muscle junction. Minor effects of these agents may be observed at the nerve-muscle junction; fading of contraction of innervated muscles may be caused by high tetanic rates of stimulation, the neuromuscular refractory period is lengthened, and high concentrations of diethyl ether and enflurane reduce twitch height.[91-94] Desensitization of the end-plate is the proposed mechanism of these actions of diethyl ether, halothane, and enflurane as well as of other inhalation anesthetics at the nerve-muscle junction.[95-97] Desensitization coupled with the competitive blockade produced by the nondepolarizing relaxants enhances the intensity of neuromuscular block. An increase in blood in the muscles seen with enflurane and isoflurane may also be important in the potentiation of nondepolarizing blockades with these two agents. This may explain why potentiation has not always been observed in isolated nerve-muscle preparations, and may be responsible for the potentiation of succinylcholine, which is observed with isoflurane only.[98,99]

The potentiation of neuromuscular blocking drugs by inhalation anesthetics has a dual aspect. Frist, the greater the depth of inhalation anesthesia, the less neuromuscular blocking drug needed to achieve the desired degree of block.[100] With 0.5, 1.0, and 1.5 MAC halothane, the amount of pancuronium needed to achieve equal twitch depression is 0.82, 0.49, and 0.35 mg/m² respectively. Second, at equipotent depth of various anesthetics, the dose of a neuromuscular blocker needed to produce identical degrees of depression of neuromuscular function depends on the inhalation anesthetic.[91,99-101] Potentiation is greatest for enflurane, isoflurane, diethyl ether, and methoxyflurane, less for halothane, and minimal for nitrous oxide. Using d-tubocu-

rarine as an example that applies to all non-depolarizing agents with a modification of dose, approximately 0.3 mg/kg produces 95% depression of twitch height with nitrous oxide, half this dose achieves equal depression with halothane, and one-third the dose is needed for enflurane at 1.25 MAC depth.[91,102,103] At equal MAC levels the amount of succinylcholine required for an equal amount of neuromuscular block is similar during halothane and enflurane anesthesia but may be up to 50% greater during halothane than during isoflurane anesthesia.[99,102]

The data on potentiation primarily involve the evaluation of the intensity of neuromuscular block. Although the effects of the interaction of neuromuscular blocking drugs and anesthetic dose on the duration of block has not been determined, a profound neuromuscular block that is induced by an overdose of relaxant in conjunction with a potentiating inhalation anesthetic agent inevitably prolongs recovery time.

Sympathomimetic amines

Inhalation anesthetics sensitize the myocardium to endogenous and exogenous sympathomimetic amines and produce arrhythmias. This sensitization is due to alterations of phase four depolarization of the heart, to an increase in the automaticity of cardiac muscle, and to the induction of hypertension.[104,105] The tendency of anesthetics to produce ventricular arrhythmias has been evaluated in numerous studies in dogs at various levels in anesthetic depth, respiratory depression, and epinephrine doses. In the dog, the order of decreasing sensitivity among common anesthetics is trichlorethylene, cyclopropane, halothane, and various halogenated ethers.[104] The extrapolation of these results to man is controversial, but such a ranking of sensitivity among anesthetics is useful in clinical practice, and studies in man indicate the basic accuracy of this approach.

Epinephrine and norepinephrine are most

likely to cause arrhythmias. The peripheral acting agents, methoxamine and phenylephrine, as well as ephedrine, mephentermine, and dopamine are not considered to be as arrhythmogenic as the first two drugs. This interaction is important because sympathomimetic amines, particularly epinephrine, produce local hemostasis when injected submucosally or subcutaneously. The greatest risk involves cyclopropane and epinephrine combinations. In one clinical series, 30% of the patients developed ventricular arrhythmias on administration of epinephrine 1:60,000, 6 ml every five minutes to a total dose of 30 ml (0.5 mg).[106] Whereas trichlorethylene is sensitizing in the dog, a clinical evaluation indicates that 1:60,000 to 1:200,000 epinephrine with a total dose not exceeding 10 ml in a ten-minute period or 30 ml per hour may be used safely.[107]

The two previously mentioned anesthetics are now seldom used but the safety of epinephrine with halothane and with the newer halogenated ethers is a topic of major concern. Studies in dogs indicate that 10/μg/kg or less of epinephrine produce ventricular extrasystoles in time.[104] With methoxyflurane, the amount of epinephrine needed to produce this amount of ventricular irritability is 14 μg/kg, with fluroxene it is over 40 μg/kg, and with isoflurane it is greater than 20μg/kg.[108-110] Earlier data concerning enflurane-epinephrine combinations in the dog indicated a 45% incidence of ventricular fibrillation with 10 μg/kg, but more recent studies suggest that a dose of 17 μg/kg is more likely to be arrhythmogenic.[109,111] Clinical studies indicate a greater sensitization with halothane-epinephrine than with either enflurane or isoflurane.[112-115] In unpremedicated patients without barbiturate induction who received epinephrine submucosally at equipotent anesthetic concentrations, three or more premature ventricular contractions were observed with 2.1 μg/kg of epinephrine in conjunction with halothane, 3.7 μg/kg with halothane anesthesia and epinephrine

mixed with lidocaine during injection, 6.7 μg/kg with isoflurane, and 10.9 μg/kg with enflurane.[113]

In spite of these differences in epinephrine dose, other clinical studies show the safety of using epinephrine (1:100,000 to 1:200,000 no more than 10 ml per ten minutes or 30 ml in an hour) during halothane and halogenated ether anesthesia, although the tolerance seems higher with the latter.[112]

There are still unresolved problems. A study suggests a lesser incidence of arrhythmias when lidocaine is mixed with epinephrine, whereas most other studies do not evaluate epinephrine-lidocaine mixtures.[113] Adequate ventilation is considered to be important in avoiding arrhythmias, although one study suggests that increasing Pa_{CO_2} will not increase the incidence of arrhythmias with halothane, isoflurane, and fluroxene.[110] The importance of anesthetic depth or of elevated arterial pressure preceding the arrhythmia in the production of ventricular irritability is not well defined.

Sympathomimetic amines are also administered during anesthesia for the treatment of hypotension. The intravenous use of epinephrine and norepinephrine is hazardous; these drugs are used only during resuscitative efforts following major cardiovascular depression with sensitizing and nonsensitizing anesthetics. In spite of their common intravenous administration, other amines have not been adequately evaluated as to their interaction with anesthetics. These agents, although occasionally given for surgical vasoconstriction, are commonly administered intravenously. Arrhythmias are caused with metaraminol and, to a lesser extent, with ephedrine intravenously in dogs during equipotent halothane and isoflurane anesthesia; the amount of amines needed is greater with isoflurane anesthesia. Phenylephrine also produces ventricular arrhythmias, but at higher doses than either ephedrine or metaraminol.[116] These effects are dose-dependent and suggest caution in the intravenous use of sympathomimetic amines during halothane anesthesia, although the peripherally acting pressor agents seem to be better tolerated.

Metabolism

The development of delayed organ toxicity following inhalation anesthesia may be related to the metabolism of the inhalation agent. Prior drug therapy induces hepatic microsomal enzymes with a resulting increase in metabolism.[117,118] Important enzyme inducers include barbiturates, ethanol, chlorpromazine, meprobamate, chlordiazepoxide, diphenylhydantoin, diphenhydramine, and various steroids.[117]

Inhalation anesthetics are also capable of enzyme induction; halothane, methoxyflurane, enflurane, and diethyl ether have induced cytochrome P-450 and have stimulated drug metabolism.[119-124] Although these inhalation anesthetics are weak inducing agents, the more soluble anesthetics remain in tissues for a length of time sufficient to produce significant induction. Anesthetic enzyme induction may increase the metabolism of the same anesthetic on subsequent administration, of other anesthetics, or of drugs administered in the postoperative period. Further work is needed in this area for a more precise definition of the problem.

Along with high levels of metabolic breakdown products, especially serum fluoride liberated with methoxyflurane or enflurane metabolism, other drugs known to cause organ toxicity may combine with lesser levels of the metabolite and produce the same toxic effect. Such a stimulation has been described in oliguric renal failure due to the administration of methoxyflurane in patients receiving tetracycline therapy.[125]

In summary, this chapter defines interactions involving inhalation anesthetics and drugs administered pre- and intraoperatively. The interactions are evaluated sufficiently to provide the anesthesiologist with important information on anesthetic management. Except in the case of monoamine oxidase inhibitors, a patient should continue to receive the benefits of previously instituted, long-term drug therapy up to the time of anesthesia. The maintenance of a stable cardiovascular system and the control of central nervous system disorders allow the patient to withstand the stress of anesthesia and operations more safely. The use of multiple agents to achieve satisfactory anesthesia carries with it the concerns of interaction among inhalation agents themselves as well as among narcotic analgesics, sedatives, neuromuscular blocking drugs, and sympathomimetic amines. These interactions are so important that they must be considered in the administration of every anesthetic.

REFERENCES

1. Hayes, A. H., and Schneck, D. W.: Antihypertensive Pharmacology. Postgrad. Med., *59*:155, 1976.
2. Foëx, P., and Prys-Roberts, C.: Anesthesia and the hypertensive patient. Br. J. Anaesth., *46*:575, 1974.
3. Goldberg, L. L.: Anesthetic management of patients treated with antihypertensive agents or levodopa. Anesth. Analg. (Cleve.), *51*:625, 1972.
4. Price, H. L., et al.: Sympathoadrenal responses to general anesthesia in man and their relation to hemodynamics. Anesthesiology, *20*:563, 1959.
5. Munson, W. M., and Jenicek, J. A.: Effects of anesthetic agents on patients receiving reserpine therapy. Anesthesiology, *23*:741, 1962.
6. Alper, M. H., Flacke, W., and Krayer, O.: Pharmacology of reserpine and its implications for anesthesia. Anesthesiology, *24*:524, 1963.
7. Katz, R. L., Weintraub, H. D., and Papper, E. M.: Anesthesia, surgery, and rauwolfia. Anesthesiology, *25*:142, 1964.
8. Hickler, R. B., and Vandam, L. D.: Hypertension. Anesthesiology, *33*:214, 1970.
9. Ominski, A. J., Wollman, H.: Hazards of general anesthesia in the reserpinized patient. Anesthesiology, *30*:443, 1969.
10. Prys-Roberts, C., Meloche, R., and Foëx, P.: Studies of anesthesia in relation to hypertension I: Cardiovascular responses of treated and untreated patients. Br. J. Anaesth., *43*:122, 1971.
11. Prys-Roberts, C., et al.: Studies of anesthesia in relation to hypertension II: Haemodynamic consequences of induction and endotracheal intubation. Br. J. Anaesth., *43*:531, 1971.
12. Prys-Roberts, C., et al.: Studies of anaesthesia in relation to hypertension V: Adrenergic *beta*-receptor blockade. Br. J. Anaesth., *45*:671, 1973.
13. Miller, R. D., Way, W. L., and Eger, E. L., II: The effects of *alpha*-methyldopa, reserpine,

guanethidine and iproniazid on minimum alveolar anesthetic requirement (MAC). Anesthesiology, *29*:1153, 1968.

14. Merin, R.G.: Anaesthetic management problems posed by therapeutic advances; III *Beta*-adrenergic blocking drugs. Anesth. Analg. (Cleve.), *51*:617, 1972.

15. Shand, D. G.: Propranolol. N. Engl. J. Med., *293*:280, 1975.

16. Craythorne, N.W.B., and Huffington, P. E.: Effects of propranolol on the cardiovascular response to cyclopropane and halothane. Anesthesiology, *27*:580, 1966.

17. Jorfeldt, L., et al.: Cardiovascular pharmacodynamics of propranolol during either anesthesia in man. Acta Anaesthesiol. Scand., *11*:159, 1967.

18. Foëx, P., et al.: Is *beta*-adrenergic blockade compatible with trichloroethylene anesthesia? Br. J. Anaesth., *46*:798, 1974.

19. Saner, C. A., et al.: Methoxyflurane and practol: a dangerous combination? Br. J. Anaesth., *47*:1025, 1975.

20. Li, T. H., Shand, M. S., and Etsten, B. E.: Decreased adrenal venous catecholamine concentration during methoxyflurane anesthesia. Anesthesiology, *29*:1145, 1968.

21. Roberts, J. G., et al.: Haemodynamic interactions of high-dose propranolol pretreatment and anaesthesia in the dog I: Halothane dose response studies. Br. J. Anaesth., *48*:315, 1976.

22. Roberts, J. G., et al.: Haemodynamic interactions of high-dose propranolol pretreatment and anesthesia in the dog II: The effects of acute arterial hypoxaemia at increasing depths of halothane anesthesia. Br. J. Anaesth., *48*:403, 1976.

23. Millar, R. A., et al.: Further studies of sympathetic actions of anesthetics in intact and spinal animals. Br. J. Anaesth., *42*:366, 1970.

24. Horan, B. F., et al.: Haemodynamic responses to enflurane anaesthesia and hypovolemia in the dog, and their modification by propranolol. Br. J. Anaesth., *49*:1189, 1977.

25. Horan, B. F., et al.: Haemodynamic responses to isoflurane anaesthesia and hypovolemia in the dog and their modification by propranolol. Br. J. Anaesth., *49*:1179, 1977.

26. Viljoen, J. F., Estafanous, G., and Kellner, G. A.: Propranolol and cardiac surgery. J. Thorac. Cardiovasc. Surg., *64*:826, 1972.

27. Kaplan, J. A., et al.: Propranolol and cardiac surgery: A problem for the anesthesiologist? Anesth. Analg. (Cleve.), *54*:571, 1975.

28. Kaplan, J. A., and Dunbar, R. W.: Propranolol and surgical anesthesia. Anesth. Analg. (Cleve.), *55*:1, 1976.

29. Kopriva, C. J., Brown, A.C.D., and Papas, G.: Hemodynamics during general anesthesia in patients receiving propranolol. Anesthesiology, *48*:28, 1978.

30. Roberts, J. G., et al.: Haemodynamic interactions of high-dose propranolol pretreatment and anaesthesia in the dog III: The effects of haemorrhage during halothane and trichloroethylene anaesthesia. Br. J. Anaesth., *48*:411, 1976.

31. Prys-Roberts, C., et al.: Interaction of anesthesia, *beta*-receptor blockade, and blood loss in dogs with induced myocardial infarction. Anesthesiology, *45*:326, 1976.

32. Evans, G. H., and Shand, D. G.: The disposition of propranolol. VI. Independent variations in steady-state circulating drug concentrations and half-life as a result of plasma binding in man. Clin. Pharmacol. Ther., *14*:494, 1973.

33. Faulkner, S. L., et al.: Time required for complete recovery from chronic propranolol therapy. N. Engl. J. Med., *289*:607, 1973.

34. Goldberg, L. I.: Dopamine—clinical uses of an endogenous catecholamine. N. Engl. J. Med., *291*:707, 1974.

35. Goldberg, L. I.: Levodopa and anesthesia. Anesthesiology, *34*:1, 1971.

36. Liu, P. L., Kronis, L. J., and Ngai, S. H.: The effect of levodopa on the norepinephrine stores in the rat heart. Anesthesiology, *34*:4, 1971.

37. Ngai, S. H.: Parkinsonism, levodopa, and anesthesia. Anesthesiology, *37*:344, 1972.

38. Katz, R. L., Lord, C. O., and Eakins, K. E.: Anesthetic-dopamine cardiac arrhythmias and their prevention by *beta*-adrenergic blockade. J. Pharmacol. Exp. Ther., *158*:40, 1967.

39. Wiklund, R. A., and Ngai, S. H.: Rigidity and pulmonary edema after Innovar in a patient on levodopa therapy: report of a case. Anesthesiology, *35*:545, 1971.

40. Williams, R. B., and Sherter, C.: Cardiac complications of tricyclic antidepressant therapy. Ann. Intern. Med. *74*:395, 1971.

41. Jenkins, L. C., and Graves, H. B.: Potential hazards of psychoactive drugs in association with anesthesia. Can. Anaesth. Soc. J., *12*:121, 1965.

42. Edwards, R., and Miller, R. D.: Personal Communication.

43. Raisfeld, I. H.: Cardiovascular complications of antidepressant therapy—interactions at the adrenergic neuron. Am. Heart J., *88*:129, 1972.

44. Campbell, G. D.: Dangers of monoamine oxidase inhibitors. Br. Med. J., *1*:750, 1963.

45. Eckenhoff, J. E., Helrich, M., and Rolph, W. D.: The effects of promethazine upon respiration and circulation in man. Anesthesiology, *18*:703, 1957.

46. Dobkin, A. B., Gilbert, R. C. G., and Melville, K. I.: Chlorpromazine review and investigation as a premedicant in anesthesia. Anesthesiology, *17*:135, 1956.

47. Dundee, J. W., et al.: Studies of drugs given before anesthesia. VI: The phenothiazine derivates. Br. J. Anaesth., *37*:332, 1965.

48. Gold, M. I.: Profound hypotension associated with preoperative use of phenothiazines. Anesth. Analg. (Cleve.), *53*:844, 1974.

49. Eggers, G. W. N., Jr., Crossen, G., and Allen, C. R.: Comparison of vasopressor responses in the presence of phenothiazine derivatives. Anesthesiology, *20*:261, 1959.

50. Graves, C. L., Downes, N. H., and Browne, A. B.: Cardiovascular effects of minimal analgesic quantities of Innovar, fentanyl, and droperidol in man. Anesth. Analg. (Cleve.), *54*:15, 1975.

51. Prys-Roberts, C., and Kelman, G. R.: The influ-

ence of drugs used in neuroleptanalgesia on cardiovascular and ventilatory function. Br. J. Anaesth., *39*:134, 1967.

52. Johnstone, R. E., Kulp, R. A., and Smith, T. C.: Effects of acute and chronic ethanol administration on isoflurane requirement in mice. Anesth. Analg. (Cleve.), *54*:277, 1975.

53. Han, Y. H.: Why do chronic alcoholics require more anesthesia? Anesthesiology, *30*:341, 1969.

54. Perisho, J. A., Buechel, D. R., and Miller, R. D.: The effect of diazepam (Valium) on minimum alveolar anesthetic requirement in man. Can. Anaesth. Soc. J., *18*:536, 1971.

55. Saidman, I. I., and Eger, E. I., II: Effect of nitrous oxide and of narcotic premedication on the alveolar concentration of halothane required for anesthesia. Anesthesiology, *25*:302, 1964.

56. Munson, E. S., Saidman, L. J., and Eger, E. I., II: Effect of nitrous oxide and morphine on the minimum anesthetic concentration of fluroxene. Anesthesiology, *26*:134, 1965.

57. Filner, B. E., and Kasliner, J. S.: Alterations of normal left ventricular performance by general anesthesia. Anesthesiology, *45*:610, 1976.

58. Rao, S., et al.: Cardiopulmonary effects of diazepam. Clin. Pharmacol. Ther., *14*:182, 1973.

59. Dalen, J. E., et al.: The hemodynamics and respiratory effects of diazepam. Anesthesiology, *30*:259, 1969.

60. Cote, P., Gueret, T., and Bourassa, M. G.: Systemic and coronary hemodynamic effects of diazepam in patients with normal and diseased coronary arteries. Circulation, *50*:1210, 1974.

61. Tweed, W. A., Minuk, M., and Mymin, D.: Circulatory responses to ketamine anesthesia. Anesthesiology, *37*:613, 1972.

61a. Johnston, R. R., Miller, R. D., and Way, W. L.: The interaction of ketamine with d-tubocurarine, pancuronium, and succinylcholine in man. Anesth. Analg. (Cleve.), *53*:496, 1974.

61b. Bidwai, A. V., et al.: The effects of ketamine on cardiovascular dynamics during halothane and enflurane anesthesia. Anesth. Analg. (Cleve.), *54*:588, 1975.

61c. White, P. F., Johnston, R. R., and Pudwill, C. R.: Interaction of ketamine and halothane in rats. Anesthesiology, *42*:179, 1975.

62. Lowenstein, E., et al.: Cardiovascular responses to large doses of intravenous morphine in man. N. Engl. J. Med., *281*:1389, 1969.

63. Tarhan, S., et al.: Hemodynamic and blood gas effects of Innovar in patients with acquired heart disease. Anesthesiology, *34*:250, 1971.

64. Wong, K. C., et al.: The cardiovascular effects of morphine sulfate with oxygen and with nitrous oxide in man. Anesthesiology, *38*:542, 1973.

65. Stoelting, R. K., and Gibbs, P. S.: Hemodynamic effects of morphine and morphine-nitrous oxide in valvular heart disease and coronary artery disease. Anesthesiology, *38*:45, 1973.

66. McDermott, R. W., and Stanley, T. H.: The cardiovascular effects of low concentrations of nitrous oxide during morphine anesthesia. Anesthesiology, *44*:89, 1974.

67. Stoelting, R. K., et al.: Circulatory effects of halothane added to morphine anesthesia in patients with coronary-artery disease. Anesth. Analg. (Cleve.), *53*:449, 1974.

68. Stoelting, R. K., et al.: Hemodynamic and ventilatory responses to fentanyl, fentanyl-droperidol, and nitrous oxide in patients with acquired valvular disease. Anesthesiology, *42*:319, 1975.

69. Saidman, L. J., and Eger, E. I., II: Effect of nitrous oxide and of narcotic premedication on the alveolar concentration of halothane required for anesthesia. Anesthesiology, *25*:302, 1964.

70. Munson, E. S., Saidman, L. J., and Eger, E. I., II: Effect of nitrous oxide and morphine on the minimum anesthetic concentration of fluroxene. Anesthesiology, *26*:134, 1965.

71. Stoelting, R. K.: The effect of nitrous oxide on the MAC of methoxyflurane needed for anesthesia. Anesthesiology, *34*:353, 1971.

72. Torri, G., Dania, G., and Fabiani, M.: Effect of nitrous oxide on the anesthetic requirement of enflurane. Br. J. Anaesth., *46*:468, 1974.

73. Stevens, W. C., et al.: Minimal alveolar concentrations (MAC) of isoflurane with and without nitrous oxide in patients of various ages. Anesthesiology, *42*:197, 1975.

74. Epstein, R. M., et al.: Influence of the concentration effect on the uptake of anesthetic mixtures: The second gas effect. Anesthesiology, *25*:364, 1964.

75. Stoelting, R. K., and Eger, E. I., II: An additional explanation for the second gas effect. Anesthesiology, *30*:273, 1969.

76. Hornbein, T. F., et al.: Nitrous oxide effects on the circulatory and ventilatory responses to halothane. Anesthesiology, *31*:250, 1969.

77. Dolan, W. M., et al.: The cardiovascular and respiratory effects of isoflurane-nitrous oxide anaesthesia. Can. Anaesth. Soc. J., *21*:557, 1974.

78. Eckenhoff, J. E., and Helrich, M.: The effect of narcotics, thiopental and nitrous oxide upon respiration and respiratory response to hypercapnia. Anesthesiology, *19*:240, 1958.

79. Eger, E. I., II, et al.: Surgical stimulation antagonizes the respiratory depression produced by Forane. Anesthesiology, *36*:544, 1972.

80. Bahlman, S. H., et al.: The cardiovascular effects of nitrous oxide-halothane anesthesia in man. Anesthesiology, *35*:274, 1971.

81. Smith, N. T., et al.: The cardiovascular and sympathomimetic responses to the addition of nitrous oxide to halothane in man. Anesthesiology, *32*:410, 1970.

82. Hill, G. E., et al.: Cardiovascular responses to nitrous oxide during light, moderate, and deep halothane anesthesia in man. Anesth. Analg. (Cleve.), *57*:84, 1978.

83. Stoelting, R. K., Reis, R. R., and Longnecker, D. E.: Hemodynamic responses to nitrous oxide-halothane and halothane in patients with vascular heart disease. Anesthesiology, *37*:430, 1972.

84. Smith, N. T., et al.: The cardiovascular responses to the addition of nitrous oxide to diethyl ether in man. Can. Anaesth. Soc. J., *19*:42, 1972.

85. Smith, N. T., et al.: The cardiovascular responses

to the addition of nitrous oxide to fluroxene in man. Br. J. Anaesth., *44*:142, 1972.

86. Smith, N. T., et al.: Impact of nitrous oxide on the circulation during enflurane anesthesia in man. Anesthesiology, *48*:345, 1978.

87. Bennett, G. M., et al.: Cardiovascular responses to nitrous oxide during enflurane and oxygen anesthesia. Anesthesiology, *46*:227, 1977.

88. Millar, R. A., Warden, J. C., and Cooperman, L. H.: Central sympathetic discharge and mean arterial pressure during halothane anesthesia. Br. J. Anaesth., *41*:918, 1969.

89. Fukunage, A. F., and Epstein, R. M.: Sympathetic excitation during nitrous oxide-halothane anesthesia in the cat. Anesthesiology, *39*:23, 1973.

90. Ngai, S. H., Hanks, E. C., and Farhie, S. E.: Effects of anesthetics on neuromuscular transmission and somatic reflexes. Anesthesiology, *26*:162, 1965.

91. Miller, R. D., et al.: Comparative neuromuscular effects of Forane and halothane alone and in combination with d-tubocurarine in man. Anesthesiology, *35*:38, 1971.

92. Epstein, R. A., and Jackson, S. H.: The effect of depth of anesthesia on the neuromuscular refractory period of anesthetized man. Anesthesiology, *32*:494, 1970.

93. Katz, R. L.: Neuromuscular effects of diethyl ether and its interaction with succinylcholine and d-tubocurarine. Anesthesiology, *27*:52, 1966.

94. Lebowitz, M. H., Bliff, C. D., and Walts, L. F.: Depression of twitch response to stimulation of the ulnar nerve during Ethrane anesthesia in man. Anesthesiology, *33*:52, 1970.

95. Gissen, A. I., Karis, H. H., and Nastuk, W. L.: The effect of halothane on neuromuscular transmission. J.A.M.A., *190*:770, 1966.

96. Karis, J. H., Gissen, A. J., and Nastuk, W. L.: Mode of action of diethyl ether in blocking neuromuscular transmission. Anesthesiology, *27*:42, 1966.

97. Waud, B. E., and Waud, D. R.: The effects of diethyl ether, enflurane, and isoflurane at the neuromuscular junction. Anesthesiology, *42*:275, 1975.

98. Vitez, T. S., et al.: Comparison in vitro of isoflurane and halothane potentiation of d-tubocurarine and succinylcholine neuromuscular blockades. Anesthesiology, *41*:53, 1974.

99. Miller, R. D., et al.: Comparative neuromuscular effects of pancuronium, gallamine, and succinylcholine during Forane and halothane anesthesia in man. Anesthesiology, *35*:509, 1971.

100. Miller, R. D., Way, W. L., and Dolan, W. M.: The dependence of pancuronium- and d-tubocurarine-induced neuromuscular blockades on alveolar concentrations of halothane and Forane. Anesthesiology, *37*:573, 1972.

101. Katz, R. L., and Gissen, A. J.: Neuromuscular and electromyographic effects of halothane and its interaction with d-tubocurarine in man. Anesthesiology, *28*:564, 1967.

102. Fogdall, R. P., and Miller, R. D.: Neuromuscular effects of enflurane, alone and in combination with d-tubocurarine, pancuronium, and succinylcholine in man. Anesthesiology, *42*:173, 1975.

103. Donlon, J. V., Ali, H. H., and Savarese, J. J.: A new approach to the study of four nondepolarizing relaxants in man. Anesth. Analg. (Cleve.), *53*:934, 1974.

104. Katz, R. L., and Gail, G. J.: Surgical infiltration of pressor drugs and their interaction with volatile anesthetics. Br. J. Anaesth., *38*:712, 1966.

105. Katz, R. L., and Epstein, R. A.: The interaction of anesthetic agents and adrenergic drugs to produce cardiac arrhythmias. Anesthesiology, *29*:763, 1968.

106. Matteo, R. S., Katz, R. L., and Papper, E. M.: The injection of epinephrine during general anesthesia with halogenated hydrocarbons and cyclopropane in man. 3. Cyclopropane. Anesthesiology, *24*:327, 1963.

107. Matteo, R. S., Katz, R. L., and Papper, E. M.: The injection of epinephrine during general anesthesia with halogenated hydrocarbons and cyclopropane in man. 1. Trichloroethylene. Anesthesiology, *23*:360, 1962.

108. Bamforth, B. J., et al.: Effect of epinephrine on the dog heart during methoxyflurane anesthesia. Anesthesiology, *22*:169, 1961.

109. Munson, E. S., and Tucker, W. K.: Doses of epinephrine causing arrhythmia during enflurane, methoxyflurane and halothane anesthesia in dogs. Can. Anaesth. Soc. J., *22*:495, 1975.

110. Joas, T. A., and Stevens, W. C.: Comparison of the arrhythmic doses of epinephrine during Forane, halothane, and fluroxene anesthesia in dogs. Anesthesiology, *35*:48, 1971.

111. McDowell, S. A., Holl, K. D., and Stephen, C. R.: Difluoro-methyl 1, 1, 2-trifluoro-2-chloroethyl ether; experiments on dogs with a new inhalational anesthetic agent. Br. J. Anaesth., *40*:511, 1968.

112. Katz, R. L., Matteo, R. S., and Papper, E. M.: The injection of epinephrine during general anesthesia with halogenated hydrocarbons and cyclopropane in man. 2. Halothane. Anesthesiology, *23*:597, 1962.

113. Johnston, R. R., Egar, E. I., II, Wilson, C.: A comparative interaction of epinephrine with enflurane, isoflurane and halothane in man. Anesth. Analg. (Cleve.), *55*:709, 1976.

114. Konchigeri, H. N., Shaker, M. H., and Winnie, A. P.: Effect of epinephrine during enflurane anesthesia. Anesth. Analg. (Cleve.), *53*:894, 1974.

115. Lippman, M., and Reisner, L. S.: Epinephrine injection with enflurane anesthesia: Incidence of cardiac arrhythmias. Anesth. Analg. (Cleve.), *53*:886, 1974.

116. Tucker, W. K., Rackstein, A. D., and Munson, E. S.: Comparison of arrhythmic doses of adrenalin, metaraminol, ephedrine, and phenylephrine during isoflurane and halothane anesthesia. Br. J. Anaesth., *46*:392, 1974.

117. Brown, B. R., Jr.: Hepatic microsomal enzyme induction. Anesthesiology, *39*:178, 1973.

118. Reynolds, E. S., Brown, B. R., Jr., and Vandam, L. D.: Massive hepatic necrosis after fluroxene anesthesia—a case of drug interaction? N. Engl. J. Med., *286*:530, 1972.

119. Linde, H. W., and Berman, M. L.: Non-specific stimulation of drug-metabolizing enzymes by in-

halation anesthetic agents. Anesth. Analg. (Cleve.), *50*:656, 1971.

120. Van Dyke, R. A.: Metabolism of volatile anesthetics III: Induction of microsomal dechlorinating and ether-cleaving enzymes. J. Pharmacol. Exp. Ther., *154*:365, 1966.

121. Berman, M. L., and Bochantin, B. S.: Nonspecific stimulation of drug metabolism in rats by methoxyflurane. Anesthesiology, *32*:500, 1970.

122. Hitt, B. A., et al.: Species, strain, sex and individual differences in enflurane metabolism. Br. J. Anaesth., *47*:1157, 1975.

123. Berman, M. L., et al.: Enzyme induction by enflurane in man. Anesthesiology, *44*:496, 1976.

124. Brown, B. R., Jr., and Sagalyn, A. M.: Hepatic microsomal enzyme induction by inhalation anesthetics: Mechanism in the rat. Anesthesiology, *40*:152, 1974.

125. Kuzucu, E. Y.: Methoxyflurane, tetracycline and renal failure. J.A.M.A., *211*:1162, 1970.

Chapter 18

Neuromuscular Blocking Agents

RONALD D. MILLER

Numerous drug interactions have been reported that involve muscle relaxants or their antagonists.[1-4] Several problems confuse the interpretation of these interactions, however. It is important to establish which interactions are clinically relevant and which are exclusively of pharmacologic or of academic interest. The difficulty of extrapolating animal data to man is nowhere more evident than in this context. The difference is not only quantitative, but is also qualitative, since interactions in man may depend on entirely different mechanisms (for example, decreased renal excretion, hypercapnia, increased anesthetic depth).

Ideally, all drug interactions should be detected clinically and should be confirmed by controlled clinical or animal studies. This discussion therefore concerns only those interactions that have been documented either clinically or in animal species known to respond similarly to man. Those drugs discussed are: (1) azathioprine, (2) furosemide, (3) antibiotics, (4) steroids, (5) inhalation anesthetics, (6) local anesthetics, (7) antiarrhythmics, (8) ketamine, (9) lithium, (10) magnesium sulfate, (11) other muscle relaxants, (12) acetylcholinesterase inhibitors, (13) pseudocholinesterase inhibitors, (14) hypotensive agents, and (15) agents used in the treatment of renal failure. Many interactions are illustrated by case reports drawn either from our experience or from the literature. Only those drugs known to interact with muscle relaxants and likely to have clinical relevance are included. The following case report describes a patient who experienced a prolonged d-tubocurarine neuromuscular blockade. In addition to renal failure, the patient received seven drugs that could have prolonged the block. Each drug is discussed after the case report.

CASE REPORT

A 38-year-old, 64-kg man with end-stage renal disease secondary to chronic glomerulonephritis was admitted to the University of California Hospitals for kidney transplantation. The patient had been treated by hemodialysis previously. Prior to operation, his arterial blood pressure was 170/100 torr, hemoglobin 6.8 gms %, serum creatinine 6.0 mg %, and serum potassium 5.3 meq/L. He was taking daily oral doses of azathioprine, 300 mg; prednisone, 120 mg; Lugol's solution, ten drops; and *alpha*-methyldopa, 250 mg.

The patient received no preanesthetic medications. Anesthesia was induced with halothane and nitrous oxide, 60%. His trachea was intubated without the use of other drugs. Neuromuscular function was monitored to allow recording of twitch height. Although the patient was anesthetized, the operation was delayed because of multiple traumatic attempts to insert a Foley catheter into the bladder. Since the trauma might have caused septicemia, gentamicin, 120 mg, was given intravenously. In spite of not having been given a relaxant previously, the patient's twitch height started to decrease immediately (Fig. 18–1) Twenty minutes later, a small dose of d-tubocurarine, 6 mg, completely abolished the twitch (Fig. 18–1). It was two hours before any further twitch began to appear. The patient started to recover from the neuromuscular block three hours after d-tubocurarine administration. Immediately before opening the vasculature to the kidney, furosemide, 80 mg, in divided doses, and mannitol, 12.5 gms, were given intravenously; neuromuscular block was augmented and prolonged (Fig. 18–2). At the end of the operation, the patient's subcutaneous tissue was irrigated with a neomycin-bacitracin solution. Despite the administration of neostigmine, 5 mg, and of atropine, 1.0 mg,

intravenously, the patient was weak and dyspneic in the recovery room. After three hours of controlled ventilation, his neuromuscular function returned, as evidenced by a vital capacity of 3.8 L and by a sustained response to a tetanic stimulus of 50 Hz, as well as by the absence of post-tetanic facilitation.

Many drugs and/or physiologic changes could have accounted for the prolonged neuromuscular blockade, including azathioprine, furosemide, mannitol, bacitracin, neomycin, gentamicin, prednisone, renal failure, and halothane. Each is discussed separately. The particular importance of monitoring neuromuscular function is also illustrated by this case. If it had not been recognized that gentamicin had caused a partial block, perhaps more than 6 mg of d-tubocurarine might have been given, which would have been an even greater overdose.

AZATHIOPRINE

Azathioprine, a derivative of mercaptopurine, is an immunosuppressant used in patients who undergo kidney transplantation. It antagonizes a nondepolarizing and augments a depolarizing neuromuscular blockade.[5] This effect is probably due to the inhibition of phosphodiesterase at the motor nerve terminal. The role of cyclic nucleotides in neuromuscular transmission has been recently emphasized by Standaert et al.[6] However, I doubt whether this interaction is important clinically. Antagonism of an existing nondepolarizing neuromuscular blockade was observed when 300 mg of aza-

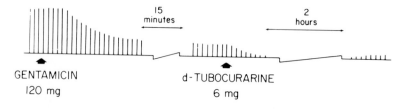

Fig. 18–1. The effect on twitch height of gentamicin, 120 mg given intravenously to a 64-kg patient who had received no previous muscle relaxants. Six milligrams of d-tubocurarine completely abolished the twitch, which resumed only after 2 hours.

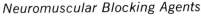

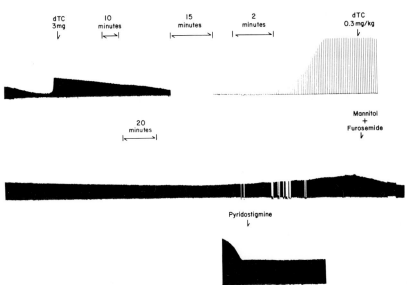

Fig. 18–2. (The panel reads from right to left) A decrease in twitch tension following intravenous administration of mannitol, 12.5 g, and furosemide, 80 mg.

thioprine were given intravenously. Azathioprine is usually given in this dose orally a few hours before anesthesia, however. In this latter situation, azathioprine is not likely to influence significantly the neuromuscular blockade from muscle relaxants.

DIURETICS

One might predict that diuretics will hasten the elimination of nondepolarizing muscle relaxants and will thereby shorten the duration of neuromuscular blockade. Diuretics, however, do no hasten the elimination of d-tubocurarine, and some may even augment and prolong its block. Elimination of muscle relaxant is not accelerated because most diuretics act at renal sites different from those that regulate the excretion of relaxants.[7] Muscle relaxants have a low molecular weight and are filtered by renal glomeruli. They are ionized, are not reabsorbed by the tubular epithelium, and hence are promptly eliminated by the kidney. Diuretics primarily affect tubular function and have little influence on glomerular filtration, which is mainly responsible for the excretion of neuromuscular blocking agents.

Although mannitol appears to have little or no effect on neuromuscular blocking agents, furosemide may augment a nondepolarizing neuromuscular blockade by a direct effect at the neuromuscular junction, possibly by displacing the relaxant from nonactive to active sites. Proof for the latter hypothesis is weak and is based on observations in one patient in whom furosemide increased the plasma concentration of d-tubocurarine even though no d-tubocurarine had been administered during the previous hour.[8] A more likely explanation is that furosemide may exert a direct depressant effect on the neuromuscular junction, probably by reducing the influx of calcium into the motor nerve terminal that is necessary for the release of acetylcholine. This reduced influx may be the result of protein kinase inhibition.[9] Clinical concentrations of furosemide apparently do not affect twitch height, but do augment a nondepolarizing blockade.[10] The ability of neostigmine to antagonize a combined nondepolarizing-furosemide block has not been established.

ANTIBIOTICS

There are more than 120 clinical reports concerning the enhancement of neuromuscular blockade by antibiotics.[11] Although most antibiotics produce a neuromuscular blockade similar to that of d-tubocurarine, their blocking actions are antagonized unpredictably by neostigmine and by pyridostigmine (Table 18–1). Calcium does not usually produce a persistent antagonism. The neuromuscular blockade from antibiotics appears to be antagonized predictably and persistently by 4-aminopyridine.[11a] To date, this drug is not available for routine clinical use in the United States.

The search for a mechanism of antibiotic-induced neuromuscular blockade probably is confused by the possibilities inherent in the variety of antibiotics that can cause blockade. One popular theory is that streptomycin, neomycin, and kanamycin, and chelate calcium produce a neuromuscular blockade by reducing serum calcium concentrations. However, determinations of ionized rather than total calcium levels have discredited this hypothesis.[11]

Attempts to clarify the mechanisms for antibiotic neuromuscular actions have frustrated me. Polymyxin B is an example. The most recent information suggests that polymyxin B exerts its primary neuromuscular effect by depressing the postjunctional membrane's response to acetylcholine.[12] If this were true we should be able at least partially to antagonize the block by increasing the acetylcholine concentration at the neuromuscular junction by means of neostigmine administration. The opposite occurs, however; neostigmine augments rather than antagonizes a polymyxin B block.[13] This is one example of inconsistency in the literature concerning antibiotic-induced neuromuscular blockade.

Of prime importance is the management of a combined muscle relaxant-antibiotic neuromuscular blockade. I arbitrarily administer neostigmine up to 5 mg/70 kg. Calcium is not given unless hypocalcemia is clearly established. Calcium is an inconsis-tent antagonist and may antagonize the antibacterial effect.[13a] The following case report, taken from an article by Fogdall, illustrates why more than 5 mg/70 kg of neostigmine or the equivalent of other drugs should not be administered to antagonize the neuromuscular block.[14]

CASE REPORT

A 76-year-old man was admitted to a hospital in 1972 for open reduction and internal fixation of a right femoral neck fracture. With the exception of congenital ocular palsies and hip fracture, physical examination disclosed no abnormality. Anesthesia was induced and maintained with nitrous oxide, 60%, in oxygen, and with an end tidal halothane concentration of 0.75%. The patient's trachea was intubated without additional drug. Neuromuscular function was evaluated by supramaximal stimulation of the ulnar nerve at the wrist, and the force of adduction of the thumb was measured by a force-displacement transducer. Thirty-five minutes after the induction of anesthesia, pancuronium bromide, 2.4 mg/m^2 (4.8 mg), was administered intravenously, resulting in 100% depression of twitch height. Fifty minutes later, when the twitch was still absent, the surgical wound was irrigated with one liter of 0.9% sodium chloride containing polymyxin B, 250,000 units, and bacitracin, 50,000 units.

Because 100% neuromuscular block still existed 103 minutes after the administration of pancuronium, and because the end of the surgical procedure was anticipated, antagonism of the neuromuscular blockade was attempted by a bolus intravenous injection of pyridostigmine, 14.5 mg, and atropine, 0.6 mg. This dose of pyridostigmine is equivalent to about 2.8 mg of neostigmine. Since 26 minutes later the twitch had returned to only 10% of the control height, 10 mg more of pyridostigmine were given.

Approximately four hours after the administration of pancuronium (and two hours after initial pyridostigmine administration), twitch had returned to only 80% of the control height, and the response to a tetanic stimulus of 50 Hz for five seconds was unsustained, with a spontaneous tidal volume of 0.35 L. Total doses of medications given were pyridostigmine, 24.5 mg, neostigmine, 1.0 mg, edrophonium, 10 mg, and calcium chloride, 1,200 mg.

Neuromuscular function was monitored continuously in the recovery room for the next two hours, during which time an additional 200 mg of calcium chloride was administered with-

Table 18–1

Interaction of Antibiotics, Muscle Relaxants, Neostigmine, and Calcium

	Neuromuscular Block from Antibiotic Alone Antagonized by		Increase in Neuromuscular Block of		Neuromuscular Block from Antibiotic and d-Tubocurarine Antagonized by	
	Neostigmine	Calcium	d-Tubocurarine	Succinylcholine	Neostigmine	Calcium
Neomycin	sometimes	sometimes	yes	yes	usually	usually
Streptomycin	sometimes	sometimes	yes	yes	usually	usually
Gentamicin	sometimes	yes x	yes	*	sometimes	yes x
Kanamycin	sometimes	sometimes	yes	yes	sometimes	sometimes
Paromomycin	yes x	yes x	yes	*	yes x	yes x
Viomycin	yes x	yes x	yes	*	yes x	yes x
Polymyxin A	no	no	yes	yes	no	no
Polymyxin B	not†	no	yes	yes	not†	no
Colistin	no	sometimes	yes	no	no	sometimes
Tetracycline	no	*	yes	*	partially	partially
Lincomycin	partially	partially	yes	*	partially	partially
Clindamycin	partially	partially	yes	*	partially	partially

* Not studied
† Block augmented by neostigmine
x In spite of this, difficulty with antagonizing the block from these antibiotics is still likely to occur

out benefit. The patient responded to vocal commands with a slight nod of the head but was able neither to lift his head off the bed nor to grip a pencil. Because the patient's spontaneous tidal volume was only 0.20 L, his ventilation was controlled. Six hours after pancuronium administration, the response to tetanus still unsustained, monitoring of neuromuscular block with the force-displacement transducer was discontinued. Thirteen hours after the administration of pancuronium, the patient's vital capacity had increased to 0.60 L, but the maximum inspiratory force was less than 20 cm H_2O. Controlled ventilation was continued.

Twenty-one hours after the administration of pancuronium, the patient was able to lift his head off the pillow for at least 20 seconds, and his bilateral grip strength was equal to that of the observer. His maximum inspiratory force was greater than 40 cm H_2O, his vital capacity was 1.0 L, and his chest roentgenogram was normal. Sustained response to a tetanic stimulus of 30 Hz for five seconds was elicited. When the patient started breathing spontaneously without an endotracheal tube, his arterial P_{O_2}, P_{CO_2}, and pH were 122 torr, 41 torr, and 7.40, respectively, with oxygen administered at a flow rate of 5 L/min through a nasal cannula. The patient recovered without further complications.

This case report illustrates the problem of repeated pharmacologic attempts to antagonize an antibiotic-relaxant neuromuscular blockade. Unknown to the anesthesiologists, including myself, neostigmine actually *augments* a polymyxin B block.[13] Thus the patient would have recovered from the neuromuscular blockade much sooner if no attempts to antagonize the block had been made. Unfortunately, it is impossible for the anesthesiologist to assess the percentage contributed to the blockade by the antibiotic, as opposed to the effect of the nondepolarizing relaxant; only the latter can be consistently antagonized by either neostigmine or pyridostigmine. For these reasons, as indicated previously, our attempts to antagonize the neuromuscular block are limited to the administration of neostigmine, 5 mg/70 kg, or of pyridostigmine, 15 mg/kg. If this fails, controlled ventilation is indicated until the neuromuscular blockade terminates spontaneously.

RENAL FAILURE

In patients who are without kidney function, the neuromuscular block from those relaxants (gallamine and decamethonium) that depend entirely on the kidney for excretion will be prolonged unless small doses are used. Churchill-Davidson et al. reported prolonged paresis following gallamine administration in seven such patients.[15] Three of these patients required hemodialysis to eliminate the gallamine. The researchers conclude that gallamine should not be given to patients with impaired renal function, and the same conclusion probably applies to decamethonium. White et al. disagree with Churchill-Davidson and suggest that gallamine "in appropriate doses" is a satisfactory relaxant in patients who are without renal function.[16] They adduce as evidence the absence of prolonged paralysis of "recurarization" in 17 patients who received gallamine (1 to 2 mg/kg). Although White et al. attempted to explain their results by suggesting that gallamine is metabolically degraded, there is a simpler and more likely explanation. I believe that they did not administer doses large enough to saturate the inactive depots. This can be quantitated by determining the volume of distribution of gallamine by a pharmacokinetic analysis. If the inactive depots are saturated, urinary excretion becomes the only route by which gallamine can be removed from plasma. Since the volume of the inactive depots is small, it does not take a large amount of a highly ionized drug such as gallamine to saturate them. Therefore, as emphasized by White et al., gallamine should be used sparingly in patients with renal failure.[16] I believe that whereas White et al. may be correct on pure pharmacologic grounds, the approach of Churchill-Davidson et al. is more practical.[15,16] Only relaxants that do not entirely depend on renal excretion for their elimination should be used in patients with renal failure.

Recent studies indicate that d-tubocurarine may be preferable to pancuronium in patients with renal failure. In man, 40% of an injected dose of d-tubocurarine is eliminated in the urine.[17] Since the remaining 60% is eliminated from the body by unidentified nonrenal routes, d-tubocurarine disappears from plasma (and from neuromuscular junction) even if renal function is absent (Fig. 18–3).[17] In contrast, the elimination of pancuronium from plasma is impaired by renal failure (Fig. 18–3).[18] From the curves in Figure 18–3 it has been calculated that 80% of an injected dose of pancuronium is eliminated in the urine, although this has not been confirmed by actual measurements.

Using a pharmacokinetic computer simulation model for d-tubocurarine excretion, Gibaldi et al. predicted that the absence of renal function should prolong the duration of action of d-tubocurarine only if large single or multiple doses are injected.[19] For example, the researchers predict that the neuromuscular blockade of d-tubocurarine, 18 mg/m² (0.4 mg/kg), will last about two hours. This agrees with the data reported by Churchill-Davidson et al.[15] Riordan et al. reported a prolonged block induced by larger and repeated doses of d-tubocurarine.[20] Thus if single doses smaller than 18 mg/m² (0.4 mg/kg) are administered, significant prolonged paralysis should not occur.

This discussion of renal failure does not deal with drug interaction as such, although any drug that depresses glomerular filtration may delay the excretion of d-tubocurarine or of pancuronium and may thereby prolong the neuromuscular blockade. For example, halothane decreases glomerular filtration by approximately 40 to 50%.[18] It is not known, however, whether halothane delays the excretion of these relaxants, because the problem has not been investigated.

PREDNISONE

Animals that have undergone adrenalectomy and hypophysectomy have a de-

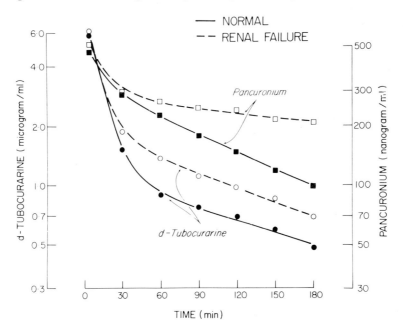

Fig. 18–3. Rates at which plasma concentrations of d-tubocurarine and pancuronium decrease in patients with normal renal function and with renal failure. Note that the decay rates (the slopes of the long lines) are about the same in patients with normal renal function. However, the decay rate is much slower in patients with renal failure receiving pancuronium than in those receiving d-tubocurarine. The data for pancuronium were obtained from McLeod et al.[90] and those for d-tubocurarine from Miller et al.[17] (From Miller, R. D.: Reversal of neuromuscular blockage. Regional Refresher Courses in Anesthesiology, 5:134, 1977.)

creased amplitude of action potentials generated from the neuromuscular junction;
this can be reversed by the administration of
cortisone or of ACTH (adrenocorticotropic
hormone). ACTH also can improve
neuromuscular function in patients with
myasthenia gravis. Recently, Meyers described the anesthetic management of a patient who received long-term cortisone
therapy.[19] After the induction of anesthesia,
the administration of pancuronium resulted
in a prolonged neuromuscular blockade that
was partially antagonized by hydrocortisone. The patient was suspected of having
inadequate replacement of adrenocortical
hormones.

The mechanism of corticosteroid action
on the neuromuscular junction is unknown.
Steroids probably have little effect at the
neuromuscular junction unless the patient is
depleted of these compounds. In this case, it
is conceivable that low prednisone levels
could have contributed to the prolonged
block described by Meyers.[19] Further
studies are required to clarify the role of
corticosteroids and neuromuscular transmission.

INHALATION ANESTHETICS

In the patient in the case report, who was
undergoing kidney transplantation,
halothane could have augmented the nondepolarizing block intraoperatively, but not
in the recovery room, when most of the
halothane should have been eliminated from
the neuromuscular junction. Inhalation anesthetics augment the neuromuscular block
from nondepolarizing relaxants in a dose-
dependent fashion (Fig. 18–4) that, surpris-
ingly, does not depend on the duration of
anesthesia.[20,21] Of the anesthetic agents
studied, inhalation anesthetics augment the
muscle relaxants in decreasing order: isoflurane and enflurane, halothane, fluroxene
and cyclopropane, and nitrous oxide–
barbiturate-narcotic anesthesia.[22–23]

There are several theories as to the mechanisms by which inhalation anesthetics pro-

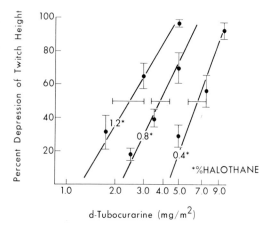

Fig. 18–4. The effects of 3 alveolar concentrations of halothane on mean depression of twitch
height by d-tubocurarine. Each solid dot represents
mean depression of twitch height.(± 1 SE) for three
patients. From these data, lines of linear regression
were determined. (From Miller, R. D., et al.: The
dependence of pancuronium and d-tubocurarine
induced neuromuscular blockades on alveolar concentrations of halothane and Forane. Anesthesiology, *37*:573, 1972.)

duce relaxation and augment the neuromuscular blockade from muscle relaxants. The
non-neuromuscular mechanisms are:

1. Central nervous system depression.
2. Increased muscle blood flow (isoflurane).
3. Decreased glomerular filtration.
4. Decreased liver blood flow.
5. Hypothermia (poikilothermic).

Neuromuscular mechanisms are as follows:

1. Some inhalation anesthetics increase
   blood flow in the muscle, which de-
   livers a greater fraction of the injected
   relaxant to the neuromuscular junction.[24] This is probably significant only
   with isoflurane, which increases muscle blood more than do other inhalation
   anesthetic agents.
2. Inhalation anesthetics induce relaxation at a site proximal to the neuromuscular junction, which site obviously is the central nervous system.[25]

3. Inhalation anesthetics decrease the sensitivity of the postjunctional membrane to depolarization.[29,30]

4. They possibly act at a site distal to the cholinergic receptor and postjunctional membrane, such as at the muscle membrane.[27,28,31]

Inhalation anesthetics do not interfere with the release of acetylcholine from the motor nerve terminal, and these agents have no demonstrable effect on the cholinergic receptor.[26-28]

Although most inhalation agents such as halothane do not decrease twitch tension, conceptually they reduce the margin of safety of neuromuscular transmission. Waud indicates that halothane acts at a site distal to the cholinergic receptor, perhaps by interfering with calcium conductance or by release from depolarization, which may interfere with muscle contraction.[28,29,31] In his excellent review, Ngai points out that inhalation anesthetics are capable of producing relaxation with minimal neuromuscular blockade by acting on the central nervous system.[31] Thus these agents can induce adequate muscle relaxation without causing neuromuscular blockade.

CASE REPORT

(Conclusion of kidney transplant case report)
Of all the possibilities, decreased renal function, antibiotics, and furosemide appear to be likely causes of the prolonged d-tubocurarine neuromuscular blockade. Azathioprine and prednisone had been given several hours before the administration of muscle relaxants and their concentration in the patient's blood was presumably low. Furthermore, azathioprine antagonizes rather than augments a nondepolarizing blockade. Halothane administration had been stopped, yet the block persisted in the recovery room. Mannitol has been shown not to affect neuromuscular transmission.

LOCAL ANESTHETICS

In large doses, most local anesthetics block neuromuscular transmission; in smaller doses they enhance the neuromuscular block from both nondepolarizing and depolarizing muscle relaxants.[32,33] Telivuo and Katz found an additional decrease in twitch height and in tidal volume from lidocaine, mepivacaine, prilocaine, and bupivacaine in patients partially paralyzed with nortoxiferine.[32] Thus local anesthetics given as antiarrhythmic agents intra- or postoperatively may augment a residual neuromuscular block.

In low doses, local anesthetics depress post-tetanic potentiation, which is thought to be a neural, prejunctional effect.[34] In higher doses, local anesthetics block acetylcholine-induced muscular contractions; this effect suggests a stabilizing of the postjunctional membrane.[35,36] Local anesthetics also have a direct effect on the muscle membrane by decreasing the strength of contraction of a denervated muscle or one that has received curare in response to a single shock.[37] Recently, procaine has been shown to displace calcium from the sarcolemma and thus to inhibit caffeine-induced contraction of skeletal muscle.[38] These mechanisms of action probably apply to all the local anesthetics. In essence, local anesthetics have actions on the presynaptic, postjunctional, and muscle membranes.

Although situations may exist in which local anesthetics and muscle relaxants are given intraoperatively, probably most common is the administration of 50 to 100 mg/70 kg of lidocaine intravenously for the treatment of ventricular irritability. Whether that amount of lidocaine augments a partial neuromuscular blockade is an important question. The following case is an example of such a situation.

CASE REPORT

A 48-year-old woman was anesthetized with fluroxene and with nitrous oxide for the insertion of a cardiac pacemaker. Unknown to us at that time, her dibucaine number was 23%. Three minutes after the administration of d-tubocurarine, 3 mg, succinylcholine, 70 mg, was administered intravenously. There was a 100% neuromuscular blockade, as evidenced by the complete abolition of any response to peripheral nerve stimulation. About 40 minutes later, the twitch recurred and the patient resumed breathing spontaneously; a Phase II (desensitization) block was present, as evidenced by a fade in response to tetanic stimulus of 50 Hz and post-tetanic facilitation. Ten minutes later twitch height had fully returned and tidal volume was estimated to be 0.4 L; however, premature ventricular contractions (6 to 8/min) appeared, for which lidocaine, 50 mg, was given intravenously. The patient immediately stopped breathing and the twitch disappeared. Approximately 45 minutes later, tidal volume was 0.45 L and the response to a tetanic stimulus (50 Hz) was sustained. The patient recovered with no further difficulty.

This case demonstrates that lidocaine given as a 50- to 100-mg bolus, or possibly by intravenous infusion, may augment a Phase II block caused by succinylcholine or a nondepolarizing block caused by either d-tubocurarine or pancuronium. The interaction between lidocaine and muscle relaxants may be particularly important in the recovery room. If a patient has a slight undetected residual neuromuscular block that does not affect tidal volume, and subsequently receives lidocaine for ventricular irritability, a profound block may occur.

ANTIARRHYTHMIC DRUGS (EXCLUDING LOCAL ANESTHETICS)

Several drugs used for the treatment of arrhythmias also augment the block caused by muscle relaxants, particularly by d-tubocurarine.[39] For example, patients have become "recurarized" after receiving quinidine in the recovery room. These cases may represent unrecognized residual effects of curare that are augmented by the administration of quinidine. Furthermore, when quinidine is administered to facilitate cardioversion in patients anesthetized with thiopental and succinylcholine, a prolonged neuromuscular blockade is likely to follow.[40] Quinidine potentiates the neuromuscular block caused by both nondepolarizing and depolarizing muscle relaxants;[41] edrophonium is ineffective in antagonizing a

nondepolarizing blockade after quinidine. In these clinical doses, quinidine appears to act at the prejunctional membrane since it does not affect acetylcholine-evoked twitch. However, large, nonclinical doses of quinidine given intra-arterially produce a depolarizing neuromuscular blockade that is augmented by edrophonium.[42]

KETAMINE

Ketamine induces inadequate muscle relaxation, although it enhances the magnitude and duration of the neuromuscular block brought about by d-tubocurarine concomitantly administered.[43] Succinylcholine neuromuscular blockade appears not to be affected. *In vivo* (cat) and *in vitro* (frog) microelectrode studies have demonstrated that ketamine reduces the postjunctional membrane sensitivity to acetylcholine.[44]

MAGNESIUM SULFATE

Microelectrode studies performed in the frog nerve-muscle preparation suggest that magnesium has both pre- and postsynaptic activity.[45] Thus magnesium (1) decreases the amplitude of the end-plate potential, (2) decreases the depolarizing action of acetylcholine applied directly and the excitability of the muscle fiber itself, and (3) decreases the amount of acetylcholine release from the motor nerve terminal through nerve impulse.

Magnesium sulfate is used for the treatment of preeclamptic and eclamptic toxemia of pregnancy; these patients may also receive muscle relaxants during anesthesia for cesarean section. The neuromuscular blocking properties of both d-tubocurarine and succinylcholine are enhanced by magnesium, probably in an additive manner.[46,47] An increased neuromuscular block from d-tubocurarine is easily explained, since magnesium reduces the output of acetylcholine from the motor nerve terminal and reduces the sensitivity of the postjunctional membrane. These factors should antagonize the block from succinylcholine, although the opposite occurs. However, succinylcholine appears to be less affected by magnesium than does d-tubocurarine.[47]

LITHIUM CARBONATE

Lithium carbonate is used with increasing frequency in psychiatric disorders. If a patient is receiving lithium, will the neuromuscular depression from muscle relaxants be prolonged? Only one case report in the literature suggests that the block from nondepolarizing muscle relaxants may be prolonged.[48] The interaction between lithium and succinylcholine has been well documented by Hill et al.; the following case report is abstracted from their article.[49]

CASE REPORT

A 38-year-old woman was anesthetized for an emergency cesarean section. She had previously received lithium carbonate by mouth daily, which resulted in a blood level of 1.2 meq/L. Anesthesia was induced with pancuronium, 0.5 mg, thiopental 350 mg, and succinylcholine, 150 mg, intravenously, followed by a succinylcholine drip (310 mg total in 120 minutes). A 5-1b 6-oz infant was delivered with no difficulty (Apgar scores were five and nine).

Postoperatively, the patient remained apneic for four hours. Stimulation of the ulnar nerve indicated probable Phase II block. After four hours of mechanical ventilation, she could raise her head; tidal volume was 0.45 L, and forced vital capacity was 0.9 L; her handgrip was strong. The patient's trachea was then extubated without further respiratory problem. Her dibucaine number was 73.

In order to explore further the interaction between succinylcholine and lithium, Hill et al. performed studies in their laboratory.[49] They found that both the time it took to reach peak effect (onset) and the duration of succinylcholine neuromuscular blockade were prolonged by the concomitant administration of clinical doses of lithium. Hence this seems to be a well-established fact. However, the delayed onset of succinylcholine deserves additional comment. If a rapid induction of anesthesia is attempted in a patient pretreated with lithium, the ten-

dency of the anesthetist will be to give repeated doses of succinylcholine because relaxation does not occur as promptly as expected. This practice will be avoided when the retardant effect of lithium is fully recognized.

The ultimate mechanism of action of lithium on the neuromuscular junction remains unknown.

INTERACTION BETWEEN NONDEPOLARIZING MUSCLE RELAXANTS AND SUCCINYLCHOLINE

Nondepolarizing (d-tubocurarine, pancuronium, and gallamine) and depolarizing (succinylcholine and decamethonium) muscle relaxants show antagonistic or additive properties depending on the method of testing.[50,51] Both types of relaxants are administered concomitantly in three clinical situations.

Succinylcholine is commonly given to facilitate intubation of the trachea and is usually followed by a longer-acting nondepolarizing relaxant such as d-tubocurarine or pancuronium. Presumably the block caused by a nondepolarizing relaxant will not be affected if the longer-acting drug is given after the block from succinylcholine has dissipated. Katz, however, reported that prior administration of succinylcholine nearly doubled the depression of twitch height induced by the same dose of pancuronium.[51] The duration of the block was similarly increased. Although succinylcholine and d-tubocurarine are supposedly antagonistic, Katz et al. have speculated that the end-plate may remain desensitized by the initial dose of succinylcholine.[51] If true, this may account for the unexpected increase in duration of nondepolarizing block induced by previous succinylcholine administration.

The second possible association is the injection of d-tubocurarine or pancuronium for prolonged relaxation, followed by the shorter-acting succinylcholine to facilitate closure of the peritoneum. The amount of succinylcholine required for adequate relaxation directly depends on the amount of residual d-tubocurarine or pancuronium blockade present. For example, if succinylcholine is added to a 65% neuromuscular block due to d-tubocurarine, the onset from succinylcholine will be delayed 150% and its duration will be decreased from nine to approximately seven minutes.[52] Although the onset of succinylcholine block will be delayed, its duration will be increased to 17 minutes (100% increase) when added to a preexisting partial pancuronium block. The mechanism by which pancuronium prolongs a succinylcholine neuromuscular blockade has not been established. Pancuronium inhibits plasma cholinesterase, although this inhibition is not clinically significant.[52] Despite the questionable pharmacologic reasoning, concomitant administration of an antagonist and agonist in appropriate doses appears to be effective.[53] Whether this is the best approach to the problem is disputed. Many anesthetists prefer either to give an additional dose of a nondepolarizer that can be easily antagonized at the end of the operation or to increase the anesthetic dose or concentration, since relaxation and augmentation of the effect of muscle relaxants depends on anesthetic dose.[20] I prefer the latter approach. (See Chapter 1.)

A small dose of a nondepolarizing agent is commonly given prior to administering succinylcholine to prevent adverse effects. Succinylcholine administration may increase intraocular and intragastric pressure, and may cause muscle pains and possibly hyperkalemia.[54-57] These adverse effects can be either attenuated or prevented by prior administration of a subparalyzing dose of d-tubocurarine or gallamine. Despite its advantages, this technique has been questioned for two reasons: (1) more succinylcholine is required for adequate relaxation, and (2) prolonged apnea may occur from a desensitization block. The latter effect has not been documented.[53] The former is well established, but it causes little difficulty clinically.[58,59] In an excellent study, Dery has provided further evidence of the safety of this approach.[60] I have only mentioned d-tubocurarine and gallamine, although theoretically pancuronium should be just as useful. However, the effectiveness of pancuronium in preventing the increase in intraocular and intragastric pressure has not been determined. In any case, the administration of d-tubocurarine, 3 mg/70 kg, or of gallamine, 20 mg/70 kg, prior to succinylcholine seems to be acceptable.

INTERACTION OF NEOSTIGMINE WITH SUCCINYLCHOLINE

The importance of the interaction between neostigmine and succinylcholine revolves around two questions: (1) Is it rational to administer succinylcholine when a nondepolarizing block has been antagonized by neostigmine? (2) Should neostigmine be used to antagonize a Phase II (desensitization) block?

The answer to the first question is that although this practice may be reasonable, one should realize that the neuromuscular block from succinylcholine will be prolonged.[61] This is because, in addition to inhibiting acetylcholinesterase at the endplate, neostigmine also inhibits plasma cholinesterase. As a result, the breakdown of succinylcholine, when administered after neostigmine, will be delayed. My experience indicates that when succinylcholine (0.75 to 1.5 mg/kg) is administered within 20 minutes after the administration of 2 to 3 mg/70 kg of neostigmine, the ensuing neuromuscular block may last as long as 60 to 90 minutes. This observation has been confirmed experimentally by Nastuk et al., who observed a reduction in the concentration of depolarizing drug required to produce paralysis in the presence of acetylcholinesterase inhibitors.[62] It is not known how much time should elapse after the administration of neostigmine before one can expect a normal response to succinylcholine. Neostigmine has a duration of action of 50 to 90 minutes, which is probably the necessary interval for the return of a normal response to succinylcholine.[63]

With regard to the second question, a well-defined Phase II block by succinylcholine can be antagonized with neostigmine. My opinion differs from that of Katz and Churchill-Davidson, who suggest that neostigmine should probably be avoided altogether in patients who manifest a prolonged response to succinylcholine.[64] This difference of opinion is based on reports that neostigmine may either antagonize or enhance a Phase II (desensitizing) block from succinylcholine.[61,65,66] How can we predict successful antagonism of a desensitizing neuromuscular block? Gissen et al. attribute importance to the presence of succinylcholine in plasma.[67] In the absence of circulating succinylcholine, anticholinesterase drugs will antagonize a desensitizing block induced by succinylcholine. In the presence of circulating succinylcholine, however, anticholinesterase drugs either will not affect or will enhance the succinylcholine-induced desensitizing block. Since no simple method for determining the succinylcholine level in plasma exists, these researchers suggest that anticholinesterase drugs should be avoided in the management of patients whose response to succinylcholine is prolonged.

As indicated above, I believe that attempts to antagonize a prolonged succinylcholine block may be appropriate in well-defined circumstances. To avoid the chance that neostigmine may prolong the block, I first use edrophonium as a diagnostic drug. If, following administration of edrophonium, tetanus becomes unequivocally sustained, post-tetanic facilitation disappears, and tidal volume, vital capacity, or inspiratory force increase for at least three to five minutes, it is reasonable to expect complete and prolonged antagonism of the succinylcholine blockade by neostigmine. Apparently, antagonism of a desensitizing neuromuscular block should not be attempted when the patient is apneic.[65] A review of reported cases with low dibucaine

numbers suggests that attempts to reverse succinylcholine desensitizing blocks before there was evidence of spontaneous muscle activity have resulted in more profound and prolonged neuromuscular blocks. Perhaps this indicates a high level of succinylcholine in the plasma. However, in those cases in which spontaneous muscle activity had begun to appear, there usually was an immediate and lasting antagonism of the neuromuscular block when an anticholinesterase was administered.[65]

DRUGS THAT PROLONG SUCCINYLCHOLINE BLOCK BY INHIBITION OF PSEUDOCHOLINESTERASE

Drugs that may prolong a succinylcholine neuromuscular blockade by inhibition of pseudocholinesterase (plasma cholinesterase) are: (1) echothiophate, (2) hexafluorenium, (3) phenelzine, (4) tetrahydroaminacrine (tacrine), and (5) cytotoxic drugs (alkylating agents) including nitrogen mustard and cyclophosphamide. Pseudocholinesterase breaks down succinylcholine by hydrolysis. If pseudocholinesterase is absent, a prolonged block may occur. The extent to which pseudocholinesterase must be reduced before a prolonged block occurs has not been defined, but it is estimated that a decrease of at least 20% is necessary. I discuss only those drugs that inhibit pseudocholinesterase sufficiently to bring about a clinically detectable effect.

Echothiophate iodide, which is used in the treatment of glaucoma, probably has received the most attention. It inhibits pseudocholinesterase, from 15 to 40%.[68] It increases the duration of succinylcholine block by 10 to 20 minutes. More details can be found in the excellent review by Pantuck and Pantuck.[68]

Phenelzine, a monoamine oxidase inhibitor, used for the treatment of mental depression, also increases the duration of a succinylcholine block by the inhibition of pseudocholinesterase. Apparently, pseudocholinesterase levels do not return to normal for two weeks after the discontinuance of phenelzine.[68] Even though phenelzine can dramatically reduce pseudocholinesterase levels in some patients, the reduction is unpredictable and sometimes nonexistent.[68] The reasons for this unpredictability are unclear.

It has been reported that cytotoxic or alkylating agents prolong succinylcholine neuromuscular block by the alkylation of pseudocholinesterase.[69,70] Recently Bennett et al. reported one case of a prolonged pancuronium neuromuscular blockade in a patient who was receiving an alkylating drug, triethylenethiophosphoramide (thio-TEPA);[71] the interaction is unrelated to changes in pseudocholinesterase. This patient, however, was affected by myasthenia gravis; the presence of this condition casts some doubt on the mechanism of the interaction. Further studies are required to confirm this observation.[71]

HYPOTENSIVE DRUGS

Ganglionic blocking drugs, particularly trimethaphan (Arfonad), can affect neuromuscular blockade by several mechanisms, namely, changes in blood flow, inhibition of pseudocholinesterase, and decreased sensitivity of the postjunctional membrane. Drugs that are used to induce hypotension deliberately can affect the neuromuscular block because of changes in blood flow to the neuromuscular junction. In general, a reduction in muscle blood flow will delay the onset and will prolong the duration of neuromuscular blockade. A study by Goat et al. presents evidence that a reduction in muscle blood flow does not prolong a nondepolarizing blockade.[72] They reported that time required to recover from the block by 25 to 75% were not prolonged, but the researchers did not actually report the duration of neuromuscular blockade. Hence it can be stated that the "slope" of recovery was not prolonged, but this study cannot provide conclusions on the duration of

neuromuscular blockade on the basis of the reported data. For example, one might ask how long it would take to achieve 25% recovery. Furthermore, changes in blood flow were induced by a roller pump through a shunt, a system that probably does not approximate the low flow conditions caused by hypotensive drugs. Therefore, this study does not discredit the theory that a neuromuscular block may be prolonged by a decrease in muscle flow.

Can the hypotensive drugs affect the neuromuscular junction directly, independent of changes in muscle blood flow? Apparently sodium nitroprusside has no direct effect.[73] Gergis et al. have proposed that trimethaphan (Arfonad) depresses the postjunctional membrane as evidenced by decreased sensitivity of the membrane to iontophoretically applied acetylcholine.[73] This would explain a prolonged nondepolarizing blockade, but not the clinical observation that neostigmine may augment, rather than antagonize, the block.[74,75] Obviously the interaction among neostigmine, trimethaphan, and the nondepolarizing relaxants needs further study, and, until more information becomes available, I use an arbitrary and empiric approach to this type of drug interaction. If a prolonged nondepolarizing block occurs in a patient who has received trimethaphan, I administer neostigmine, 2.5 to 5.0 mg/70 kg, or pyridostigmine, 10 to 15 mg/70 kg. If the block is not antagonized, the patient's ventilation should be controlled until the block terminates spontaneously, since the administration of additional anticholinesterase may augment neuromuscular blockade.[73,75]

In addition to altering the effect of muscle relaxants by decreasing blood flow and by directly affecting the neuromuscular junction, trimethaphan inhibits pseudocholinesterase activity.[75] Sklar et al. have estimated that pseudocholinesterase activity is suppressed by trimethaphan to such an extent that the duration of action from succinylcholine is doubled.[76] However, sodium nitroprusside does not alter pseudocholinesterase activity.[76] In summary, trimethaphan alters the action of muscle relaxants in several ways, whereas sodium nitroprusside appears only to decrease muscle blood flow.

DRUG INTERACTIONS INVOLVING THE CARDIOVASCULAR EFFECTS OF d-TUBOCURARINE AND PANCURONIUM

CASE REPORT

A 69-year-old man was anesthetized with halothane and nitrous oxide (60%) for total hip arthroplasty. Halothane was maintained at an end-tidal concentration of 0.75 volume %. The patient's systolic blood pressure was 130 torr. Three minutes after the administration of d-tubocurarine 12 mg/m² (21 mg total), his systolic blood pressure began to decrease. Ten minutes later, the systolic blood pressure was 70 torr. Halothane was discontinued and ephedrine, 15 mg, was administered intravenously. The patient's systolic blood pressure promptly increased to 120 torr. Halothane was gradually reinstituted without further difficulty with blood pressure.

Hypotension in this case appears to be related to the administration of d-tubocurarine. Although ephedrine administration was successful in reversing the hypotension, this approach can be dangerous. Ephedrine, which elicits both direct and indirect sympathetic responses, increases the incidence of arrhythmias with halothane; this drug interaction is discussed in Chapter 6.

Hypotension from d-tubocurarine is probably due to histamine release and to ganglionic blockade.[77,78] The magnitude of hypotension probably depends on several factors, the most important of which are depth of anesthesia (Fig. 18–5), dose of d-tubocurarine administered, age, and intravascular volume.[79,80] The most likely situation in which hypotension might develop is in an elderly, bedridden patient who is deeply anesthetized, and who is receiving a large dose of d-tubocurarine. In my experience, hypotension is rare when d-tubocurarine is used in doses of less than 9 mg/m² (15 mg/70 kg) (Fig. 18–5). Since doses larger

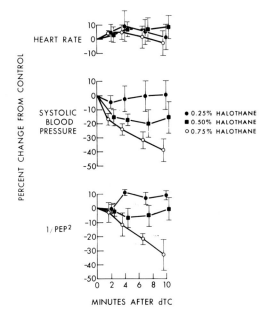

Fig. 18–5. Effects of alveolar halothane concentration on systolic blood pressure, heart rate, and myocardial inotropy (1/PEP²) following administration of d-tubocurarine 12 mg/m², as an intravenous bolus. Each point represents the mean of values for five patients (± 1 SE). All patients also received nitrous oxide, 60%. (From Munger, W. L., Miller, R. D., and Stevens, W. C.: The dependence of d-tubocurarine hypotension on alveolar concentration of halothane, dose of d-tubocurarine, and nitrous oxide. Anesthesiology, *40*:442, 1974.)

than this are not necessary for adequate relaxation during halothane anesthesia, hypotension from d-tubocurarine should not be a problem.

Why is hypotension from d-tubocurarine more severe with higher concentrations of halothane? This may be because both drugs block ganglionic transmission in a dose-dependent manner and both may have an additive effect.[80,81] With deeper levels of halothane, the onset of d-tubocurarine ganglionic blockade occurs at lower doses; the opposite is also true. This situation probably applies to anesthetic agents other than halothane.

CASE REPORT

A 48-year-old 60-kg woman was scheduled for a radical mastectomy. She was anesthetized with halothane and nitrous oxide,

60%, after the administration of thiopental, 150 mg. After the induction of anesthesia, her systolic blood pressure was 130 torr and her heart rate was 90 beats per minute. Pancuronium, 6 mg, was then administered intravenously. Within three minutes the patient's heart rate was approximately 180 beats per minute and her systolic blood pressure was 90 torr. Administration of lidocaine, 100 mg, intravenously had no effect. Neostigmine, 1.5 mg, was administered intravenously. This resulted in a prompt decrease in heart rate to 80 beats per minute and in a systolic blood pressure of 120 torr. The neuromuscular blockade was also antagonized. Anesthesia and the operation proceeded without any further difficulty. Postoperatively the patient was interviewed more thoroughly for possible drug intake information missed on the preoperative visit. It was then learned that she had been taking imipramine for over a year.

This case report represents a triple drug interaction—pancuronium, tricyclic antidepressants, and halothane. Pancuronium administration induces a transient tachycardia and slight hypertension.[82] The tachycardia is probably due to the vagolytic action of pancuronium, but the stimulation of the sympathetic nervous system has been suggested as a cause of tachycardia. Specifically, the negative chronotropic and inotropic actions of cholinergic drugs such as acetylcholine and carbachol are blocked by pancuronium. These actions support the theory of pancuronium's vagolytic mechanism of action.[83] Furthermore, the prior administration of atropine will attenuate the tachycardia from pancuronium (Fig. 18–6).[82] However, Seed and Chamberlain have found that pancuronium exerts a positive inotropic effect that is independent of an increase in heart rate.[84] Furthermore, reports of an increase in the plasma concentration of catecholamine following pancuronium and of a block of the reuptake of myocardial catecholamines suggest sympathetic activation.[85,86] The evidence supports a primarily vagolytic action. Even though Zsigmond et al. did not find an increase in plasma catecholamine concentrations, all other evidence points to a secondary stimulation of the sympathetic nervous system.[87]

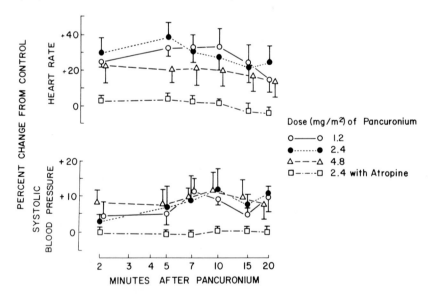

Fig. 18–6 Relationship between percentage increase in heart rate, systolic blood pressure, and time after pancuronium, 1.2, 2.4, or 4.8 mg/m². One group of patients received atropine, 0.33 mg/m², prior to pancuronium administration. Each symbol represents the mean −1 SE for five patients. (From Miller, R. D., et al.: Pancuronium-induced tachycardia in relation to alveolar halothane, dose of pancuronium, and prior atropine. Anesthesiology, *42*:352, 1975.)

A combined vagolytic and sympathomimetic effect are compatible with the observations in this case. It is well known that halothane "sensitizes" the myocardium to catecholamines. As a result, arrhythmias such as ventricular extrasystoles or atrioventricular dissociation are more likely to occur with the administration of either atropine or vasopressors during halothane anesthesia.[82,88] Such arrhythmias also are more likely when pancuronium is given during halothane anesthesia.[82] The propensity to cardiac arrhythmias is further increased by tricyclic antidepressants, such as imipramine, which are known to block the reuptake of catecholamines.[89] Recent work in our laboratory indicates that such arrhythmias are less likely to occur if one uses anesthetic agents that do not sensitize the myocardium to catecholamines, such as enflurane or nitrous oxide-narcotic anesthesia.[89a]

Therefore, we use a muscle relaxant other than pancuronium or gallamine when a patient has taken tricyclic antidepressants. Conversely, if pancuronium is administered, we use anesthetics that do not sensitize the myocardium to catecholamines.

DRUGS THAT ALTER THE REQUIRED DOSES OF NEOSTIGMINE OR OF PYRIDOSTIGMINE

Several antibiotics increase the dose of neostigmine or of pyridostigmine required for antagonism, but these antibiotics also make it impossible for complete antagonism to occur no matter what dose of neostigmine is given. There are probably other drugs that act similarly, but they have not been identified. Those drugs that may interfere with the neostigmine–d-tubocurarine interaction are likely to intensify the neuromuscular blockade from nondepolarizing relaxants such as d-tubocurarine. Thus when a neuromuscular blockade cannot be antagonized it is difficult to know whether the block is too intense to be antagonized or

whether a specific problem with the neostigmine-relaxant interaction exists.

Even though no other drugs are known to alter specifically the neostigmine-relaxant interaction, some drugs can create secondary conditions that interfere with the reversal of neuromuscular blockade. These conditions are: (1) neuromuscular blockade that is too intense (hypothermia and renal failure), (2) antibiotics, (3) respiratory acidosis, (4) metabolic alkalosis (hypokalemia and hypocalcemia). In the case of the last three conditions, not only is more neostigmine required, but also it is impossible to antagonize the block completely unless the antibiotic is eliminated or unless the acid-base abnormality is corrected.

Narcotics have little or no effect on a nondepolarizing neuromuscular blockade as such. However, if respiratory acidosis ensues from their administration, complete antagonism by neostigmine is difficult and often impossible.[91,92] This is a spurious effect of the narcotic.

There are other drugs that may have little direct effect on neuromuscular transmission, but that cause secondary changes that may have important consequences. Chronic diuretic therapy causes hypokalemia, which augments a nondepolarizing neuromuscular blockade and increases the dose of neostigmine required for neuromuscular blockade.[93] General anesthetic agents, particularly halothane and enflurane, decrease renal and liver function as well as the patient's ability to maintain normal body temperature. Diminished renal function and hypothermia delay the excretion of muscle relaxants (Figs. 18–3 and 18–7).[17,90,94–97] Administration of sodium bicarbonate sufficient to increase arterial pH above 7.5 creates a situation in which a d-tubocurarine or pancuronium neuromuscular blockade cannot be antagonized completely by neostigmine.[91,92] One may mistakenly conclude that the incomplete antagonism is due to the elevated pH; however, the administration of sodium bicarbonate also decreases plasma

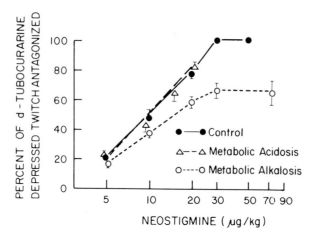

Fig. 18–7. Correlation by dose of neostigmine and percentage of dTC-depressed twitch antagonized. Each symbol represents the mean ±1 SE. (From Miller, R. D., et al.: The effect of acid-base balance on neostigmine antagonism of d-tubocurarine-induced neuromuscular blockade. Anesthesiology, *42*:377, 1975.)

calcium and potassium levels. When plasma calcium and potassium levels are normal, an elevated pH has no effect on a nondepolarizing blockade or on its antagonism by neostigmine.[98]

Generally, neostigmine, 2.5 to 5.0 mg/70 kg, or pyridostigmine, 10 to 20 mg/kg, should antagonize a nondepolarizing neuromuscular blockade. What should be done if these doses fail? In this situation, additional antagonist should not be given unless certain questions have been answered:[99]

1. Has enough time been allowed for the neostigmine or pyridostigmine to act fully?
2. Is the neuromuscular blockade too intense to be antagonized?
3. What is the acid-base and electrolyte status of the patient?
4. What is the patient's temperature?
5. Is the patient receiving any drug that might interfere with reversal?

The answers to these questions may help to correct conditions that prevent prompt, complete reversal of neuromuscular blockade by either neostigmine or pyridostigmine.

REFERENCES

1. Miller, R. D.: Antagonism of neuromuscular blockade. Anesthesiology, *44*:293, 1976.
2. Foldes, F. F.: Factors which alter the effects of muscle relaxants. Anesthesiology, *20*:464, 1959.
3. Miller, R. D.: Factors affecting the action of muscle relaxants. *In* Muscle Relaxants. Edited by R. L. Katz. Amsterdam, Excerpta Medica, North Holland Publishing Co., 1975.
4. Ali, H. H., and Savarese, J. J.: Monitoring of neuromuscular function. Anesthesiology, *45*:216, 1976.
5. Dretchen, K. L., et al.: Azathioprine: effects on neuromuscular transmission. Anesthesiology, *45*:604, 1976.
6. Standaert, F. G., Dretchen, K. L., and Skirboll, L. R.: A role of cyclic nucleotides in neuromuscular transmission. J. Pharmacol. Exp. Ther., *199*:553, 1976.
7. Matteo, R. S., et al.: Urinary excretion of d-tubocurarine in man—effect of osmotic diuretic. *In* Abstracts of Scientific Papers, Chicago, American Society of Anesthesiology, 1975.
8. Miller, R. D., Sohn, Y. J., and Matteo, R.: Enhancement of d-tubocurarine neuromuscular blockade by diuretics in man. Anesthesiology, *45*:442, 1976.
9. Scapaticci, K. A., et al.: Effects of furosemide on the motor nerve terminal. Fed. Proc. (In press.)
10. Ham, J., et al.: Effects of furosemide on neuromuscular transmission. (In press.)
11. Pittinger, C. B., and Adamson, R.: Antibiotic blockade of neuromuscular function. Annu. Rev. Pharmacol., *12*:169, 1972.
11a. Foldes, F. F.: Personal communication.
12. Wright, J. M., and Collier, B.: The site of the neuromuscular block produced by polymyxin B

and rolitetracycline. Can. J. Physiol. Pharmacol., *54*:926, 1976.

13. Van Nyhuis, L. S., Miller, R. D., and Fogdall, R. P.: The interaction between d-tubocurarine, pancuronium, polymyxin B, and neostigmine on neuromuscular function. Anesth. Analg. (Cleve.), *55*:237, 1976.

13a.Giesecke, A. H.: Personal communication.

14. Fogdall, R. P., and Miller, R. D.: Prolongation of a pancuronium-induced neuromuscular blockade by polymyxin B. Anesthesiology, *40*:84, 1974.

15. Churchill-Davidson, H. C., Way, W. L., and de Jong, R. H.: The muscle relaxants and renal excretion. Anesthesiology, *28*:540, 1967.

16. White, R. D., De Weerd, J. H., and Dawson, B.: Gallamine in anesthesia for patients with chronic renal failure undergoing bilateral nephrectomy. Anesth. Analg. (Cleve.), *50*:11, 1971.

17. Miller, R. D., et al.: Influence of renal failure on the pharmacokinetics of d-tubocurarine in man. J. Pharmacol. Exp. Ther., *202*:1, 1977.

18. Deutsch, S., et al.: Effects of halothane anesthesia on renal function in normal man. Anesthesiology, *27*:793, 1966.

19. Meyers, E. F.: Partial recovery from pancuronium neuromuscular blockade following hydrocortisone administration. Anesthesiology, *46*:148, 1977.

20. Miller, R. D., et al.: The dependence of pancuronium and d-tubocurarine induced neuromuscular blockades on alveolar concentrations of halothane and Forane. Anesthesiology, *37*:573, 1972.

21. Miller, R. D., Criqui, M., and Eger, E. I., II: The influence of duration of anesthesia on a d-tubocurarine neuromuscular blockade. Anesthesiology, *44*:207, 1976.

22. Miller, R. D., et al.: Comparative neuromuscular effects of pancuronium, gallamine, and succinylcholine during Forane and halothane anesthesia in man. Anesthesiology, *35*:509, 1971.

23. Fogdall, R. P., and Miller, R. D.: Neuromuscular effects of enflurane alone and in combination with d-tubocurarine, pancuronium, and succinylcholine in man. Anesthesiology, *42*:173, 1975.

24. Vitez, T. S., Miller, R. D., and Eger, E. I., II: An in vitro comparison of halothane and isoflurane potentiation of neuromuscular blockade. Anesthesiology, *41*:53, 1974.

25. Ngai, S. H., Hanks, E. C., and Farhie, S. E.: Effects of anesthetics on neuromuscular transmission and somatic reflexes. Anesthesiology, *26*:162, 1965.

26. Gergis, S. D., et al.: Effect of anesthetics on acetylcholine release from the myoneural junction. Proc. Soc. Exp. Biol. Med., *141*:629, 1972.

27. Waud, B. E., and Waud, D. R.: The effects of diethyl ether, enflurane, and isoflurane at the neuromuscular junction. Anesthesiology, *42*:275, 1975.

28. Waud, B. E., and Waud, D. R.: Comparison of drug-receptor dissociation constants at the mammalian neuromuscular junction in the presence and absence of halothane. J. Pharmacol. Exp. Ther., *187*:40, 1973.

29. Karis, J. H., Gissen, A. J., and Nastuk, W. L.: Mode of action of diethyl ether in blocking neuromuscular transmission. Anesthesiology, *27*:42, 1966.

30. Gissen, A. J., Karis, J. H., and Nastuk, W. L.: Effect of halothane on neuromuscular transmission. J.A.M.A., *197*:770, 1966.

31. Ngai, S. H.: Action of general anesthetics in producing muscle relaxation: interaction of anesthetics and relaxants. *In* Muscle Relaxants. Edited by R. L. Katz. Amsterdam, Excerpta Medica, North-Holland Publishing Co., 1975.

32. Telivuo, L., and Katz, R. L.: The effects of modern intravenous local analgetics on respiration during partial neuromuscular block in man. Anaesthesia, *25*:30, 1970.

33. Usubiaga, J. E., et al.: Interaction of intravenously administered procaine, lidocaine, and succinylcholine in anesthetized subjects. Anesth. Analg. (Cleve.), *46*:39, 1967.

34. Usubiaga, J. E., and Standaert, F.: The effects of local anesthetics on motor nerve terminals. J. Pharmacol. Exp. Ther., *159*:353, 1968.

35. Steinback, A. B.: Alteration by xylocaine (lidocaine) and its derivatives on the time course of end plate potentials. J. Gen. Physiol., *52*:144, 1968.

36. Kordas, M.: The effect of procaine on neuromuscular transmission. J. Physiol., *209*:689, 1970.

37. Gesler, R. M., and Matsuba, M.: Neuromuscular blocking actions of local anesthetics. J. Pharmacol. Exp. Ther., *103*:314, 1951.

38. Thorpe, W. R., and Seeman, P.: The site of action of caffeine and procaine in skeletal muscle. J. Pharmacol. Exp. Ther., *179*:324, 1971.

39. Harrah, M. D., Way, W. L., and Katzung, B. G.: The interaction of d-tubocurarine with antiarrhythmic drugs. Anesthesiology, *33*:406, 1970.

40. Grogono, A. W.: Anesthesia for atrial defibrillation. Effect of quinidine on muscle relaxation. Lancet, *2*:1039, 1963.

41. Miller, R. D., Way, W. L., and Katzung, B. G.: The potentiation of neuromuscular blocking agents by quinidine. Anesthesiology, *28*:1036, 1967.

42. Miller, R. D., Way, W. L., and Katzung, B. G.: The neuromuscular effects of quinidine. Proc. Soc. Exp. Biol. Med., *129*:215, 1968.

43. Johnston, R. R., Miller, R. D., and Way, W. L.: The interaction of ketamine with neuromuscular blocking drugs. Anesth. Analg. (Cleve.), *53*:496, 1974.

44. Cronnelly, R.: Interaction of ketamine HCl with neuromuscular agents. Fed. Proc., *31*:535, 1972.

45. Del Castillo, J., and Engback, L.: The nature of the neuromuscular block produced by magnesium. J. Physiol., *124*:370, 1954.

46. Giesecke, A. H., et al.: Of magnesium, muscle relaxants, toxemic parturients, and cats. Anesth. Analg. (Cleve.), *47*:689, 1968.

47. Ghoneim, M. M., and Long, J. P.: The interaction between magnesium and other neuromuscular blocking agents. Anesthesiology, *32*:23, 1970.

48. Borden, H., Clarke, M., and Katz, H.: The use of pancuronium bromide in patients receiving lithium carbonate. Can. Anaesth. Soc. J., *21*:79, 1974.

49. Hill, G. E., Wong, K. C., and Hodges, M. R.: Potentiation of succinylcholine neuromuscular blockade by lithium carbonate. Anesthesiology, *44*:439, 1976.

50. Walts, L. F., and Dillon, J. B.: Clinical studies of the interaction between d-tubocurarine and succinylcholine. Anesthesiology, *31*:39, 1969.

51. Katz, R. L.: Modification of the action of pancuronium by succinylcholine and halothane. Anesthesiology, *35*:602, 1971.

52. Ivankovich, A. D., et al.: Dual action of pancuronium on a succinylcholine block. Can. Anaesth. Soc. J., *24*:228, 1977.

53. Miller, R. D.: The advantages of giving d-tubocurarine before succinylcholine. Anesthesiology, *37*:569, 1972.

54. Miller, R. D., Way, W. L., and Hickey, R. L.: Inhibition of succinylcholine induced increased intraocular pressure by nondepolarizing muscle relaxants. Anesthesiology, *29*:123, 1968.

55. Miller, R. D., and Way, W. L.: Inhibition of succinylcholine induced increased intragastric pressure by nondepolarizing muscle relaxants and lidocaine. Anesthesiology, *34*:185, 1971.

56. Lamoreaux, L. F., and Urback, K. F.: Incidence and prevention of muscle pain following administration of succinylcholine. Anesthesiology, *21*:394, 1960.

57. Birch, A. A. B., Mitchell, G. D., and Playford, G. A.: Changes in serum potassium response to succinylcholine following trauma. J.A.M.A., *210*:490, 1969.

58. Miller, R. D., and Way, W. L.: The interaction between succinylcholine and subparalyzing doses of d-tubocurarine and gallamine in man. Anesthesiology, *35*:567, 1971.

59. Cullen, D. J.: The effect of pretreatment with nondepolarizing muscle relaxants on the neuromuscular blocking action of succinylcholine. Anesthesiology, *35*:572, 1971.

60. Dery, R.: The effects of precurarization with a protective dose of d-tubocurarine in the conscious patient. Can. Anaesth. Soc. J., *21*:68, 1974.

61. Baraka, A.: Suxamethonium-neostigmine interaction in patients with normal or atypical cholinesterase. Br. J. Anaesth., *49*:479, 1977.

62. Nastuk, W. L., and Gissen, A. J.: Actions of acetylcholine and other quaternary ammonium compounds at the muscle postjunctional membrane. *In* Muscle. Edited by W. M. Paul and E. C. Daniel. Oxford, Pergamon Press, Ltd., 1967.

63. Miller, R. D., et al.: Comparative time to peak effect and duration of neostigmine and pyridostigmine. Anesthesiology, *41*:27, 1974.

64. Churchill-Davidson, H. C., and Katz, R. L.: Dual, phase II, or desensitization block? Anesthesiology, *27*:546, 1966.

65. Vickers, M. D. A.: The mismanagement of suxamethonium apnea. Br. J. Anaesth., *35*:260, 1963, 1966.

66. Katz, R. L., and Katz, G. J.: Clinical use of muscle relaxants. *In* Advances in Anesthesiology: Muscle Relaxants. Edited by L. C. Clark and E. M. Papper. New York, Hoeber, 1967.

67. Gissen, A. J., Katz, R. L., and Karis, J. H.: Neuromuscular block in man during prolonged arterial infusion with succinylcholine. Anesthesiology, *27*:242, 1966.

68. Pantuck, E. J., and Pantuck, C. B.: Cholinesterases and anticholinesterases. *In* Muscle Relaxants. Edited by R. L. Katz. Amsterdam, Excerpta Medica, North-Holland Publishing Co., 1975.

69. Zsigmond, E. K., and Robbins, G.: The effect of a series of anticancer drugs on plasma cholinesterase activity. Can. Anaesth. Soc. J., *19*:75, 1972.

70. Wang, R. I. H., and Ross, C. A.: Prolonged apnea following succinylcholine in cancer patients receiving AB-132. Anesthesiology, *24*:363, 1963.

71. Bennett, E. J., et al.: Muscle relaxants, myasthenia, and mustards? Anesthesiology, *46*:220, 1977.

72. Goat, V. A., et al.: The effect of blood flow upon the activity of gallamine triethiodide. Br. J. Anaesth., *48*:69, 1976.

73. Gergis, S. D., Sokoll, M. D., and Rubbo, J. T.: Effect of sodium nitroprusside and trimethaphan on neuromuscular transmission in the frog. Can. Anaesth. Soc. J., *24*:220, 1977.

74. Wilson, S. L., et al.: Prolonged neuromuscular blockade associated with trimethaphan: a case report. Anesth. Analg. (Cleve.), *55*:353, 1976.

75. Deacock, A. R., and Davis, T. D. W.: The influence of certain ganglionic blocking agents on neuromuscular transmission. Br. J. Anaesth., *30*:217, 1958.

76. Sklar, G. S., and Lanks, K. W.: Effects of trimethaphan and sodium nitroprusside on hydrolysis of succinylcholine *in vitro*. Anesthesiology, *47*:31, 1977.

77. Norman, N., and Lofstrom, B.: Interaction of d-tubocurarine, ether, cyclopropane, and thiopental on ganglionic transmission. J. Pharmacol. Exp. Ther., *114*:231, 1955.

78. Westgate, H. D., and Van Bergen, F. H.: Changes in histamine blood levels following d-tubocurarine administration. Can. Anaesth. Soc. J., *9*:497, 1962.

79. Stoelting, R. K., and Longnecker, D. E.: Influence of end-tidal halothane concentration on d-tubocurarine hypotension. Anesth. Analg. (Cleve.), *51*:364, 1972.

80. Munger, W. L., Miller, R. D., and Stevens, W. C.: The dependence of d-tubocurarine hypotension on alveolar concentration of halothane, dose of d-tubocurarine, and nitrous oxide. Anesthesiology, *40*:442, 1974.

81. Price, H. L., and Price, M. L.: Has halothane a predominant circulatory action? Anesthesiology, *27*:764, 1966.

82. Miller, R. D., et al.: Pancuronium-induced tachycardia in relation to alveolar halothane, dose of pancuronium, and prior atropine. Anesthesiology, *42*:352, 1975.

83. Saxena, P. R., and Bonta, I. L.: Specific blockade of cardiac muscarinic receptors by pancuronium bromide. Arch. Intern. Pharmacodyn., *189*:410, 1971.

84. Seed, R. F., and Chamberlain, J. H.: Myocardial stimulation by pancuronium bromide. Br. J. Anaesth., *49*:401, 1977.

85. Nana, S., Cardan, E., and Domokos, M.: Blood

catecholamine changes after pancuronium. Acta Anaesthesiol. Scand., *17*:83, 1973.

86. Domenech, J. S., et al.: Pancuronium bromide: an indirect sympathomimetic agent. Br. J. Anaesth., *48*:1143, 1976.

87. Zsigmond, E., et al.: The effect of pancuronium bromide on plasma norepinephrine and cortisol concentrations during thiamylal induction. Can. Anaesth. Soc. J., *21*:147, 1974.

88. Jones, R. E., Deutsch, S., and Turndorf, H.: Effects of atropine on cardiac rhythm in conscious and anesthetized man. Anesthesiology, *22*:67, 1961.

89. Axelrod, J., Whitby, L. G., and Hertting, G.: Effect of psychotropic drugs on the uptake of H³-norepinephrine by tissues. Science, *133*:383, 1961.

89a. Edwards, R., et al.: Unpublished data.

90. McLeod, K., Watson, M. J., and Rawlines, M. D.: Pharmacokinetics of pancuronium in patients with normal and impaired renal function. Br. J. Anaesth., *48*:341, 1976.

91. Miller, R. D., and Roderick, L.: Acid-base and a pancuronium neuromuscular blockade and its antagonism by neostigmine. Br. J. Anaesth., *50*:317, 1978.

92. Miller, R. D., et al.: The effect of acid-base balance on neostigmine antagonism of d-tubocurarine-induced neuromuscular blockade. Anesthesiology, *42*:377, 1975.

93. Miller, R. D., and Roderick, L.: Diuretic-induced hypokalemia and a pancuronium neuromuscular blockade and its antagonism by neostigmine. Br. J. Anaesth., *50*:541, 1978.

94. Miller, R. D., Van Nyhuis, L. S., and Eger, E. I., II: The effect of temperature on a d-tubocurarine neuromuscular blockade and its antagonism by neostigmine. J. Pharmacol. Exp. Ther., *195*:237, 1975.

95. Miller, R. D., and Roderick, L.: Pancuronium-induced neuromuscular blockade and its antagonism by neostigmine at 29, 37, and 41°C. Anesthesiology, *46*:333, 1977.

96. Ham, J., et al.: The effect of temperature on the pharmacodynamics and pharmacokinetics of d-tubocurarine. Anesthesiology, *49*:324, 1978.

97. Miller, R. D., et al.: Hypothermia and the pharmacodynamics and pharmacokinetics of pancuronium in the cat. J. Pharmacol. Exp. Ther., *207*:532, 1978.

98. Miller, R. D., Agoston, S., and Van der Pool, F.: Is the effect of matabolic alkalosis on a pancuronium neuromuscular blockade and its antagonism by neostigmine a pH effect? (In preparation).

99. Miller, R. D.: Reversal of neuromuscular blockade. Regional Refresher Courses in Anesthesiology, *5*:134, 1977.

The editorial advice of Dorothy Urban and Trudy Garrettson is greatly appreciated.

Local Anesthetics

EDWIN S. MUNSON

A drug interaction occurs when the effects of one drug are modified by the prior or concurrent administration of another drug. Interactions arising from the administration of local anesthetic drugs may result from alterations in absorption, distribution, or elimination of one drug by another; or from the combination of their actions on various organ systems. The discussion of chemical or physical incompatibilities among drugs, their preservatives, or their containers is beyond the scope of this chapter.

ABSORPTION

CASE REPORT

A healthy 36-year-old woman was admitted to the hospital for repair of a severely deviated nasal septum. Preoperatively she received meperidine, 100 mg, pentobarbital, 100 mg, and atropine, 0.4 mg, intramuscularly. Anesthesia was induced with thiopental, 250 mg, and maintained with nitrous oxide, 60%, and halothane, 1%. Cocaine flakes, 100 mg, and 1 ml of 1:1,000 epinephrine (1,000 μg) were mixed together and placed on three cotton pledgets within the nasal cavity for three minutes; they were then removed. During the three minutes, 20 ml of a 2% lidocaine solution, which contained 0.5 ml of 1:1,000 epinephrine (500 μg), was prepared; 3 ml of this solution was injected into the dorsum of the nose and infraorbital areas. When the skin incision was made, the blood was noted to be dark; after a few minutes the anesthetist reported an irregular pulse and hypotension. Cardiac asystole occurred and resuscitative efforts were unsuccessful.

This report illustrates the potential hazards of using large doses (>1,000 μg) of epinephrine combined with cocaine and an inhalation anesthetic agent known to possess the potential for inducing cardiac arrhythmias. The use of cocaine and epinephrine with these inhalation anesthetic agents (particularly halothane and cyclopropane) may increase the incidence of catecholamine-induced arrhythmias.

Cocaine

Cocaine, 10%, applied to the nasal mucosa in human beings, may delay its own absorption because of concomitant vasoconstriction. Van Dyke et al. found that, although plasma levels of cocaine reached a peak (0.12 to 0.47 μg/ml) from 15 to 60 minutes after administration, the drug persisted in the plasma for four to six hours.[1] Since residual cocaine was detectable on the nasal mucosa for as long as three hours, absorption probably continued, which resulted in persistent plasma levels. Also, plasma cocaine levels are higher and last longer in dental patients with cardiovascular disease. The possibility of potentiating sympathomimetic amines administered during the course of anesthesia and surgical procedures should be anticipated. In addition, drugs such as cocaine that interfere with intraneural uptake of catecholamines can facilitate the development of epinephrine-induced arrhythmias during halothane anesthesia.[2]

Epinephrine

The addition of epinephrine to local anesthetic solutions reduces plasma local anesthetic concentrations and prolongs the block, and it has little, if any, effect on a delayed onset time of analgesia. Scott et al. showed that the addition of 1:200,000 epinephrine to a 2% lidocaine solution lowered plasma levels when 400 mg of lidocaine was injected for various block procedures (Fig. 19–1).[3]

Whenever solutions containing epinephrine are administered in the presence of an inhalation anesthetic agent, the possibility of increased arrhythmogenicity should be considered. The halothane-epinephrine interaction is well documented (see Chapter 6, "Sympathomimetic Drugs"). Johnston et al. found that the addition of an 0.5%

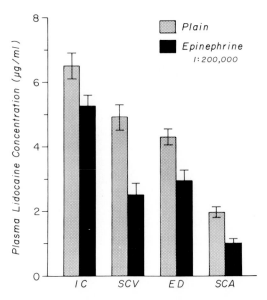

Fig. 19–1. Mean (± SE) maximum plasma concentrations following the injection of 400 mg lidocaine for intercostal (IC), subcutaneous vaginal (SCV), epidural (ED), and subcutaneous abdominal (SCA) block. The addition of epinephrine significantly (P<0.01) reduced lidocaine plasma levels in each instance. (Redrawn from Scott, D. B., et al.[3])

lidocaine solution made the use of epinephrine safer during halothane anesthesia.[4]

Sodium bisulfite, a reducing agent, is added to local anesthetic-epinephrine solutions by the manufacturer. Although oxidative decomposition of epinephrine is prevented, sodium bisulfite is strongly acidic and increases tissue buffer demands.[5] Clinically, compared with the stabilizer-free solution, a greater initial concentration of local anesthetic is required to attain the same effectiveness. When epinephrine is administered, ampules of local anesthetic-epinephrine solutions containing a single dose and no chemical stabilizers, or freshly prepared epinephrine solutions, should be employed.

Carbon dioxide

Bromage et al. have shown that carbonated solutions of lidocaine and prilocaine produce a 20 to 40% more rapid onset and intensity of block than do the hydrochloride salts.[6] The investigators suggest that the addition of carbon dioxide, a fast membrane penetrator and acidifying agent, improves the distribution of the anesthetic drug in the various components of nerve tissue. Carbon dioxide more readily converts the local anesthetic amide to the more active ammonium ion by lowering the pH *inside* the membrane. This effect of carbon dioxide is opposite to that of tissue acidosis, such as that produced from tissue infection or from the injection of sodium bisulfite, both of which increase *extramural* buffer demands.

Dextran

The addition of low molecular weight dextran 40 to local anesthetic solutions prolongs the effectiveness of the anesthetic agent by decreasing its rate of absorption.[7-9] This technique offers particular advantage during intercostal nerve block for prolonged and postoperative analgesia. Kaplan et al. showed that the duration of nerve block with bupivacaine, 0.75%, and dextran 40 was 36 hours, as compared with 12 hours produced by bupivacaine and saline solutions in combination.[9]

DISTRIBUTION
CASE REPORT

A 27-year-old, 60-kg man with chronic glomerular nephritis and congestive heart failure was hospitalized for repair of an arteriovenous shunt previously established to facilitate long-term hemodialysis. A nerve block of the left brachial plexus was attempted by the axillary approach using 30 ml of lidocaine, 1.5%, with 1:200,000 epinephrine. Since satisfactory anesthesia was not obtained, additional lidocaine was injected into the axillary space, raising the initial dosage of 450 mg to a total of 1,400 mg within one hour. The patient developed twitching of the face and extremities, and oxygen was administered immediately by face mask. Seizure activity promptly subsided, but the patient remained drowsy and unresponsive. There were no appreciable changes in any of the vital signs during this episode. Small amounts of procaine were then administered locally for placement of a new shunt in the same arm. The patient's recovery was uneventful.[10]

This report describes a toxic reaction to an overdose of lidocaine in a patient whose cardiac and renal functions were compromised. In addition to excessively large doses of local anesthetic, decreases in the volume of drug distribution and renal clearance probably also contributed to the patient's reaction.

Cardiac failure

Lidocaine metabolism is decreased in patients with cardiac failure and cardiogenic shock after myocardial infarction.[11,12] In heart failure, both the volume of distribution and the plasma clearance of lidocaine are reduced. The plasma concentration of lidocaine during intravenous infusion is higher in patients with cardiac failure; the terminal plasma half-life may be prolonged as much as three- to sixfold. The administration of an amide-type local anesthetic for regional block procedures in these patients can produce potentially toxic levels of local anesthetics in the plasma, particularly if, in addition, lidocaine has been administered to control cardiac arrhythmias. In patients with cardiovascular disease, levels of cocaine in the plasma after intranasal application are also higher, and their duration is more prolonged, than are cocaine levels in healthy dental patients.[1]

Hemorrhage

Lidocaine plasma levels are higher in animals during hemorrhage than in normovolemic animals.[13] Elevated blood levels reflect a decrease in both rates of clearance and volumes of distribution. The elevated blood concentrations are similar to those observed in patients with congestive heart failure.

Vasopressors

The administration of sympathomimetic drugs during lidocaine infusion may influence lidocaine blood concentrations. Hepatic blood flow is increased by isoproterenol and is decreased by norepinephrine.[13] Steady-state lidocaine blood levels are directly related to changes in hepatic blood flow (Fig. 19–2). Alterations in the clearance of local anesthetic relate to change in hepatic blood flow rather than to an altered extraction ratio. Decreased lidocaine clearance after the administration of propranolol also has been described by Branch et al. in dogs.[14] Clinically, the administration of norepinephrine might induce lidocaine toxicity in patients with previously stable levels of local anesthetic drugs in plasma.

The use of vasopressor drugs for the treatment of arterial hypotension also may increase the toxicity of local anesthetics. Mather et al. found that whereas intravenous ephedrine relieved cardiovascular depression following epidural block, lidocaine levels in plasma were elevated.[15] This increased systemic absorption from the epidural site would also shorten the period of cardiovascular depression.

Protein binding

Tucker and colleagues have shown that the ranking of local anesthetics according to their ability to bind with plasma proteins is as follows: bupivacaine > mepivacaine > lidocaine.[16] Furthermore, this order correlates well with the blocking action (potency) of these drugs. Since the binding of drugs to plasma proteins is reversible and nonspecific, drugs can compete with one

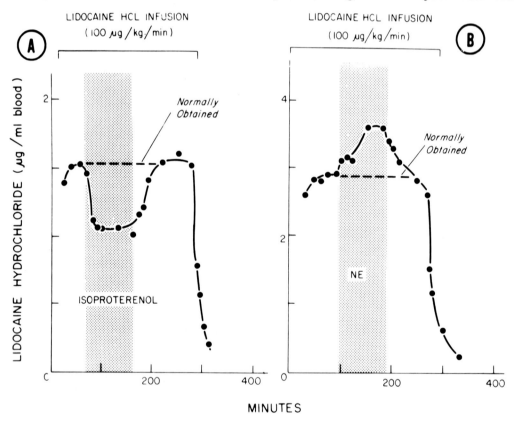

Fig. 19–2. The effects of isoproterenol and norephinephrine (NE) on steady-state arterial lidocaine concentrations in the rhesus monkey. The vasopressors were administered over the time period shown by the shaded area. Dashed lines indicate the lidocaine plasma levels normally obtained in the absence of vasopressors. (From Benowitz, N., et al.: Lidocaine disposition kinetics in monkey and man. II. Effects of hemorrhage and sympathomimetic drug administration. Clin. Pharmacol. Ther., *16*:99, 1974.)

another for binding sites. Also, since protein binding influences drug distribution and elimination, changes in binding, either as the result of physiologic changes or from other drugs, may modify the action and duration of local anesthetics. For example, the addition of phenytoin (diphenylhydantoin), quinidine, meperidine, or desipramine to normal human plasma causes a displacement of bupivacaine.[17] If this effect occurs *in vivo*, patients receiving these drugs may have a four- to sixfold increase in unbound or active bupivacaine. Although drug interactions of this type have not been reported clinically, the possibility of increased toxicity of local anesthetics exists.

Blood pH may also alter the binding of local anesthetics to plasma proteins.[18] Lidocaine protein binding is decreased when plasma pH is lowered from 7.6 to 7.0. This decrease suggests that the concentration of available (active) drug is greater in the presence of acidosis. Since acidosis usually accompanies central nervous system (CNS) and cardiovascular depression, metabolic and respiratory acidosis should be corrected to lessen toxicity and to interrupt this self-perpetuating effect.

ELIMINATION
CASE REPORT

A 22-year-old woman was scheduled for dental extractions. A few minutes after the injection of procaine, she became weak and felt nauseated and dyspneic; she subsequently became cyanotic and lost consciousness. The patient was resuscitated successfully by ventilation with oxygen and by the administration of vasopressors. Seven years later, the same patient manifested prolonged apnea following the administration of succinylcholine. Subsequent examinations showed that she was an atypical homozygote with a dibucaine number of 18 and thus had reduced hydrolysis rates for benzylcholine and procaine. The family history revealed that the patient's sister had had cardiovascular collapse after the administration of 320 mg of procaine for pudendal nerve block anesthesia. Subsequent testing showed that her plasma cholinesterase activity and dibucaine number were also abnormally low.[19]

The occurrence of concomitant CNS and neuromuscular toxicity in the same patient is unusual. However, since ester-type local anesthetics and succinylcholine are both hydrolyzed by plasma pseudocholinesterase, a competitive phenomenon occurs whenever these drugs are administered together. The occurrence of prolonged apnea following the use of succinylcholine should alert the clinician to the possibility of atypical plasma cholinesterase. Hence the use of large amounts of ester-type local anesthetics may result in severe systemic toxicity in such patients. Many other drugs and disease states may also modify the elimination of local anesthetics.

Enzymatic hydrolysis

Anticholinergic Drugs. Neostigmine and pyridostigmine are frequently used to reverse the neuromuscular blockade produced by nondepolarizing muscle relaxants. In addition to inhibiting acetylcholinesterase, neostigmine and pyridostigmine inhibit plasma cholinesterase.[20] The depression of plasma cholinesterase activity may last as long as two hours after the administration of pyridostigmine (Fig. 19–3). Patients who receive neostigmine or pyridostigmine should be given succinylcholine and ester-type local anesthetic agents in reduced amounts.

Echothiophate Iodide. Patients with glaucoma frequently are treated with echothiophate iodide eye drops. This organophosphorous compound is a long-acting inhibitor of both acetylcholinesterase and pseudocholinesterase. Although reported drug interactions involve increased neuromuscular blockade after the administration of succinylcholine, a potential interaction with ester-type local anesthetics exists.[21] Similar considerations should be given to patients subjected to related alkylphosphate compounds, such as diisopropyl fluorophosphate (DFP). These compounds are still present in many insecticides.

Glucocorticoids. Foldes et al. reported that butylcholinesterase activity in plasma de-

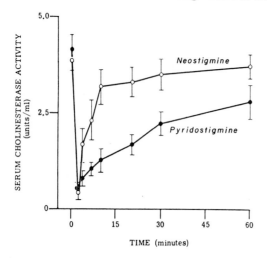

Fig. 19–3. Mean (± SE) serum cholinesterase activity values were significantly (P < 0.05) reduced for five minutes after administration of neostigmine and for at least 120 minutes after pyridostigmine. (From Stoelting, R. K.: Serum cholinesterase activity following pancuronium and antagonism with neostigmine or pyridostigmine. Anesthesiology, *45*:674, 1976.)

creases about 50% in patients who receive large doses of prednisone.[22] Subsequent studies in dogs showed that both methylprednisolone and dexamethasone decrease cholinesterase activity (pseudocholinesterase) in plasma. The cholinesterase enzyme is responsible for the hydrolysis of both succinylcholine and the ester-type local anesthetics such as procaine and tetracaine. A decrease in cholinesterase by glucocorticoids may be caused by inhibition of hepatic protein synthesis and also is expected to increase the systemic toxicity of procaine-related drugs.

Chemotherapeutic Drugs. Cholinesterase activity may be lower in patients suffering from certain types of cancer than in healthy persons.[23] In addition, prolonged apnea resulting from the use of succinylcholine in two patients receiving an antitumor drug was described by Wang and Ross.[24] The cancer chemotherapeutic agent AB-132, that is, ethyl-N-(bis [2-2-diethylenimido] phosphoro) carbamate, has been shown to inhibit both plasma and erythrocyte cholin-

esterases. The warning that succinylcholine should be administered with caution to patients who receive this chemotherapeutic agent also applies to the ester-type local anesthetics. A similar drug interaction should be expected between hydrolyzable local anesthetics administered in the presence of other chemotherapeutic agents that inhibit cholinesterase activity in plasma.

Pregnancy. Cholinesterase activity in plasma decreases during pregnancy and the immediate postpartum period. Most reports of prolonged apnea during cesarean section have been attributed to a reduced rate of enzymatic hydrolysis. However, Blitt et al. found that no correlation exists between cholinesterase activity in the plasma and the duration of paralysis from succinycholine.[25] Similarly, Finster demonstrated that the rate of hydrolysis of chloroprocaine in parturient patients did not differ from that of either men or nonpregnant women.[26] However, the sensitivity of infants to ester local anesthetics may be increased, since Reidenberg has shown that newborn infants hydrolyze procaine much more slowly than do healthy adults.[27]

Enzyme induction

Drugs that induce hepatic microsomal enzyme systems (for example, phenobarbital) may alter the rate of metabolism of amide local anesthetics and may increase the rate at which metabolites of lidocaine are formed. Pretreating dogs with phenobarbital increases the hepatic clearance of lidocaine from 25 to 50% (Fig. 19–4).[28] Plasma lidocaine levels in seven epileptic patients treated with phenobarbital were also lower than those in control subjects receiving the same intravenous dose of lidocaine (Fig. 19–5).[29] Although four of the seven patients had taken regular doses of some barbiturate for periods ranging from one to four years, almost all of them had also received phenytoin, as well as other drugs known to have enzyme-inducing properties. Patients who receive agents that induce drug-metaboliz-

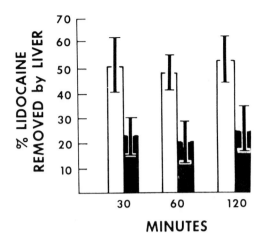

Fig. 19–4. Mean (± SD) hepatic extraction fractions of lidocaine in dogs pretreated with phenobarbital (open bars) were significantly increased as compared with control animals (closed bars). (From DiFazio, C. A., and Brown, R. E.: Lidocaine metabolism in normal and phenobarbital-pretreated dogs. Anesthesiology, 36:238, 1972.)

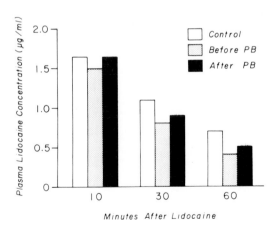

Fig. 19–5. Mean venous plasma lidocaine levels in untreated control subjects (open bars) and in epileptic patients (gray and black bars) before and after administration of phenobarbital (PB). Lidocaine plasma levels in both epileptic groups were significantly (P < 0.01) lower than in control subjects at 30 and 60 minutes. However, the addition of phenobarbital to other anticonvulsant medications taken before the experiment did not result in further enzyme induction or in lowering of lidocaine levels in the blood. (Drawn from the data of Heinonen; ‡., et al.[29])

ing enzymes may have an increased tolerance to the systemic effects of repeated doses of lidocaine. However, this may not be apparent in patients with chronic liver disease because of their inability to respond to microsomal enzyme-inducing drugs.[30]

Hepatic elimination

Liver Disease. Clearance of lidocaine from plasma is reduced in patients with liver disease.[11,30] Central nervous system toxicity developed in a patient with liver disease who was given lidocaine at a rate usually well tolerated by patients with healthy livers.[31] Forrest et al. reported that lidocaine elimination is prolonged in patients with chronic liver disease.[30] The mean (± SE) half-life of orally administered lidocaine in 19 of 21 patients with liver disease was 6.6 ± 1.1 hours, as compared with values in healthy subjects of 1.4 ± 0.3 hours.[30] Since lidocaine and other amide-type local anesthetics are eliminated primarily by hepatic metabolism, removal from plasma depends on blood flow through the liver. Impaired lidocaine elimination in patients with liver disease results from decreased hepatic blood flow secondary to cirrhosis and increased portosystemic shunting.[32]

The plasma half-lives of lidocaine, antipyrine, and paracetamol showed that significant correlations are related to serum albumin concentration. Of the three drugs studied, the prolonged half-life of lidocaine was the most sensitive indicator of hepatic dysfunction. In patients with liver disease who are known to have taken drugs capable of causing microsomal enzyme induction, drug half-lives were not significantly different from those of other patients with a similar degree of hepatic disease, as judged by routine liver function tests.[30] The severity of hepatic dysfunction should be taken into account when one considers lidocaine dosage in patients with chronic liver disease.

General Anesthesia. Decreased hepatic removal of local anesthetics should be anticipated when patients are anesthetized with potent inhalation agents. The hepatic elimination of lidocaine in animals anesthetized with halothane was slower than in animals receiving nitrous oxide and curare.[28,33] Reduced elimination may be related to decreased hepatic blood flow and to depressed hepatic microsomes induced by halothane. Clinical studies in volunteers and patients anesthetized with a combination of nitrous oxide and gallamine, with or without halothane, have shown that general anesthesia delays the rise of lidocaine concentration in the plasma after oral administration of the drug.[34] This delay in absorption is accompanied by a delayed disappearance of lidocaine from the plasma, which suggests that the metabolism of lidocaine is retarded during halothane anesthesia (Fig. 19–6).

Propranolol. The administration of propranolol in animals anesthetized with morphine and chloralose prolongs lidocaine plasma half-life by about 50%.[14] Beta-adrenergic blockade, in addition to decreasing both cardiac output and hepatic blood flow, reduces lidocaine clearance with little alteration in the rate of hepatic lidocaine extraction. This interaction results in higher plasma lidocaine levels than would be expected in patients not exposed to *beta-*adrenergic blocking drugs.

Renal excretion

The kidney is the major route of elimination for local anesthetic drugs and their metabolites. The ester-type drugs are hydrolyzed by plasma pseudocholinesterase, but the primary metabolite of procaine, para-aminobenzoic acid, is excreted by the kidney. Amide-type drugs, which have a small capacity for protein binding, such as prilocaine, have greater rates of renal clearance.[35] Renal clearance is inversely related to urine pH; hence any clinical situation that promotes renal acidification enhances the elimination of local anesthetics. Patients with impaired renal function hydrolyze procaine more slowly than do healthy adults.[27] Although the degree of slowing of procaine hydrolysis in patients with renal disease is proportional to blood urea nitrogen levels, the mechanism is related to decreased levels of enzyme activity rather than to competitive enzyme inhibition. Ester local anesthetics should be administered, in reduced dosage, to patients who have kidney disease.

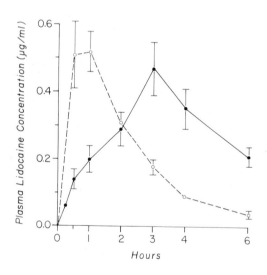

Fig. 19–6. Mean (± SE) plasma lidocaine concentration in seven awake subjects (open circles) and 12 anesthetized patients (closed circles) following ingestion of lidocaine, 400 mg. Note the marked delay in the rise of plasma lidocaine concentrations in the anesthetized patients, indicating delayed absorption. The decreased rate of drug disappearance from the plasma suggests impaired drug metabolism during anesthesia. (Drawn from the data of Adjepon-Yamoah, K. K., et al.[34])

PHARMACOLOGIC INTERACTIONS
CASE REPORT

An 8-year-old boy weighing 25 kg was admitted to the hospital for an intravenous pyelogram and a renal biopsy. He received meperidine, 50 mg, and pentobarbital, 50 mg, intramuscularly 60 minutes before the placement of a catheter in a peripheral vein. Inadvertently, instead of radiopaque dye, mepivacaine, 300 mg (without epinephrine), was administered rapidly. Generalized seizures developed immediately and were terminated quickly by the administration of oxygen by mask and of intravenous diazepam, 10 mg. Ventilation was supported, and one hour later the child was alert and conversing normally.

Two days later diagnostic studies were performed without incident; the patient was discharged from the hospital the next day.[36]

This report of gross mepivacaine overdosage (12 mg/kg) in a child illustrates several points: (1) commonly used premedicant drugs offer little, if any, protection against the development of central nervous system toxicity; (2) diazepam is an effective and rapidly acting anticonvulsant agent that has minimal secondary effects on circulation and ventilation; and (3) recovery from the administration of a single large dose of a local anesthetic is rapid, provided proper attention is given to the maintenance of the patient's ventilation and circulation.

The brain, the heart, and the neuromuscular system are particularly sensitive to the action of local anesthetics, which generally depress excitable membranes. Therefore, the use of other depressant drugs in clinical practice may result in significant drug interactions.

Anticonvulsant drugs

Although barbiturates have long been known as anticonvulsant drugs, the benzodiazepine derivative diazepam shows specific antagonism through its action on the limbic system of the brain. Clinically, compared with barbiturates, local anesthetic overdosage treated with diazepam appears to have less residual depression and, therefore, recovery is quicker. The lethal dose of lidocaine is increased by the administration of pentobarbital in animals.[37] Pretreatment of animals with diazepam has also been shown to increase both the seizure dosage and the plasma concentration of lidocaine at which seizures occur.[38,39] Although diazepam elevates seizure threshold, it may also mask the signs of impending toxicity. When seizures develop in animals pretreated with diazepam, larger doses of the anticonvulsant drug are required to control seizures than are necessary when diazepam premedication is not given. Diazepam is recommended to control seizure activity, but seizures induced by the administration of local anesthetics can be treated effectively by other intravenous, as well as inhalation, anesthetic agents. Epileptic patients receiving long-term therapy with barbiturates and/or with other anticonvulsant medication may show an increased tolerance to local anesthetic drugs, since enzyme induction may be present (see the "Enzyme Induction" section of this chapter and Figure 19–5).

Blood gases and acid-base disturbances

Oxygen. The arterial oxygen tension level (>60 torr) is not critical to the development of local anesthetic CNS toxicity. Although oxygen inhalation does not prevent CNS seizure activity, hyperoxemia after the onset of seizures is beneficial.[40]

Carbon Dioxide. The seizure dosage for lidocaine has been demonstrated in anesthetized cats to be inversely related to the arterial carbon dioxide tension.[41] Other investigators have confirmed this relationship in dogs, but not in monkeys.[42,43] The effect of hypercapnia may be related to the role of carbon dioxide in increasing cerebral blood flow and therefore may increase the rate of delivery of the local anesthetic to the central nervous system.

Hydrogen Ion. Increased hydrogen ion concentration also increases cerebral toxicity.[42] Also, protein binding of lidocaine is reduced during acidosis, which increases the active portion of lidocaine and thereby augments toxicity.[18] The use of hyperventilation to reduce cerebral seizure threshold and to increase protein binding is recommended during the treatment of any seizure induced by local anesthetics. It should be noted that the cardiovascular responses to lidocaine in animals did not correlate to changes in arterial carbon dioxide tension (12 to 73 torr) and in pH (7.69 to 7.11).[44]

Inhalation anesthetic agents

Local anesthetic toxicity may be modified by inhalation anesthetic agents. The administration of nitrous oxide or of low concentrations of other agents protects against seizures induced by lidocaine, procaine, or tetracaine.[45,46] De Jong et al. were able to increase the seizure threshold of lidocaine by 50% in cats breathing nitrous oxide, 70% (Fig. 19–7).[45] I have made similar observations with nitrous oxide in rhesus monkeys. However, the inhalation of high concentrations of halothane, fluroxene, or methoxyflurane enhanced the lethal effects of both amide and ester-type drugs.[46] Increases in toxicity probably occur through an interaction of the depressive actions of these drugs on the cardiorespiratory systems. Studies in dogs show that blood levels of local anesthetics resulting from equal doses during anesthesia descend in the following order: diethyl ether, chloroform, thiopental. In addition, the lethal dose of procaine in dogs anesthetized with ether is approximately one-half that observed with chloroform.[47]

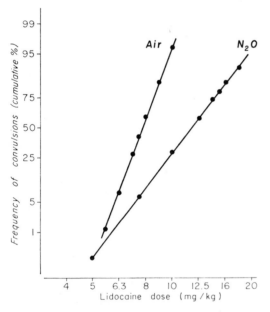

Fig. 19–7. Dose-response lines of awake cats (left) and those anesthetized with nitrous oxide, 70% (right) show that the lidocaine seizure threshold was elevated 50% in anesthetized animals. (From de Jong, R. H., Heavner, J. E., and de Oliveira, L. F.: Effects of nitrous oxide on the lidocaine seizure threshold and diazepam protection. Anesthesiology, 37:299, 1972.)

The administration of lidocaine during diethyl ether anesthesia in man and during enflurane anesthesia in dogs results in ventilatory depression.[48,49] Since lidocaine also proportionally reduces anesthetic requirement (MAC), enhanced depression of ventilation can be avoided by reducing the concentration of the inhalation anesthetic.[49]

Local anesthetic mixtures

Local anesthetic drugs frequently are combined with one another to produce rapid onset and prolonged duration of anesthesia. Although the administration of large doses of multiple drugs is considered to be an important cause of local anesthetic toxicity, clinical reports indicate that local anesthetic solutions containing amide- and ester-type drugs can be used without an apparent increase in toxicity. However, studies in rhesus monkeys show that mixtures of lidocaine-etidocaine and lidocaine-tetracaine in equipotent doses have approximately the same CNS toxicity in rhesus monkeys when given intravenously as either drug has when administered alone. That is, anesthetic toxicity is additive.[50]

Other reports indicate that repeated administration of local anesthetics cannot by itself alter seizure dosage or threshold.[39,51] The toxicity of mixtures of ester-type local anesthetics would be expected to be at least additive, since these drugs all depend on serum cholinesterase for their inactivation. However, the addition of tetracaine to procaine and to chloropropane has been shown to increase toxicity during constant-rate intravenous infusions in rats.[52]

In contrast to accidental rapid intravenous injections, the clinical tolerance of a mixture of local anesthetic drugs can be increased further following regional block procedures if the compounded drugs have different kinetic or metabolic characteristics. For example, the duration and high levels in the blood of ester derivatives such as procaine and tetracaine are limited by the activity of serum cholinesterase. In contrast, the decay of blood levels of amide derivatives such as lidocaine are subject to slower processes of redistribution, hepatic metabolism, and elimination.

Delirium induced by the combination of lidocaine and procaine amide has been reported, and bupivacaine and other amide local anesthetics (etidocaine) also have inhibited the hydrolysis of chloroprocaine by serum cholinesterase.[53,54] If these drugs are to be given concurrently, dosage should be reduced. Amide-ester mixtures containing chloroprocaine also may reduce the active (uncharged) amount of amide available in the solution. This phenomenon is related to the low pH (3.5) of chloroprocaine and may result in tachyphylaxis to the local anesthetic solution after repeated administrations to areas, such as the epidural space, with limited buffering capacities.[55]

Muscle relaxant drugs

The combined use of local anesthetic agents and other drugs that share common metabolic pathways may cause significant drug interactions. Prolonged apnea or severe systemic toxicity, or both, may occur if succinylcholine and the procaine-like ester drugs (including cocaine) are administered together, since serum cholinesterase is required for the hydrolysis and the inactivation of both types of compounds.[56] Other compounds known to possess anticholinesterase properties are pancuronium, hexafluorenium, and the hypotensive agent trimethaphan.[57-59]

DeKornfeld and Steinhaus reported that the apneic period produced by a dose of succinycholine ten minutes after the administration of lidocaine in dogs was almost twice as long as would have been anticipated if lidocaine had been omitted.[60] In addition, the administration of lidocaine following a subapneic dose of succinylcholine caused apnea in all animals studied. Whereas it is possible that this effect involves a drug interaction at the neuromuscular junction, these investigators suggested that the prolonged apnea is related to competition between the two drugs for plasma cholines-

terase. A lidocaine dose of 10 mg/kg was employed in these animals anesthetized with pentobarbital. Although this dosage is greater than would be employed clinically, any combination of the two drugs should be used cautiously, since the duration of the succinylcholine-induced apnea is likely to be longer in the presence of lidocaine.

The nondepolarizing muscle relaxants gallamine and d-tubocurarine elevate both the seizure dosage and the threshold of lidocaine in nonmedicated monkeys, whereas succinylcholine does not.[51] However, Acheson, Bull, and Glees found that the prior administration of succinylcholine (1 mg/kg) reduced the seizure dosage of lidocaine from 10 to 5 mg/kg in cats anesthetized with nitrous oxide.[61] In a related work, DeKornfeld and Steinhaus found that lidocaine (10 mg/kg) produced apnea in anesthetized dogs pretreated with subapneic doses of succinylcholine.[60] No reasonable explanation for these interactions has been proposed.

Telivuo and Katz have shown that the intravenous administration of lidocaine, mepivacaine, prilocaine, and bupivacaine in man results in a small neuromuscular blocking action and in a depression of ventilation.[62] These studies and those using inhalation anesthesia agents suggest that the major cause of respiratory depression by local anesthetics, in the absence of muscle relaxants, is primarily related to a direct action on the central nervous system. More recently, Matsuo et al. using the rat's phrenic nerve-hemidiaphragm showed that neuromuscular blocking agents and local anesthetics increase the neuromuscular blocking effects of one other.[63] This interaction should be considered when administering intravenous lidocaine to surgical patients for the treatment of cardiac arrhythmias when these patients have also received muscle relaxants.

Tricyclic antidepressant drugs

The seizure threshold of lidocaine appears to be indirectly related to levels of 5-hydroxytryptophan in the cerebrum.

Treatment of cats with 5-hydroxytryptophan decreases the seizure threshold of lidocaine and prolongs the duration of seizure activity.[64] In other studies, the increase of cerebral 5-hydroxytryptamine content by administering 5-hydroxytryptophan, and the decrease of 5-hydroxytryptamine content by giving P-chloro-p-phenylalanine resulted in increased and decreased cerebral sensitivities to lidocaine, respectively.[65] This observation is interesting in regard to the sensitivity of the amygdala, a portion of the limbic system and an area of the brain known to have a high content of 5-hydroxytryptophan.

Local anesthetic solutions containing catecholamines may interact with tricyclic antidepressant drugs to cause hypertension and tachycardia. Lidocaine and mepivacaine solutions containing norepinephrine

have produced severe headache in two dental patients who were given protriptyline.[66] A similar norepinephrine-desmethylimipramine interaction has been demonstrated in dogs.[67] The observed cardiovascular changes are related to the interaction of catecholamines and monoamine oxidase inhibitors. Other tricyclic agents that increase levels of norepinephrine at nerve terminals and the ester-type local anesthetic cocaine are likely to show a similar action.

Local anesthetic drug metabolites

Pharmacologically active metabolites of lidocaine may contribute to CNS toxicity in some patients. Strong et al. demonstrated that monoethylglycinexylidide and glycinexylidide are present in patients receiving lidocaine for the treatment of cardiac

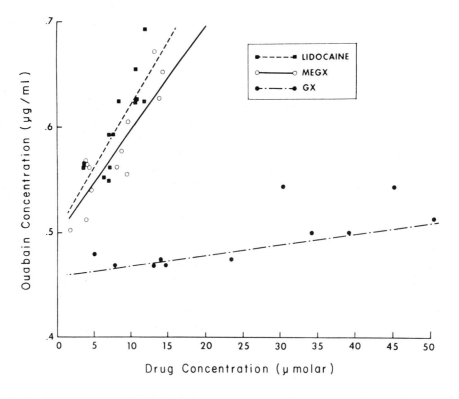

Fig. 19–8. The protective effects of lidocaine and monoethylglycinexylidide (MEGX) against ouabain-induced arrhythmias in isolated guinea pig atria. Lidocaine and MEGX potency are nearly identical, whereas glycinexylidide (GX) potency is about one-tenth that of the parent compound. (From Burney, R. G., et al.: Anti-arrhythmic effects of lidocaine metabolites. Am. Heart J., 88:765, 1974.)

arrhythmias.[68] Since some patients who showed signs of CNS toxicity had plasma concentrations of lidocaine within the accepted therapeutic range (less than 2.8 μg/ml), perhaps these metabolites are active and contribute to the observed toxicity. This speculation is supported by animal studies showing that lidocaine and monoethylglycinexylidide have equal potential for inducing convulsions.[69]

Monoethylglycinexylidide, the primary metabolite of lidocaine, is approximately 80% as potent as the parent compound in protecting against ouabain-induced arrhythmias in guinea pig atria (Fig. 19–8). Glycinexylidide is only one-tenth as potent.[70] Plasma concentrations of these metabolites, as well as those of lidocaine, should be considered when evaluating lidocaine therapy and local anesthetic toxicity. These principles might also apply when administering lidocaine or other amide-type local anesthetics to patients who have received prolonged lidocaine therapy.

Evidence also indicates that nontoxic doses of para-aminobenzoic acid, the primary metabolite of procaine, as well as sodium and ammonium benzoate, increase the lethal dosages of procaine and lidocaine in rats. Molgo et al. suggest that the mechanisms for these actions are directly related to cellular effects rather than to the inactivation of local anesthetic metabolism.[71] Electrocardiographic studies performed on patients who received a variety of anesthetic agents (including cyclopropane and cocaine) indicate that the intravenous administration of diethylaminoethanol reduces the incidence and the severity of cardiac arrhythmias produced at the time of endotracheal intubation.[72]

Circadian rhythm

Central nervous system responses of experimental animals to lidocaine may vary independent of drug dosage.[73] The responses are rhythmic and are closely related to the cyclic periods of light and darkness in the day. The importance and applicability of this phenomenon to clinical practice are unknown.

REFERENCES

1. Van Dyke, C., et al.: Cocaine: plasma concentrations after intranasal application in man. Science, *191*:859, 1976.
2. Koehntop, D. E., Liao, J. C., and Van Bergen, F. H.: Effects of pharmacologic alterations of adrenergic mechanisms by cocaine, tropolone, aminophylline, and ketamine on epinephrine-induced arrhythmias during halothane-nitrous oxide anesthesia. Anesthesiology, *46*:83, 1977.
3. Scott, D. B., et al.: Factors affecting plasma levels of lignocaine and prilocaine. Br. J. Anaesth., *44*:1040, 1972.
4. Johnston, R. R., Eger, E. I. II, and Wilson, C.: A comparative interaction of epinephrine with enflurane, isoflurane, and halothane in man. Anesth. Analg. (Cleve.), *55*:709, 1976.
5. De Jong, R. H., and Cullen, S. C.: Buffer-demand and pH of local anesthetic solutions containing epinephrine. Anesthesiology, *24*:801, 1963.
6. Bromage, P. R., et al.: Quality of epidural blockade. III. Carbonated local anaesthetic solutions. Br. J. Anaesth., *39*:197, 1967.
7. Loder, R. E.: A local anesthetic solution with longer action. Lancet, *2*:346, 1960.
8. Chinn, M. A., and Wirjoatmadja, K.: Prolonging local anesthesia. Lancet, *2*:834, 1967.
9. Kaplan, J. A., Miller, E. D., Jr., and Gallagher, E. G., Jr.: Postoperative analgesia for thoracotomy patients. Anesth. Analg. (Cleve.), *54*:773, 1975.
10. Marx, G. F., et al.: Drug overdose in axillary block of brachial plexus. N.Y. State J. Med., *68*:304, 1968.
11. Thomson, P. D., et al.: Lidocaine pharmacokinetics in advanced heart failure, liver disease, and renal failure in humans. Ann. Intern. Med., *78*:499, 1973.
12. Prescott, L. F., Adjepon-Yamoah, K. K., and Talbot, R. G.: Impaired lignocaine metabolism in patients with myocardial infarction and cardiac failure. Br. Med. J., *1*:939, 1976.
13. Benowitz, N., et al.: Lidocaine disposition kinetics in monkey and man. II. Effects of hemorrhage and sympathomimetic drug administration. Clin. Pharmacol. Ther., *16*:99, 1974.
14. Branch, R. A., et al.: The reduction of lidocaine clearance by *dl*-propranolol: An example of hemodynamic drug interaction. J. Pharmacol. Exp. Ther., *184*:515, 1973.
15. Mather, L. E., et al.: Hemodynamic drug interaction: peridural lidocaine and intravenous ephedrine. Acta Anaesthesiol. Scand., *20*:207, 1976.
16. Tucker, G. T., et al.: Binding of anilide-type local anesthetics in human plasma: I. Relationships between binding, physiochemical properties, and anesthetic activity. Anesthesiology, *33*:287, 1970.
17. Ghoneim, M. M., and Pandya, H.: Plasma protein binding of bupivacaine and its interaction with other drugs in man. Br. J. Anaesth., *46*:435, 1974.

18. Burney, R. G., DiFazio, C. A., and Foster, J.: Effects of pH on protein binding of lidocaine. Anesth. Analg. (Cleve.), *57*:478, 1978.

19. Zsigmond, E. K., and Eilderton, T. E.: Abnormal reaction to procaine and succinylcholine in a patient with inherited atypical plasma cholinesterase: case report. Can. Anaesth. Soc. J., *15*:498, 1968.

20. Stoelting, R. K.: Serum cholinesterase activity following pancuronium and antagonism with neostigmine or pyridostigmine. Anesthesiology, *45*:674, 1976.

21. Pantuck, E. J.: Ecothiopate iodide eye drops and prolonged response to suxamethonium. A case report. Br. J. Anaesth., *38*:406, 1966.

22. Foldes, F. F., et al.: The influence of glucocorticoids on plasma cholinesterase (38219). Proc. Soc. Exp. Biol. Med., *146*:918, 1974.

23. Kaniaris, P., et al.: Serum cholinesterase levels in patients with cancer. Anesth. Analg. (Cleve.), *58*:82, 1979.

24. Wang, R. I. H., and Ross, C. A.: Prolonged apnea following succinylcholine in cancer patients receiving AB-132. Anesthesiology, *24*:363, 1963.

25. Blitt, C. D., et al.: Correlation of plasma cholinesterase activity and duration of action of succinylcholine during pregnancy. Anesth. Analg. (Cleve.), *56*:78, 1977.

26. Finster, M.: Toxicity of local anesthetics in the fetus and the newborn. Bull. N.Y. Acad. Med., *52*:222, 1976.

27. Reidenberg, M. M., James, M., and Dring, L. G.: The rate of procaine hydrolysis in serum of normal subjects and diseased patients. Clin. Pharmacol. Ther., *13*:279, 1972.

28. DiFazio, C. A., and Brown, R. E.: Lidocaine metabolism in normal and phenobarbital-pretreated dogs. Anesthesiology, *36*:238, 1972.

29. Heinonen, J., Takki, S., and Jarho, L.: Plasma lidocaine levels in patients treated with potential inducers of microsomal enzymes. Acta Anaesthesiol. Scand., *14*:89, 1970.

30. Forrest, J. A. H., et al.: Antipyrine, paracetamol, and lignocaine elimination in chronic liver disease. Br. Med. J., *1*:1384, 1977.

31. Selden, R., and Sasahara, A. A.: Central nervous system toxicity induced by lidocaine. Report of a case in a patient with liver disease. J.A.M.A., *202*:908, 1967.

32. Stenson, R. E., Constantino, R. T., and Harrison, D. C.: Inter-relationships of hepatic blood flow, cardiac output, and blood levels of lidocaine in man. Circulation, *43*:205, 1971.

33. Burney, R. G., and DiFazio, C. A.: Hepatic clearance of lidocaine during N_2O anesthesia in dogs. Anesth. Analg. (Cleve.), *55*:322, 1976.

34. Adjepon-Yamoah, K. K., Scott, D. B., and Prescott, L. F.: Impaired absorption and metabolism of oral lignocaine in patients undergoing laparoscopy. Br. J. Anaesth., *45*:143, 1973.

35. Eriksson, E., and Granberg, P. O.: Studies on the renal excretion of Citanest and Xylocaine. Acta Anesthesiol. Scand. (Suppl.), *16*:79, 1965.

36. Mepivacaine overdosage in a child. (Discussion, E. S. Munson.) Anesth. Analg. (Cleve.), *52*:422, 1973.

37. Richards, R. K., Smith, N. T., and Katz, J.: The effects of interaction between lidocaine and pentobarbital on toxicity in mice and guinea pig atria. Anesthesiology, *29*:493, 1968.

38. De Jong, R. H., and Heavner, J. E.: Diazepam prevents and aborts lidocaine convulsions in monkeys. Anesthesiology, *41*:226, 1974.

39. Ausinsch, B., Malagodi, M. H., and Munson, E. S.: Diazepam in the prophylaxis of lignocaine seizures. Br. J. Anaesth., *48*:309, 1976.

40. Munson, E. S., Pugno, P. A., and Wagman, I. H.: Does oxygen protect against local anesthetic toxicity? Anesth. Analg. (Cleve.), *51*:422, 1972.

41. De Jong, R. H., Wagman, I. H., and Prince, D. A.: Effect of carbon dioxide on the cortical seizure threshold to lidocaine. Exp. Neurol., *17*:221, 1967.

42. Englesson, S., and Grevsten, S.: The influence of acid-base changes on central nervous system toxicity of local anaesthetic agents II. Acta Anaesthesiol. Scand., *18*:88, 1974.

43. Munson, E. S., and Wagman, I. H.: Acid-base changes during lidocaine induced seizures in *Macaca mulatta*. Arch. Neurol., *20*:406, 1969.

44. Yakaitis, R. W., Thomas, J. D., and Mahaffey, J. E.: Cardiovascular effects of lidocaine during acid-base imbalance. Anesth. Analg. (Cleve.), *55*:863, 1976.

45. De Jong, R. H., Heavner, J. E., and de Oliveira, L. F.: Effects of nitrous oxide on the lidocaine seizure threshold and diazepam protection. Anesthesiology, *37*:299, 1972.

46. Staniweski, J. A., and Aldrete, J. A.: The effects of inhalation anaesthetic agents on convulsant (LD–50) doses of local anaesthetics in the rat. Can. Anaesth. Soc. J., *17*:602, 1970.

47. Hulpieu, H. R., and Cole, V. V.: The effects of thiopental sodium, chloroform, and diethyl ether on the metabolism and toxicity of procaine. J. Pharmacol. Exp. Ther., *99*:370, 1950.

48. Siebecker, K. L., et al.: Effect of lidocaine administered intravenously during ether anesthesia. Acta Anaesthesiol. Scand., *4*:97, 1960.

49. Himes, R. S., Jr., Munson, E. S., and Embro, W. J.: Enflurane requirement and ventilatory response to carbon dioxide during lidocaine infusion in dogs. Anesthesiology, *51*:131, 1979.

50. Munson, E. S., Paul, W. L., and Embro, W. J.: Central-nervous-system toxicity of local anesthetic mixtures in monkeys. Anesthesiology, *46*:179, 1977.

51. Munson, E. S., and Wagman, I. H.: Elevation of lidocaine seizure threshold by gallamine in rhesus monkeys. Arch. Neurol., *28*:329, 1973.

52. Daos, F. G., Lopez, L., and Virtue, R. W.: Local anesthetic toxicity modified by oxygen and by combination of agents. Anesthesiology, *23*:755, 1962.

53. Ilyas, M., Owens, D., and Kvasnicka, G.: Delirium induced by a combination of anti-arrhythmic drugs. Lancet, *2*:1368, 1969.

54. Lalka, D., et al.: Bupivacaine and other amide local anesthetics inhibit the hydrolysis of chloroprocaine by human serum. Anesth. Analg. (Cleve.), *57*:534, 1978.

55. Brodsky, J. B., and Brock-Utne, J. G.: Mixing local anaesthetics (Correspondence). Br. J. Anaesth., *50*:1269, 1978.

56. Jatlow, P., et al.: Cocaine and succinylcholine sensitivity: A new caution. Anesth. Analg. (Cleve.), *58*:235, 1979.

57. Stovner, J., Oftedal, N., and Holmboe, J.: The inhibition of cholinesterase by pancuronium. Br. J. Anaesth., *47*:949, 1975.

58. Bennett, E. J., et al.: Pancuronium and the fasciculations of succinylcholine. Anesth. Analg. (Cleve.), *52*:892, 1973.

59. Poulton, T. J., James, F. M., and Lockridge, O.: Prolonged apnea following trimethaphan and succinylcholine. Anesthesiology, *50*:54, 1979.

60. DeKornfeld, T. J., and Steinhaus, J. E.: The effect of intravenously administered lidocaine and succinylcholine on the respiratory activity of dogs. Anesth. Analg. (Cleve.), *38*:173, 1959.

61. Acheson, F., Bull, A. B., and Glees, P.: Electroencephalogram of the cat after intravenous injection of lidocaine and succinylcholine. Anesthesiology, *17*:802, 1956.

62. Telivuo, L., and Katz, R. L.: The effects of modern intravenous local analgesics on respiration during partial neuromuscular block in man. Anaesthesia, *25*:30, 1970.

63. Matsuo, S., et al.: Interaction of muscle relaxants at the neuromuscular junction. Anesth. Analg. (Cleve.), *57*:580, 1978.

64. de Oliveira, L. F., Heavner, J. E., and de Jong, R. H.: 5-hydroxytryptophan intensifies local anesthetic-induced convulsions. Arch. Int. Pharmacodyn. Ther., *207*:333, 1974.

65. de Oliveira, L. F., and Bretas, A. D.: Effects of 5-hydroxytryptophan, iproniazid and p-chlorophenylalanine on lidocaine seizure threshold of mice. Eur. J. Pharmacol., *29*:5, 1974.

66. Dornfest, F. D.: Drug interaction (Letter to the editor). S. Afr. Med. J., *46*:1104, 1972.

67. Goldman, V., Astrom, A., and Evers, H.: The effect of a tricyclic antidepressant on the cardiovascular effects of local anaesthetic solutions containing different vasoconstrictors. Anaesthesia, *26*:91, 1971 (abstract).

68. Strong, J. M., Parker, M., and Atkinson, A. J., Jr.: Identification of glycinexylidide in patients treated with intravenous lidocaine. Clin. Pharmacol. Ther., *14*:67, 1973.

69. Blumer, J., Strong, J. M., and Atkinson, A. J., Jr.: The convulsant potency of lidocaine and its N-dealkylated metabolites. J. Pharmacol. Exp. Ther., *186*:31, 1973.

70. Burney, R. G., et al.: Anti-arrhythmic effects of lidocaine metabolites. Am. Heart J., *88*:765, 1974.

71. Molgo, J., Montoya, G., and Guerrero, S.: Influencia del benzoato de sodio, benzoato de amonio y acido p-aminobenzoico sobre la dosis letal media de procaina y lidocaina en la rata macho. Arch. Biol. Med. Exp. (Santiago), *9*:50, 1973.

72. Burstein, C. L., Zaino, G., and Newman, W.: Electrocardiographic studies during endotracheal intubation. III. Effects during general anesthesia and intravenous diethylaminoethanol. Anesthesiology, *12*:411, 1951.

73. Lutsch, E. F., and Morris, R. W.: Circadian periodicity in susceptibility to lidocaine hydrochloride. Science, *156*:100, 1967.

Chapter **20**

Drugs and Anesthetic Depth

DAVID J. CULLEN

CASE REPORT

A 33-year-old white woman with a history of ulcerative colitis was admitted to the hospital, complaining of abdominal pain, bloody diarrhea, and anorexia. In 1971, she had undergone exploration for a possible toxic megacolon; her colon had not been removed but an appendectomy had been performed. Anesthesia, consisting of halothane, nitrous oxide, oxygen, and curare, had been uneventful at that time, as had been the patient's postoperative course. Medications had included sulfadiazine, prednisone 30 mg/day, tincture of opium with belladona, diazepam, iron, and Fiorinal.

On admission to the hospital, the patient's hematocrit was 35% and her white blood count was 8,900/mm.[3] An abdominal film showed large loops of distended colon and elevation of the left hemidiaphragm from a large dilated splenic flexure. She required meperidine 75 to 100 mg q3h to control pain from increasing distension and toxicity. Three days after hospital admission, the patient underwent surgical exploration for toxic megacolon and possible colonic perforation.

After 1.5 ml of Innovar intravenously, thiopental 250 mg and succinylcholine 100 mg were administered IV. The patient's trachea was intubated rapidly and easily. Anesthesia was maintained with nitrous oxide, 4 L in combination with oxygen, 2 L. Additional thiopental (50 mg) and Innovar (1.5 ml) were given followed by pancuronium (4 mg) prior to incision. Approximately 30 minutes after the incision, fentanyl was given incrementally to a total of 0.15 mg. Total medication prior to abdominal closure was thiopental, 300 mg, Innovar, 3 ml, fentanyl, 0.15 mg, and pancuronium, 6 mg.

The patient was 5 ft. 4 in. tall and weighed 130 lbs. Prior to the induction of anesthesia, her pulse was 140 and her blood pressure was 120/60. After induction, her pulse slowed to 120; her blood pressure remained between 100 and 120 systolic throughout the operation. Her temperature fell from 37.5° to 36°C during the three-hour procedure. Respiration was controlled. According to the anesthetist, pupillary dilatation, tearing, perspiration, grimacing,

287

movement, hypertension, rise in heart rate, or any other signs of light anesthesia were not evident.

The patient's postoperative course, with two exceptions, was uncomplicated. She was discharged from the hospital three weeks later. Complications:

I. On the first postoperative day, the surgeon noted that "patient reports rather accurately the remembrance of sensations during the procedure, including the memory of hearing a 'four-letter word' that was used when the colon was entered at its place of perforation into the diaphragm." The anesthetist reported that the patient recalled conversation, abdominal discomfort, inability to move, and details of various manipulations. Although the patient was not unduly upset by her experience, her state of awareness during the procedure went unnoticed by the anesthetist when the usual clinical signs were used. She had no tearing, her eyeballs were fixed without conjugate movements, and her pupils were constantly constricted to 2 mm without dilating to stimuli. Although a persistent tachycardia was present, hyperventilation and hypertension were not.

II. On admission to the recovery room, a chest roentgenogram was obtained in order to determine the location of the central venous pressure (CVP) line. A total pneumothorax was seen, which means that the diaphragm must have been entered inadvertently when the colonic perforation was dissected. The patient was awake and in no respiratory distress. She was neither hyperpneic nor cyanotic. After the insertion of a chest tube, the patient's lung was fully expanded. Prior to inserting the chest tube, her respiratory rate was 20 to 24 per minute, her CVP 7 to 9 cm H_2O, her blood pressure 120/70 torr, and her apical pulse 100 per minute and regular. Following insertion of the chest tube, the patient's vital signs did not change. Blood gases were not obtained prior to the insertion of the chest tube. Pa_{O_2} (on room air five hours after the chest tube was placed) was 82 torr, Pa_{CO_2} 39 torr, pH 7.44.

One year later, the patient had an arthrodesis under enflurane-nitrous oxide and oxygen anesthesia. One month after the arthrodesis, she underwent total knee replacement under halothane, nitrous oxide, and oxygen anesthesia. Both anesthetic courses were uneventful. One year after the latter procedure, the patient had a total knee replacement on the other side. Again, the anesthesia was uneventful, even though only 4 ml of Innovar, 7 mg of morphine, and 42 mg of curare were used. She had taken no narcotic during the previous two years.

The patient is a pleasant, intelligent, articulate person who has a realistic view of her illness and hospital experiences. During her hospitalization for colectomy, the events of which she recalled, she was interviewed by her anesthetist, who recorded the following conversation:

" 'Tell me how you felt when you first came down to the operating room.'

'I would say when I first came down to the operating room I was extremely apprehensive. I wasn't rested because I hadn't had any drugs in advance of the operation, and I was so tense, I didn't know what to expect quite. My spirits were good though, I won't say they weren't. I was quite optimistic. I wasn't in a worried state at all and I felt that I was looking forward to the surgery only in so far as I knew that it would be a tremendous relief to the pain that I was having.'

'Can you remember the skin incision at all from the start of the surgery?'

'I can remember the skin incision. Only in my words, I wouldn't have put it that way. As I said earlier, I felt as if somebody had a pair of hedgeclippers and was going to clip a little bit at a time and decided not enough grass had been mowed back and took the lawnmower and started pushing a bit harder from the right side to the left side. And they kept going through this process and they would get about half way across my stomach and the lawnmower would kind of sink a bit deeper and cause a tremendous amount of undue pressure and pain which I was trying to express but had no way of doing so. I wanted to move my arms or my legs or speak, and I literally had no power within me to do that.'

'What specific conversation can you recall while you were asleep?'

'One of the things I believe I remember during the course of the surgery, I remember two or three people saying, do you think the machinery is working properly? I don't know whether this was just something that was in my mind or whether I had heard somebody say it and I just projected upon it. I began to get nervous in a way, laying there thinking that the machinery wasn't working because I was feeling so much pain and I was wondering whether anyone else was aware of this or not.'

'Can you recall any of the surgeons speaking specifically?'

'I do from time to time remember comments between the various surgeons—not necessarily all business, but just comments about what they were doing as far as passing instruments and checking that my blood pressure was up to par and things along this line. I think at one point I remembered someone saying how much longer is it going to be, but I'm not quite sure about that.'

'Do you remember anything that I did to you at all, touching you or anything like that?'

'I do remember that quite well. I remember you were trying to open my eyes many times and they just wouldn't stay open. By opening my eyes, I wanted to tell you something, that I was in this tremendous pain, and yet I had no way of communicating with you really. I didn't know if you could understand how I felt or not. I wasn't sure if the monitor that you must have had attached to me showed this pain or not, but I was in pain and I wanted to say something all the time by either some eye movement or wrist movement. But, since my arms were spread apart so far, it was just a complete lack of coordination to get my message across. But I did almost feel at one state, almost in a state of panic because I felt that maybe you were losing your grip on me for some reason.'

'Can you describe the character of your pain, was it sharp, or was it dull, was it constant, did it come and go?'

'I would have to say that the pain came and went and it would start off slowly and then a tremendous pain wave would come. And then this (I use lawnmower for goodness knows why) as it got to going up hill again, the pain was released, and then as it came back down again, because of the area where obviously the incision must have been, the pain would intensify so much more again. But I was definitely in pain which I hadn't anticipated. I literally felt as though I lived through the whole operation. If I had known what I know now, I probably would have been too afraid to go under it and to undergo the operation, that is because of all the feeling of pain that I felt as I went under it, feeling that I would be out of my misery somehow. It didn't happen and when I woke up finally, I was absolutely exhausted and I felt, I didn't feel relaxed or relieved at all and in fact, I don't think I really slept very much after the operation. I was awake more than anything else.'

'Were things fuzzy at all during the operation?'

'They were quite fuzzy. One of the things that is rather peculiar to me is everybody sort of knows me as an organized person and I always have this little black book with me. It's like a little bible; somehow, everything important ends up in it. I can remember laying on the operating table and having one book in one hand and one in the other and trying to itemize everything that you were doing to me so that when I came around, I could discuss these things because I was interested in them. I wanted to form an objective point of view but after a while, so many things happened, one upon another, that the whole sequence became lost.'

'Would you be frightened to undergo another anesthesia procedure at all?'

'No, I would not. It hasn't destroyed my faith in so called medicine, and because in fact, I anticipate having another operation in a couple of months I realize that it was just one of those freaks of nature that do happen. I have the feeling that one of the reasons that I didn't go under as deep is because, perhaps, I wasn't prepared early enough. So many patients are prepared hours before and given sedatives and I don't think I had that much time to relax and I think that may have had a bearing on it. But I definitely would say I wouldn't hesitate to have surgery again if I had to have it.' "

General anesthesia is defined as a state of general insensibility to pain and other sensations. In order for the anesthesiologist to realize that the patient perceives pain or other sensations, the patient must be able to respond to various noxious stimuli. This case illustrates that, by definition, general anesthesia was not in effect. Yet the patient was unable to tell the anesthesiologist by either somatic or sympathetic responses that she perceived pain or other sensations. Only in retrospect is it clear that the patient was not anesthetized.

The most likely explanation for this patient's state of awareness was the relatively small dose of narcotic administered with nitrous oxide to provide analgesia in the presence of a potent surgical stimulus. Additionally, the prior three-day use of meperidine for the relief of pain from toxic megacolon probably increased the patient's tolerance to the narcotics received intraoperatively. Finally, muscle relaxants, used to facilitate the abdominal operation, rendered her unable to communicate her state of awareness to the anesthesiologist.

Anesthesia can be quantitated by using the MAC concept. MAC is the Minimum Alveolar Concentration of anesthetic at one atmosphere that produces immobility in 50% of those patients or animals exposed to a noxious stimulus. MAC was chosen to measure anesthesia because it is a reliable, reproducible, visible index of potency.[1] Its end point, the abolition of movement, is of clinical importance. MAC can be applied to all inhalation anesthetics and relates the observation of movement or nonmovement in response to a painful stimulus to the partial pressure of anesthetic at the anesthetic site of action in the brain (assuming that the alveolar partial pressure has equilibrated with brain concentration). Once MAC was determined for various inhalation anesthetics, variables that alter MAC or depth of anesthesia were identified.[2] A drug that reduces MAC 30% indicates that the drug provides 30% of the anesthesia, even though that drug may not be an anesthetic itself. Many of the currently known modifiers of anesthetic depth are drugs. Their effects on the depth of anesthesia are discussed in this chapter and are related to clinical management whenever possible. In addition, common pathophysiologic changes that may alter anesthetic depth are mentioned.

QUANTITATING DEPTH OF ANESTHESIA

In 1965, Eger et al. described MAC and began to outline factors that affect MAC in animals.[2] These investigators defined one point on a dose-response curve where the dose was alveolar anesthetic concentration and the response was the reaction of the patient to a surgical incision (Table 20–1). The starting point of this curve is the awake, nonanesthetized state. Whether or not these two points can be connected by a straight line is not known.

Recently, de Jong and Eger have estimated the dose of anesthetic that anesthetizes not 50%, but 95% of the patient population (AD_{95}) (Fig. 20–1).[3] This concept is important because no clinician attempts to anesthetize patients with a concentration at which there is a 50% chance of moving during a skin incision. The anesthesiologist requires a higher probability that patients will not move. For some of the inhalation anes-

Table 20–1

Three well-defined end points describing alveolar anesthetic concentration and the response of the patient

	AWAKE MAC[39]		MAC[1–3]		ED_{95}[3]	
	(alveolar concentration)	(% of MAC)	(alveolar concentration)	(% of MAC)	(alveolar concentration)	(% of MAC)
Halothane	0.41	55	0.74	100	0.90	122
Methoxyflurane	0.081	51	0.16	100	0.22	138
Ether	1.41	73	1.92	100	2.22	116
Fluroxene	2.2	65	3.4	100	3.57	105

The awake MAC and Effective Dose (ED_{95}) of four anesthetics are listed as alveolar concentrations and as per cent of the MAC value, expressed as 100%.

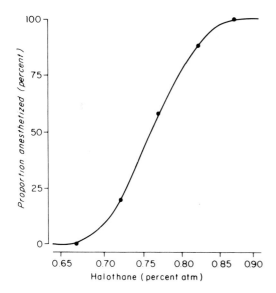

Fig. 20–1. Halothane log dose-response curve. Percentage of subjects anesthetized (i.e., not responding to skin incision) within each of five halothane dose ranges is on the vertical axis. The horizontal axis is scaled to the logarithm of the alveolar halothane concentration. Note the curve symmetry around the median (50% response) points. (From de Jong, R.H., and Eger, E. I., II: MAC expanded: AD_{50} and AD_{95} values of common inhalation anesthetics in man. Anesthesiology, *42*:386, 1975.)

thesiologists give serious attention to assessing "depth" of anesthesia because:

in any patient, only that level of anesthesia needed to meet the surgical requirements should be established. We hold the basic premise that the less the involvement of the patient's critical organs and system (i.e. the lower the concentration of the agent, or the less "deep" the anesthesia), the less will be the damage to the patient, whether this be temporary or perhaps permanent. We emphasize, however, that we firmly believe in providing sufficient anesthesia to meet the surgical requirements. We believe that anesthesia that is "light" enough so that response to surgical stimuli such as hypertension, tachycardia, recollection of stimuli and increased muscle tension may result in unnecessary harm. Consequently, it is essential that the anesthesiologist learn how to assess the various responses of the patient that give clues to the depth of anesthesia. All patients are not the same. In major surgical procedures, the condition of most patients is not the same during or at the end as at the beginning. Further, all surgeons are not the same, all surgical requirements are not the same, and all operating conditions are not the same. We submit that, if there are these many variables in an anesthetic situation, the anesthetist must learn to recognize and respond to those subtle as well as obvious changes that take place in the individual patient. Fortunately, many patients have responses that are peculiar to them. For example, some patients move a hand in response to a stimulus, other patients wrinkle an eyebrow, and other patients make more gross effort such as leg movement; other patients respond by elevation of blood pressure, increase or decrease in pulse rate, perspiration, tearing, and pupillary changes, while still others have characteristic respiratory patterns.[7]

thetics, the AD_{95} is close to the AD_{50}, or MAC concentration, whereas for other anesthetics, the AD_{95} is farther from MAC (Table 20–1). Assessing anesthetic depth is difficult since a given increase in inspired concentration does not yield a comparable increase in alveolar concentration and anesthetic depth because of uptake and distribution variables.[4]

De Jong et al. and Freund et al. suggest that anesthetic "depth" is also a function of the impact of anesthetics on the central nervous system (Fig. 20–2). They demonstrated an almost linear response of monosynaptic pathways and the susceptibility of the H-reflex to increasing concentrations of anesthetic agents. They also documented that anesthesia *is a continuum*, not an all or none response.[5,6]

Cullen and Larson have urged that anes-

Administration of anesthesia must be individualized, with the patient serving as his own control. Although Cullen and Larson have described clinical signs of light, moderate, and deep anesthesia, these signs vary greatly with the anesthetic agent and are not generally applicable.[8]

The clinical tools used to assess depth of anesthesia include: heart rate, blood pressure, pupil diameter, pupillary reactivity to light, tearing, eye movement, tidal volume, respiratory rate, and abdominal muscle

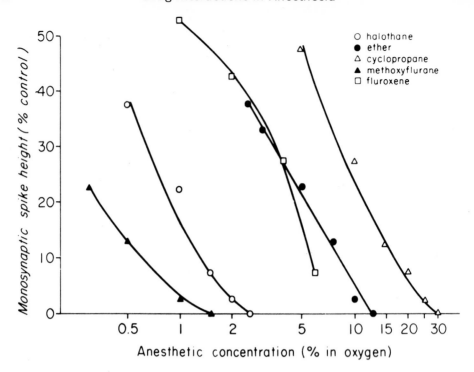

Fig. 20–2. Mean monosynaptic spike heights are plotted against inspired concentrations of five commonly used anesthetics on a semilog scale. As anesthetic concentration rose, the amplitude of the spike began to fall. Thus depression of synaptic transmission was inversely proportional to the log of the anesthetic concentration. (From de Jong, R.H., et al.: Anesthetic potency determined by depression of synaptic transmission. Anesthesiology, 29:1142, 1968.)

tone. Most of these clinical signs define the depth of anesthesia for only specific inhalation anesthetics.[8] For example, falling blood pressure indicates deepening halothane anesthesia whereas rising blood pressure indicates deepening fluroxene anesthesia (Fig. 20–3). Since similar examples abound, it is impossible to use blood pressure as the sole guide to anesthetic depth. To confuse matters further, many factors other than anesthetic depth alter the common signs of anesthesia. These factors include: preanesthetic medication; induction agents; a patient's illness, age, and general health; the site and extent of surgical stimulation; the use of muscle relaxants and/or controlled ventilation; a patient's body temperature; Pa_{CO_2}; and the duration of anesthesia. Our data related the clinical signs of anesthesia to the concentration of several inhaled anesthetics

in human volunteers in whom all of the variables mentioned were controlled.[8] Although guidelines emerged to evaluate anesthetic depth specific to each anesthetic drug, each clinical situation will undoubtedly modify many of the signs of anesthesia.

For clinical purposes, it is most important to assess depth of anesthesia just prior to incision, at the time of incision, and at various times during the surgical procedure when surgical stimulation may increase or decrease. *Anesthetic depth must always be considered in the context of the surgical stimulus.*

Clinical experience indicates that predicting the vigor of the subsequent response to an operation is extremely difficult on the basis of clinical signs prior to surgical incision. It is more practical to use the response to surgical incision as the focal point for

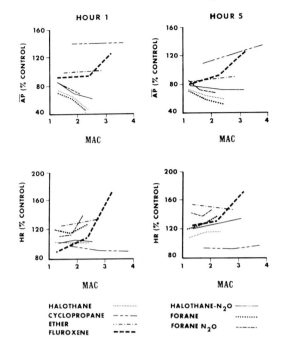

Fig. 20-3. Mean arterial pressure ($\overline{AP}$) and heart rate (HR) responses to several concentrations of seven anesthetics are shown. To permit comparison of anesthetic agents at equipotent concentrations, the horizontal axis represents multiples of MAC. The fine horizontal line is the awake control value. Note that $\overline{AP}$ responses vary widely from one anesthetic to another and that for the same agent $\overline{AP}$ response changes with prolonged anesthesia.

determining anesthetic depth. Prior to incision, the anesthesiologist determines tidal volume and respiratory rate (if he allows the patient to breathe spontaneously), blood pressure and heart rate, eye position, pupillary diameter, presence or absence of tearing, perspiration, and, if possible, abdominal muscle tone. Three possible responses to a surgical incision can be described (known as the "Goldilocks" assessment): (1) if anesthesia is *too light*, the patient moves, coughs, and bucks on the endotracheal tube (a phenomenon common with enflurane) or shows a dramatic rise in blood pressure and heart rate; (2) if *too deep*, the patient does not move, but also, more important, has no autonomic reflex response to incision, that is, no tachycardia, blood pressure increase, pupillary dilatation, deepening tidal volume,

or faster respiratory rate; and (3) when "*just right*," the patient does not move in response to incision, but rather shows reflex awareness that a painful stimulus has been applied. The pupils may dilate, heart rate and blood pressure usually increase 10 to 20%, and the patient's respiratory rate may increase whereas tidal volume definitely increases (Fig. 20-4). Interestingly, two min-

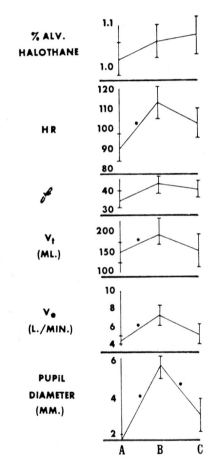

Fig. 20-4. The effects of skin incision on clinical signs of anesthesia are shown in eight healthy patients. Values at point A were obtained immediately prior to incision; B, immediately after incision; and C, twelve minutes after incision while the operation continued. The asterisk (*) denotes significant change from previous values. Note that immediately after incision, heart rate (HR), tidal volume ($\dot{V}_T$), minute ventilation ($\dot{V}_E$) and pupil diameter increased significantly, whereas respiratory rate (f) failed to change significantly. These values had returned toward control levels 12 minutes after incision although the operations continued.

utes after skin incision, during an operation, the reflex changes in clinical signs abate and in most cases return to the preincision state, indicating the importance of the skin incision as compared with other surgical stimuli. During the surgical procedure, it is helpful to reduce inspired anesthetic concentration gradually to evoke mild reflex responses in order to determine that anesthesia is indeed at the appropriate level. Since a constant inspired concentration results in a rising alveolar concentration, a patient will become more deeply anesthetized unless the inspired concentration is reduced.[4] Testing for the appearance of clinical responses will show when further reduction of inspired concentration is unwise.

EFFECT OF DRUGS ON ANESTHETIC DEPTH (TABLE 20–2)

Aside from the expected potentiation of general anesthetics by sedatives and narcotics, only one other major drug group has been shown to interact with general anesthesia. These are drugs that alter central nervous system catecholamine function. Those drugs that increase central nervous system norepinephrine levels increase MAC; conversely, drugs that decrease central norepinephrine levels decrease MAC.

Antagonism of general anesthesia

Iproniazid: Miller et al. administered iproniazid phosphate 125 mg/kg intraperitoneally in rats and observed an 8% increase in cyclopropane MAC, a statistically significant change.[9]

Amphetamine: Amphetamine is a sympathomimetic drug that stimulates central nervous system function and, more important, releases norepinephrine within the central nervous system. When dextroamphetamine 0.1, 0.5, and 1 mg/kg was administered during halothane anesthesia, MAC, determined one hour later, rose by 19%, 67%, and 96% respectively. Yet, when dextroamphetamine was administered re-

peatedly, MAC decreased by 22%. Short-term dextroamphetamine administration releases catecholamines from nerve terminals, which stimulate the central nervous system and lead to the subsequent increase in MAC. Long-term dextroamphetamine administration depletes central nervous system catecholamines and subsequently decreases MAC. Thus patients who are recent amphetamine users may require more than normal concentrations of halothane to produce anesthesia, whereas long-term amphetamine users may require less than normal amounts of anesthesic drugs.[10]

The amphetamine studies were extended to show that two drugs that reduce brain catecholamine levels, reserpine and *alpha*-methyl-para-tyrosine (AMT), minimize the increase in MAC from dextroamphetamine. Instead of a 90% increase in halothane MAC, dogs pretreated with reserpine, 2 mg/kg, or with *alpha*-methyl-p-tyrosine, 100 mg/kg, increased MAC by 50% and 17% respectively following dextroamphetamine, 1 mg/kg. To delineate the mechanism of action further, parachlorophenylalanine (350 mg/kg), a drug that increases central nervous system levels of serotonin, did not block the effect of dextroamphetamine on MAC as well as reserpine or AMT, both of which reduce central catecholamine levels. This work further supports the hypothesis that central nervous system catecholamines may modify the response to general anesthetics.[11]

Cocaine: Cocaine inhibits catecholamine reuptake at cerebral nerve endings. Stoelting et al. determined that cocaine increased halothane MAC in dogs by 27%. This study lends further support to the concept that anesthetic depth is influenced by central nervous system catecholamine concentration.[12]

Naloxone: Finck et al. antagonized anesthesia with naloxone (10 mg/kg IV) in rats that were anesthetized with either halothane or enflurane, but the mechanism remains to be demonstrated.[13]

Hypernatremia: Although not drug-

Table 20-2
Drugs that change anesthetic requirement

Drug	Dose	Anesthetic	MAC % Change	Species	Reference #
Alpha-methyldopa	50 to 600 mg/kg IV x 3 days	Halothane	↓ 16 to 31	Dogs	9
Amphetamine	Acute-0.5 mg/kg IV	Halothane	↑ 67	Dogs	10
	Chronic-2.5 mg/kg IM b.i.d. x 7 days	Halothane	↓ 22	Dogs	10
Atropine	0.015 mg/kg IP	Cyclopropane	No change	Rats	29
Cocaine	2 or 4 mg/kg IV	Halothane	↑ 27	Dogs	12
Diazepam	0.2 mg/kg IV	Halothane	↓ 35	Man	27
Guanethidine	15 mg/kg/day IV x 3 days	Halothane	No change	Dogs	9
Iproniazid	125 mg/kg IP	Cyclopropane	↑ 8	Rats	9
Isoproterenol	0.8 µg/ml IV to increase HR 80%	Halothane	No change	Dogs	18
Ketamine	50 mg/kg IV	Halothane	↓ 56	Rats	21
Levodopa	10 mg/kg IV	Halothane	↓ 52	Dogs	20
Levodopa	50 mg/kg IV	Halothane	↑ 41	Dogs	20
Lidocaine	To yield plasma conc. > 3 µg/ml	Halothane	↓ 45	Dogs	24
Morphine	8 to 15 mg subcutaneously	Halothane	↓ 10	Man	25
Morphine	10 to 12 mg IM	Fluroxene	↓ 20	Man	26
Naloxone	10 mg/kg IV	Halothane	↑ qualitatively	Rats	13
	10 mg/kg IV	Enflurane	↑ qualitatively	Rats	13
	10 mg/kg IV	Cyclopropane	↑ qualitatively	Rats	13
Phenobarbital	10 mg/kg PO x 10 days	Halothane	No change	Dogs	40
Propranolol	2 mg/kg, then 10 mg/kg IV	Halothane	No change	Dogs	18
Reserpine	0.2 to 8 mg/kg IM	Halothane	↓ 14 to 33	Dogs	9
Scopolamine	0.48 mg/kg	Cyclopropane	↓ 14	Rats	29
Tetrahydrocannabinol	1 mg/kg IP	Cyclopropane	↓ 15	Rats	30
	2 mg/kg IP	Cyclopropane	↓ 25	Rats	30
	0.5 mg/kg IV	Halothane	↓ 32	Dogs	31

Table 20–3
Pathophysiologic states that change anesthetic requirement

State	Anesthetic	MAC (% change)	Species	Reference #
Hypernatremia			Dogs	14
(Serum Na$^+$ 179 meq/L)	Halothane	↑ 43	Dogs	15
Hyperthermia (37° to 42°C)	Halothane	↑ 8°C	Dogs	32
Hypoxia (Pa$_{O_2}$ 30 torr)	Halothane	↓ Progressively towards 0	Dogs	34
Hypercapnia (Pa$_{CO_2}$ 95 to 245 torr)	Halothane	↓ Progressively to 0	Dogs	35
Hypocapnia (Pa$_{CO_2}$ 10 torr)	Halothane	No change	Pregnant Ewes	37
Pregnancy	Halothane	↓ 25	Pregnant Ewes	35
Pregnancy	Methoxyflurane	↓ 32	Pregnant Ewes	37
Pregnancy	Isoflurane	↓ 40	Dogs	41
Hypotension (mean AP 40 to 50 torr)	Halothane	↓ 20		

induced, changes in anesthetic depth may result from changes in electrolyte concentrations. Tanifuji and Eger showed that hypernatremia to a serum sodium of 179 meq/L, sufficient to increase cerebrospinal fluid (CSF) sodium to 181 meq/L, increased halothane MAC in dogs 43%. Mannitol, which increased osmolarity, increased MAC because dehydration raised CSF Na$^+$ to 176 meq/L. Hyperosmolarity not associated with increased CSF Na$^+$ did not raise MAC. Potassium changes had no effect on MAC[14] (Table 20–3).

Hyperthermia: Steffey and Eger showed that halothane MAC in dogs increased as their temperatures rose from 37 to 42°C, after which MAC decreased (Fig. 20–5, Table 20–3). The rate of increase to 42°C was 8%/°C. Assuming clinical extrapolation, febrile patients will require more halothane to maintain anesthesia.[15]

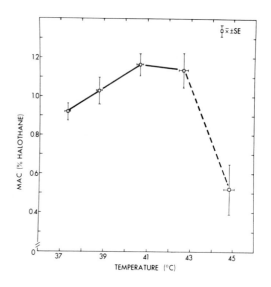

Fig. 20–5. The effect of hyperthermia on halothane MAC. Note the increase in halothane MAC until approximately 41°C. Death occurred at a mean temperature of 45.9°C. (From Steffey, E. P., and Eger, E. I., II.: Hyperthermia and halothane MAC in the dog. Anesthesiology, *41*:393, 1974.)

Potentiation of general anesthesia

Depletion of brain norepinephrine and dopamine without change in brain serotonin concentration decreases halothane MAC by a small but significant amount.[16] Similarly, drugs that decrease brain serotonin without altering norepinephrine or dopamine concentrations also decrease halothane MAC to a small degree. However, this effect was not seen in rats exposed to cyclopropane. Mueller suggested that only anesthetics such as halothane that progressively depress neuronal activity are affected by central catecholamine levels; whereas a drug such as cyclopropane, which initially excites neurones, is not affected by central catecholamines.[16]

Roizen et al. destroyed specific areas of brain that contain high concentrations of norepinephrine or of serotonin and achieved a maximal 40% reduction in halothane MAC.[17]

In a clinically applicable report, Miller, Way, and Eger observed that patients who received 1 to 6 gm/day of *alpha*-methyldopa (AMD) required lower concentrations of inhalation anesthesia to maintain adequate surgical anesthesia.[9] The researchers postulated that *alpha*-methyldopa displaces central nervous system norepinephrine and that it might potentiate anesthetic depth. In dogs, *alpha*-methyldopa and reserpine, which are drugs that reduce central and peripheral norepinephrine levels, reduced MAC in dose-related fashion by approximately 30% (Fig. 20–6). Guanethidine, which only depletes peripheral catecholamines, did not affect MAC.

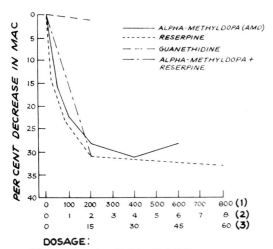

DOSAGE:

(1) AMD, mg/kg/DAY x 3 DAYS

(2) RESERPINE, mg/kg (TOTAL DOSE)

(3) GUANETHIDINE, mg/kg/DAY x 3 DAYS

Fig. 20–6. Administration in dogs of *alpha*-methyldopa, reserpine, or *alpha*-methyldopa with reserpine decreased MAC in dose-related fashion. There was no change in halothane MAC with guanethidine. (From Miller, R. D., Way, W. L., and Eger, E. I., II.: The effects of *alpha*-methyldopa, reserpine, guanethidine and iproniazide on minimum alveolar anesthetic concentration (MAC). Anesthesiology, 29:1156, 1968.)

Isoproterenol and Propranolol: Tanifuji and Eger reported that both isoproterenol, in doses sufficient to double the heart rate, and propranolol, 2 or 10 mg/kg IV, had no effect on halothane MAC in dogs.[18] Isoproterenol has not been reported to enter the CNS in significant amounts. Although propranolol crosses the blood-brain barrier, it does not alter brain norepinephrine.[19]

Levodopa: Since levodopa increases dopamine content (a neuroinhibitory transmitter) in the basal ganglia and since it is a precursor for the synthesis of central nervous system catecholamines, Johnston et al. postulated that this agent may reduce MAC. Lower doses of L-dopa—5, 10 or 25 mg/kg IV—decreased halothane MAC in dogs by as much as 52% (Fig. 20–7). However, L-dopa, 50 mg/kg, increased MAC by 41% for the first and second hours, but by the third and fourth hours, MAC decreased to 37% below control. Long-term administration of levodopa yielded variable results. The authors suggested that smaller doses of levodopa would increase dopamine levels, which, by inhibiting neurotransmission, were consistent with the reduction in MAC. However, larger doses of levodopa might displace noreprinephrine from nerve terminals in the central nervous system. This suggestion is thus consistent with the researchers' previous findings; that is, that increased central norepinephrine levels increased MAC.[20]

Ketamine: Ketamine (50 mg/kg IM [intramuscularly]) produced a dose-dependent reduction in halothane MAC in rats (Fig. 20–8). MAC remained low for several hours, and this demonstrated ketamine's long-lasting effect.[21]

Lidocaine: Lidocaine has been used as an adjunct to general anesthesia.[22] Its effects, however, were not quantitated until DiFazio reported that lidocaine linearly reduced cyclopropane MAC up to 42% in rats as plasma concentrations rose to 1 μg/ml.[23] Recently, DiFazio et al. reported that plasma lidocaine concentrations of 2 to 6 μg/ml during nitrous oxide anesthesia in man contributed 0.13 to

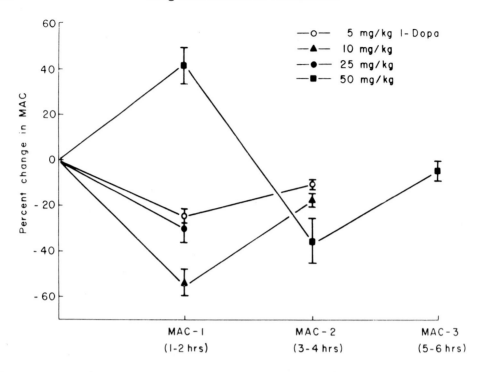

Fig. 20–7. Changes in halothane MAC with time following intravenous levodopa in dogs. Note the decrease in MAC with the lower doses of L-dopa and the 41% increase in MAC with the high dose L-dopa in the first two hours. All values are mean ±1 SE. (From Johnston, R. R., et al.: Effect of levodopa on halothane anesthetic requirement. Anesth. Analg. (Cleve.), *54*:179, 1975.)

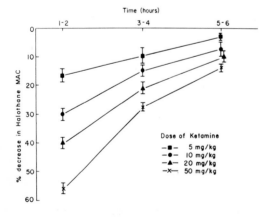

Fig. 20–8. Change in halothane MAC with time after intramuscular injection of ketamine. All values are mean ±1 SE. (From White, P. F., Johnston, R. R., and Pudwill, C. R.: Interaction of ketamine and halothane in rats. Anesthesiology, *42*:183, 1975.)

0.28 of the anesthetic requirement.[24] The ED_{50} (median effective dose) in these studies was 3.2 μg/ml. In dogs anesthetized with halothane, MAC decreased up to 45% when plasma and CSF lidocaine was higher than 3 μg/ml (Figs. 20–9A & 20–9B). In view of this decrease, the anesthetist might reduce the concentration of depressant anesthetics such as halothane when lidocaine is used to suppress coughing in such procedures as bronchoscopy, pulmonary resection, and tracheal reconstruction.

Morphine: When administered as a preanesthetic medication, morphine slightly reduces MAC. Morphine sulfate, 8 to 15 mg subcutaneously, about 1.5 hours prior to an operation, reduced halothane MAC from 0.75% to 0.68% (Fig. 20–10).[25] Morphine-

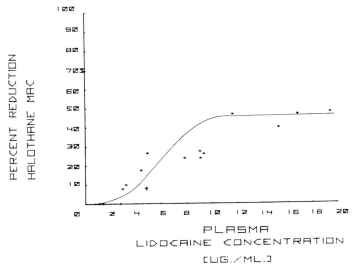

PLOT OF REDUCTION IN HALOTHANE MAC AGAINST INCREASING PLASMA LIDOCAINE CONCENTRATIONS

A

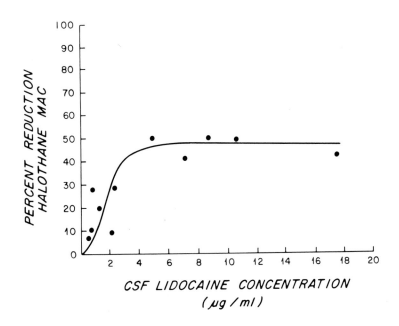

B

Fig. 20–9. *A* (From DiFazio, C. A., Burney, R. G., and Himes, R. S., Jr.: Alterations in general anesthetic requirements with lidocaine. *In* Abstracts of Scientific Papers. San Francisco, American Society of Anesthesiologists, 1976.) *B* Plot of reduction in halothane MAC against increasing CSF lidocaine concentration. (From DiFazio, C. A., Burney, R. G., and Himes, R. S., Jr.: Alterations in general anesthetic requirements with lidocaine. *In* Abstracts of Scientific Papers. San Francisco, American Society of Anesthesiologists, 1976.)

Drug Interactions in Anesthesia

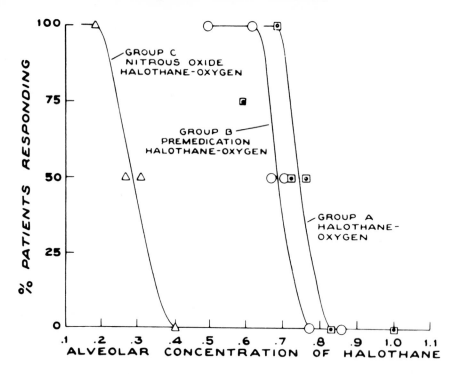

Fig. 20–10. The percentage of patients moving within each group of four is plotted on the vertical axis against the average alveolar concentration of the four which is plotted on the horizontal axis. Note that premedication with morphine sulfate, 8 to 15 mg subcutaneously, yielded a small reduction in MAC (Group B). Nitrous oxide administered with halothane resulted in a large reduction in MAC (Group C). (From Saidman, L. J., and Eger, E. I., II: Effect of nitrous oxide and of narcotic pre-medication on the alveolar concentration of halothane required for anesthesia. Anesthesiology, 25:304, 1964.)

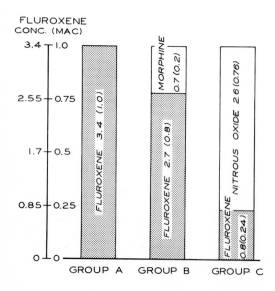

Fig. 20–11. Fluroxene concentration in volumes per cent with equivalent fractional MAC values are shown on the vertical axis. The concentration of fluroxene and MAC value are written within the bars. In group A, 3.4% fluroxene represents MAC 1.0. In group B, morphine is equivalent to 0.7% fluroxene (0.2 MAC). In group C, nitrous oxide (72% alveolar concentration) is equivalent to 2.6% fluroxene (0.76 MAC). (From Munson, E. S., Saidman, L. J., and Eger, E. I., II.: Effect of nitrous oxide and morphine on the minimum anesthetic concentration of fluroxene. Anesthesiology, 26:137, 1965.)

sulfate, 10 to 12 mg IM, given approximately 1.5 hours prior to surgical incision reduced fluroxene MAC from 3.4% to 2.7% (Fig. 20–11).[26]

Diazepam: Diazepam, 0.2 mg/kg IV, 15 to 30 minutes prior to an operation reduced halothane MAC in man from 0.73% to 0.48%, a 35% reduction.[27] Diazepam, 0.4 mg/kg IV, further reduced halothane MAC, but that dose is too large for routine clinical use.

Nitrous Oxide: Nitrous oxide reduces MAC for halothane, fluroxene (Fig. 20–11), and isoflurane by approximately 1% for each per cent of nitrous oxide administered.[25,26,28]

Atropine and Scopolamine: Although atropine has not been shown to affect MAC, large doses of scopolamine, 0.48 mg/kg, cause a maximal decrease in MAC of 14% in rats.[29] Clinical relevance is lacking because much smaller doses of scopolamine are used for premedication in man.

Tetrahydrocannabinol: Vitez et al. calculated that cyclopropane MAC fell by 15% and 25% in rats given tetrahydrocannabinol (THC), 1 or 2 mg/kg IP (intraperitoneally), respectively.[30] THC, 0.5 mg/kg, decreases MAC by 32% one hour after injection with a return to control after three hours in dogs (Fig. 20–12).[31] This short-lived effect is compatible with clinical observations that analgesia, sedation, and prolonged barbiturate sleeping time occur following THC injections. Whether these effects are clinically important to man, in whom 0.05 mg/kg of THC yields the desired euphoria, cannot be determined.

INTERACTION OF ANESTHETIC DEPTH AND PATHOPHYSIOLOGIC CHANGES (TABLE 20–3)

Hypoxia reduces halothane MAC in dogs rapidly and progressively, beginning at Pa_{O_2} 38 torr (Fig. 20–13).[32] This Pa_{O_2} is close to the level of 35 torr in man, at which level consciousness is lost as a result of acute hypoxia. MAC decreases as metabolic acidosis develops when Pa_{O_2} is held constant

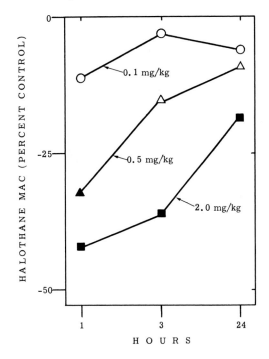

Fig. 20–12. Alterations in MAC after administration of tetrahydrocannabinol plotted as percentage of change from control. (From Stoelting, R. K., et al.: Effects of *delta*-9-tetrahydrocannabinol on halothane MAC in dogs. Anesthesiology, *38*:523, 1973.)

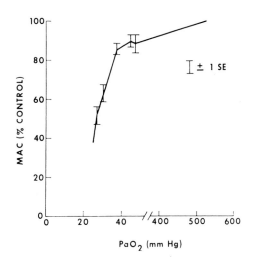

Fig. 20–13. MAC did not change significantly until arterial Pa_{O_2} decreased below 38 torr. Thereafter, a precipitous decrease in MAC developed.

at 30 torr.[32] To explore the mechanism responsible for the reduction of MAC, brain surface electrodes were applied to the cerebral cortex of dogs during hypoxia. Cerebral extracellular fluid (ECF) P_{O_2} decreased to a range of 1 to 10 torr when hypoxia to Pa_{O_2} 30 torr began (Fig. 20–14). After two hours of hypoxia, cerebral ECF pH decreased to 6.93 and cerebral ECF bicarbonate decreased to about 10 meq/L (Fig. 20–15). Cerebral

metabolic demand appears to exceed supply at this level of hypoxia, which in turn depresses MAC.[33]

Carbon dioxide

Within clinically relevant ranges, CO_2 has no effect on MAC. Until Pa_{CO_2} levels above 95 torr were achieved, MAC remained constant.[34] Above 95 torr, Pa_{CO_2} progressively reduced MAC and was completely anesthetic at 245 torr (Fig. 20–16). When CSF pH fell below 7.1, MAC began to decrease; CO_2 became fully anesthetic at CSF pH of 6.8. However, low CSF pH is not why CO_2 became anesthetic. Hypoxia studies showed that even when brain ECF pH was as low as 6.3, halothane MAC was above zero.[33] Perhaps CO_2 itself is an anesthetic at high concentrations. Despite the similarity of their physical properties, CO_2 is more potent than nitrous oxide, of which slightly more than one atmosphere is required for general anesthesia.

Hypocapnia to Pa_{CO_2} 10 torr, which maximally reduces cerebral blood flow, does not significantly reduce MAC,[35] despite the clin-

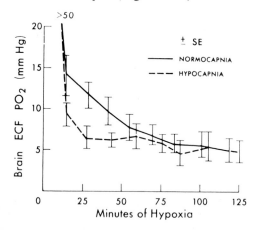

Fig. 20–14. Cerebral ECF P_{O_2} decreased at Pa_{O_2} 30 torr and corresponded to a decrease in halothane MAC.

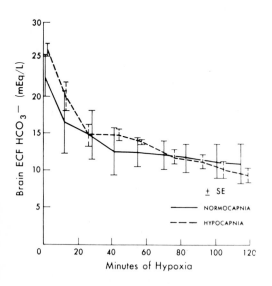

Fig. 20–15. Cerebral ECF bicarbonate values fell rapidly at Pa_{O_2} 30 torr in both hypocapnic and normocapnic dogs, and corresponded to a decrease in halothane MAC.

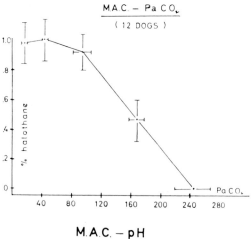

Fig. 20–16. Up to Pa_{CO_2} 95 torr, MAC is relatively constant. Above Pa_{CO_2} 95 torr, MAC declines progressively until CO_2 becomes fully anesthetic. (From Eisele, J. H., Eger, E. I., II, and Muallem, M.: Narcotic properties of carbon dioxide in the dog. Anesthesiology, *28*:858, 1967.)

ical impression that hyperventilated patients appear to be more deeply anesthetized than do spontaneously breathing patients. Assuming equivalent alveolar anesthetic concentrations and time for cerebral equilibration, a possible mechanism for this observation is that hypocapnia abolishes spontaneous activity of the reticular formation, reducing afferent impulses to the cerebral cortex and to the phrenic nerve.[36]

Pregnancy

Although not a pathophysiologic disorder, pregnancy decreases the requirements for inhaled anesthetic agents.[37] Halothane MAC decreased 25%, methoxyflurane MAC 32%, and isoflurane MAC 40% in pregnant ewes. The decreased MAC may be related to the large increase in progesterone levels during late pregnancy. Of clinical importance is that, in addition to decreased MAC, uptake and distribution are more rapid in pregnant patients. If an anesthetic state is reached at a lower alveolar concentration, the dangers of aspiration and of airway obstruction are increased.

In summary, many drugs and clinical situations reduce the anesthetic requirement. Those few that increase the anesthetic requirement increase CNS catecholamine levels. When all the variables that affect anesthetic requirement, such as age,[38] preoperative medication, anesthetic adjuvants, patient's illness, type of procedure, acid-base balance, oxygenation, temperature, and imprecise delivery systems, are taken into account, clinical signs of anesthesia must be closely observed to avoid anesthetic overdose or inadequate anesthesia. The time to test the depth of anesthesia is at the moment of surgical incision, when clearcut responses are visible, particularly in the nonparalyzed patient. Once an adequate anesthetic depth is assured, a relaxant can be given, if necessary, and inspired anesthetic concentration can be gradually reduced until signs of light anesthesia appear. By observing the patient's clinical signs and by carefully manipulating the inspired concentration accordingly, the appropriate depth of anesthesia can be maintained despite the factors that affect MAC. These factors provide a frame of reference to guide the anesthetist, but the ultimate criterion is the patient's unique response to the balance between anesthetic depression and surgical stimulation.

REFERENCES

1. Eger, E. I., II: Anesthetic Uptake and Action. Baltimore, Williams & Wilkins, 1974.
2. Eger, E. I., II, Saidman, L. J., and Brandstater, B.: Minimum alveolar anesthetic concentration: A standard of anesthetic potency. Anesthesiology, 26:756, 1965.
3. De Jong, R. H., and Eger, E. I., II: MAC expanded: AD_{50} and AD_{95} values of common inhalation anesthetics in man. Anesthesiology, 42:384, 1975.
4. Eger, E. I., II: Anesthetic Uptake and Action. Baltimore, Williams & Wilkins, 1974.
5. De Jong, R. H., et al.: Anesthetic potency determined by depression of synaptic transmission. Anesthesiology, 29:1139, 1968.
6. Freund, F. G., Martin, W. E., and Hornbein, T. F.: The H reflex as a measure of anesthetic potency in man. Anesthesiology, 30:642, 1969.
7. Cullen, S. C., and Larson, C. P., Jr.: Essentials of Anesthetic Practice. Chicago, Yearbook Medical Publishers, 1974.
8. Cullen, D. J., et al.: Clinical signs of anesthesia. Anesthesiology, 36:21, 1972.
9. Miller, R. D., Way, W. L., and Eger, E. I., II: The effects of *alpha*-methyldopa, reserpine, guanethidine and iproniazide on minimum alveolar anesthetic requirement (MAC). Anesthesiology, 29:1153, 1968.
10. Johnston, R. R., Way, W. L., and Miller, R. D.: Alteration of anesthetic requirement by amphetamine. Anesthesiology, 36:357, 1972.
11. Johnston, R. R., Way, W. L., and Miller, R. D.: The effects of CNS catecholamine-depleting drugs on dextroamphetamine-induced elevation of halothane MAC. Anesthesiology, 41:57, 1974.
12. Stoelting, R. K., Creasser, C. W., and Martz, R. C.: Effect of cocaine administration on halothane MAC in dogs. Anesth. Analg. (Cleve.), 54:422, 1975.
13. Finck, A. D., Ngai, S. H., and Berkowitz, B. A.: Antagonism of general anesthesia by naloxone in the rat. Anesthesiology, 46:241, 1977.
14. Tanifuji, Y., and Eger, E. I., II: Effect of brain sodium, potassium and osmolality on anesthetic requirements. *In* Abstracts of Scientific Papers. San Francisco, American Society of Anesthesiologists, 1976.
15. Steffey, E. P., and Eger, E. I., II: Hyperthermia and halothane MAC in the dog. Anesthesiology, 41:392, 1974.

16. Mueller, R. A., et al.: Central monaminergic neuronal effects on minimum alveolar concentrations (MAC) of halothane and cyclopropane in rats. Anesthesiology, *42*:143, 1975.

17. Roizen, M. F., et al.: The effect of destructive lesions in several key serotonin or norepinephrine brainstem areas on halothane and cyclopropane MAC. *In* Abstracts of Scientific Papers. San Francisco, American Society of Anesthesiologists, 1976.

18. Tanifuji, Y., and Eger, E. I., II: Effect of isoproterenol and propranolol on halothane MAC in dogs. Anesth. Analg. (Cleve.), *55*:383, 1976.

19. Laverty, R., and Taylor, K. M.: Propranolol uptake into the central nervous system and the effect on rat behavior and amine metabolism. J. Pharm. Pharmacol., *20*:605, 1968.

20. Johnston, R. R., et al.: Effect of levodopa on halothane anesthetic requirement. Anesth. Analg. (Cleve.), *54*:178, 1975.

21. White, P. F., Johnston, R. R., and Pudwill, C. R.: Interaction of ketamine and halothane in rats. Anesthesiology, *42*:179, 1975.

22. Blancata, L. S., Peng, A. T. C., and Alonsabe, D.: Intravenous lidocaine: adjunct to general anesthesia for endoscopy. N.Y. State J. Med., *70*:1659, 1970.

23. DiFazio, C. A., Niederlehner, J. R., and Burney, R. G.: The anesthetic potency of lidocaine in the rat. Anesth. Analg. (Cleve.), *55*:818, 1976.

24. DiFazio, C. A., Burney, R. G., and Himes, R. S., Jr.: Alterations in general anesthetic requirements with lidocaine. *In* Abstracts of Scientific Papers. San Francisco, American Society of Anesthesiologists, 1976.

25. Saidman, L. J., and Eger, E. I., II: Effect of nitrous oxide and of narcotic pre-medication on the alveolar concentration of halothane required for anesthesia. Anesthesiology, *25*:302, 1964.

26. Munson, E. S., Saidman, L. J., and Eger, E. I., II: Effect of nitrous oxide and morphine on the minimum anesthetic concentration of fluroxene. Anesthesiology, *26*:134, 1965.

27. Perisho, J. A., Buechel, D. R., and Miller, R. D.: The effect of diazepam (Valium) on minimum alveolar anesthetic requirement (MAC) in man. Can. Anaesth. Soc. J., *18*:536, 1971.

28. Stevens, W. C., et al.: Minimum alveolar concentrations (MAC) of isoflurane with and without nitrous oxide in patients of various ages. Anesthesiology, *42*:197, 1975.

29. Eger, E. I., II: Anesthetic Uptake and Action. Baltimore, Williams & Wilkins, 1974.

30. Vitez, T. S., et al.: Effects of *delta*-9-tetrahydrocannabinol on cyclopropane MAC in the rat. Anesthesiology, *38*:525, 1973.

31. Stoelting, R. K., et al.: Effects of *delta*-9-tetrahydrocannabinol on halothane MAC in dogs. Anesthesiology, *38*:521, 1973.

32. Cullen, D. J., and Eger, E. I., II: Effects of hypoxia and isovolemic anemia on the halothane requirement (MAC) of dogs. I: The effect of hypoxia. Anesthesiology, *32*:28, 1970.

33. Cullen, D. J., et al.: The effects of hypoxia and isovolemic anemia on the halothane requirement (MAC) of dogs. II: The effects of acute hypoxia on halothane requirement and cerebral-surface P_{O_2}, P_{CO_2}, pH, and bicarbonate. Anesthesiology, *32*:35, 1970.

34. Eisele, J. H., Eger, E. I., II, and Muallem, M.: Narcotic properties of carbon dioxide in the dog. Anesthesiology, *28*:856, 1967.

35. Cullen, D. J., and Eger, E. I., II: The effect of extreme hypocapnea on the anesthetic requirement (MAC) of dogs. Br. J. Anaesth., *43*:339, 1971.

36. Bonvallet, M., Hugelin, A., and Dell, P.: Sensibilité comparée du système réticule activateur ascendant et du centre respiratoire aux gaz du sang et à l'adrenaline. J. Physiol. (Paris), *47*:651, 1955.

37. Palahniuk, R. J., Shnider, S. M., and Eger, E. I., II: Pregnancy decreases the requirement for inhaled anesthetic agents. Anesthesiology, *41*:82, 1974.

38. Gregory, G. A., Eger, E. I., II, and Munson, E. S.: The relationship between age and halothane requirement in man. Anesthesiology, *30*:488, 1969.

39. Stoelting, R. K., Longnecker, D. E., and Eger, E. I., II: Minimum alveolar concentrations in man on awakening from methoxyflurane, halothane, ether, and fluroxene anesthesia. MAC awake. Anesthesiology, *33*:5, 1970.

40. Viegas, O., and Stoelting, R. K.: Halothane MAC in dogs unchanged by phenobarbital. Anesth. Analg. (Cleve.), *55*:677, 1976.

41. Tanifuji, Y., and Eger, E. I., II: Effect of arterial hypotension on anesthetic requirement in dogs. Br. J. Anaesth., *48*:947, 1976.

Chapter 21

Agents in Obstetrics: Mother, Fetus, and Newborn

MILTON H. ALPER

Perinatal pharmacology is basically complex, since it involves mother, fetus, placenta, labor, and neonatal adjustment to extrauterine life. Despite this complexity and the increased awareness of drug interactions, information on drug interactions in this area is limited. This is surprising because factors in pregnancy and parturition may dispose a patient to untoward drug reactions and interactions. These factors include:

1. Multiplicity of drugs, both prescription and over-the-counter, consumed by pregnant patients. In one study, the mean number of drugs taken was 10.3, with a range of 3 to 29, excluding anesthetic agents, intravenous fluids, vitamins, iron, cigarette smoking, and exposure to pesticides, paint, or chemicals.[1] The drugs most frequently ingested included analgesics (chiefly salicylates), diuretics, antihistamines, antibiotics, antiemetics, antacids, and sedatives. That the unexpected may occur is exemplified by one patient who had been ingesting 25 five-grain tablets (7.5 gm) of salicylate daily during pregnancy and who experienced respiratory arrest after receiving "a routine dose of sedative and analgesic agent" during labor. During the postpartum period profuse uterine bleeding necessitated a hysterectomy.

2. Physiologic changes in pregnancy, particularly in hormonal, cardiovascular, renal, and hepatic function, which may lead to alterations in drug disposition. Thus drug effects during pregnancy may be different from those in nonpregnant patients.

3. Differences in fetal and neonatal drug sensitivity and pharmacokinetics in comparison to the mature organism.

Despite these factors, descriptions of drug interactions in pregnancy, in parturition, or in neonatal life are sparse. In this chapter, the physiologic and pharmacologic milieu of the perinatal period will not be reviewed in detail. Rather, I shall present several case reports of documented or suspected drug interactions that pertain specifically to the practice of obstetric analgesia and anesthesia. In each instance, the pharmacologic and physiologic background of the interaction will be reviewed.

OXYTOCICS, VASOPRESSORS, AND ANESTHESIA

Oxytocic agents are commonly used in obstetric patients for inducing or augmenting labor, for facilitating placental expulsion, and for enhancing contractions of the uterus postpartum to reduce bleeding or to treat atony.[2-5] The clinically useful drugs are oxytocin and two ergot alkaloids, ergonovine and methylergonovine. The ergot alkaloids are less often used today because of the greater incidence of complications and because of insufficient evidence of their superiority to oxytocin.

Oxytocin (Pitocin) is a synthetic octapeptide, identical to the one normally present in and released from the posterior lobe of the pituitary gland, but free from contamination by other polypeptide hormones and proteins found in earlier natural preparations. Many of the complications described in the earlier literature were the result of the admixture of oxytocin with vasopressin (ADH), a potent octapeptide vasopressor and coronary artery vasoconstrictor. Pure synthetic oxytocin has some cardiovascular effects, but fewer than ADH, and is a specific augmentor of frequency and intensity of uterine contraction.

Ergonovine maleate (Ergotrate) and methylergonovine maleate (Methergine) dif-

fer from oxytocin in their effects on the uterus. Although the uterine effects of oxytocin closely resemble normal contractions, those induced by the ergot derivatives are of longer duration. Uterine tonus or baseline contractile intensity is also increased. The use of ergot preparations therefore is limited to the postpartum period.

Oxytocin is more safely administered as an intravenous infusion, which can be prepared by diluting 10 IU (1.0 ml) in 1,000 ml of infusion fluid. During labor, infusion rates vary from 1 mU/min to 10 mU/min, administered with an infusion pump and with careful monitoring to detect signs of fetal distress. Postpartum, rates of 20 mU to 100 mU/min may be used. Effects appear within three minutes, are maximal at about 20 minutes, and disappear within 15 to 20 minutes after discontinuing the infusion.

The ergot alkaloids are commonly given intramuscularly in a dose of 0.2 mg for the management of postpartum bleeding and of uterine atony. Onset of activity occurs within 10 minutes and increased uterine activity persists for two to six hours. The following report illustrates an interaction between oxytocics and a commonly administered vasopressor, ephedrine.

CASE REPORT

A 23-year-old woman received spinal anesthesia with tetracaine for an uncomplicated, low-forceps delivery. Prior to the administration of the anesthetic, she was given ephedrine, 25 mg, intramuscularly (IM) to prevent hypotension. Her blood pressure was stable during delivery, at 110/70. Following the birth of a healthy child, she was given Methergine, 0.2 mg IM, in addition to a slow intravenous infusion of dilute oxytocin solution. Her blood pressure was 120/80 as she left the delivery room. Twenty minutes later, the patient complained of severe, throbbing fronto-occipital headache. Her systolic blood pressure was over 220 torr. She was treated with serial injections of 2.5 mg of chlorpromazine intravenously to a total of 10 mg over 20 minutes. Her blood pressure decreased to 140/80, and her headache disappeared. She recovered uneventfully.

Cardiovascular effects of oxytocics

The cardiovascular side effects of oxytocic drugs in the obstetric patient have long been recognized. For example, in 1949 Greene and Barcham observed an increase in systolic blood pressure of 50 to 100 torr in patients receiving both a vasopressor and an oxytocic agent.[6] In fact, one patient suffered hemiplegia. The most extensive report is that of Casady et al., who studied 741 women who received continuous caudal analgesia, prophylactic methoxamine when the block was initiated, and an oxytocic drug (either ergonovine or methylergonovine and/or oxytocin) at the time of delivery of the placenta.[7] Thirty-four of the 741 patients (4.6%) developed systolic blood pressures over 140 torr postpartum. One patient experienced a ruptured intracranial aneurysm. This led to the abandonment of the routine use of prophylactic vasopressor therapy.

Hypertension following the combined use of vasopressors and oxytocics is a serious drug interaction, although it is not totally predictable. All commonly used vasopressors, including ephedrine, at present, the drug of choice in obstetrics, and both the ergot and posterior pituitary oxytocics have been incriminated. Severe hypertension is particularly likely to occur in patients who are already mildly hypertensive and who receive an ergot alkaloid postpartum. It is less frequently observed after the dilute intravenous infusion of oxytocin.

Most ergot alkaloids exert complex actions on the cardiovascular system; of chief concern is peripheral vasoconstriction by direct action on vascular smooth muscle. The ergot alkaloids display a spectrum of activity characteristic of partial agonists in that they may both stimulate and block *alpha*-adrenergic receptors. Ergonovine and methylergonovine are devoid of *alpha* receptor blocking activity and are weak vasoconstrictors, but they are additive in their effects with the vasopressors ephedrine and phenylephrine.[8]

Oxytocin also has complex cardiovascular effects, including vasoconstriction and thereby hypertension, which is more pronounced after surgical or chemical blockade of sympathetic pathways.[9] This block is an inevitable concomitant of major conduction anesthesia.

It is wise to avoid the routine use of vasopressors, particularly since they are rarely necessary. Hypotension may often be prevented by intravenous fluid therapy and by uterine displacement. Persistent hypotension can be treated with ephedrine, which will not decrease uterine blood flow. If any vasopressor has been used, ergot alkaloids are best avoided in favor of a slow intravenous infusion of dilute oxytocin with careful monitoring of blood pressure to detect the first sign of hypertension. If the use of ergot alkaloids is necessary postpartum, intramuscular rather than intravenous injection is advisable. If hypertension does occur, therapy should be promptly begun. Chlorpromazine has proven to be both safe and effective when given intravenously in a dose of 2.5 mg every 15 to 20 seconds until acceptable levels of blood pressure are reached; the total dose required is usually 10 to 15 mg. Nitroprusside should be effective, but it has not had the extensive clinical use that chlorpromazine has had.

In addition to the well-defined hazards associated with their use with vasopressors, oxytocics may also interact dangerously with anesthetic agents. Lipton and co-workers in 1962 demonstrated the lack of significant cardiovascular effects when *dilute* synthetic oxytocin was administered during general anesthesia.[10] This observation has been confirmed in both animals and human beings. In contrast, concentrated intravenous bolus injections of either natural or synthetic oxytocin may cause hypotension, tachycardia, and arrhythmias, particularly with halothane.[11-15] These effects are transient, lasting five to ten minutes, and are due to peripheral vasodilatation. Although usually well tolerated by healthy patients, these cardiovascular responses may be dangerous to patients with hypovolemia or with intrinsic heart disease.[13,14]

By contrast, the intravenous injection of ergonovine or of methylergonovine has been associated with more serious reactions from intense vasoconstriction, such as hypertension, convulsions, cerebrovascular accidents, and retinal detachment.[7,13,16,17] These drugs should not be used in patients with preeclampsia, hypertension, or cardiac disease.

Recently, Moodie and Moir could detect no difference in blood loss in parturient patients who were receiving either ergonovine or oxytocin during continuous lumbar epidural analgesia.[18] The incidence of nausea, vomiting, or retching was 46% after ergonovine and nil after oxytocin. These data combined with the cardiovascular side effects described suggest that oxytocin is most safely administered by dilute intravenous infusion by a pump rather than by intravenous bolus injection, and that the use of ergot alkaloids should be restricted, probably to the management of postpartum uterine atony.

Other effects of oxytocin

The possibility of a different type of interaction involving oxytocin has been suggested by Davies and his co-workers, who observed that total bilirubin levels were higher in two- and five-day-old infants whose mothers had had labor artificially induced by amniotomy followed immediately by intravenous oxytocin infusion.[19] In contrast, infants born after spontaneous labor augmented by oxytocin and those born after spontaneous labor without oxytocin did not have elevated levels. The researchers postulated that the elevated bilirubin levels were due to the higher incidence of drug administration during artificially induced labor and delivery. They were particularly concerned about nitrazepam, a benzodiazepine sedative, and bupivacaine, for epidural analgesia. Although no direct association between the use either of these drugs or of oxytocin and neonatal hyperbilirubinemia is known, labor of spontaneous onset is associated with higher umbilical cord cortisol levels than is induced labor.[20] Epidural block in labor prevents the usual rise in maternal cortisol levels.[21] Perhaps the liver enzymes induced by corticosteroids are low also in artificially induced labor followed by epidural analgesia, which may leave the fetal liver at a metabolic disadvantage with respect to the action of hepatic enzymes required to cope with the early postnatal bilirubin load. This interesting and provocative hypothesis requires further study.

Finally, Hodges and his associates in 1959 observed prolonged neuromuscular blockade from succinylcholine in a group of patients who had received oxytocin infusions for from eight hours to five days.[22] They suggested that the effects of succinylcholine are enhanced in such patients, possibly as the result of oxytocin-induced redistribution of potassium at the neuromuscular junction. Experiments in animals and in man failed to confirm Hodges's observations, although slightly elevated potassium levels were measured in man.[23,24] It seems likely that the altered response to succinylcholine resulted from other changes associated with prolonged labor rather than from the use of oxytocin.

MAGNESIUM SULFATE AND ANESTHESIA

The hypertensive disorders of pregnancy are hazardous to both mother and fetus. Despite intensive investigation and detailed characterization of the pathophysiology of preeclampsia and eclampsia, their cause remains unknown and their treatment empirical.[25,26] Toxemia probably occurs in 6 to 7% of pregnancies and is responsible for about 20% of all maternal deaths and for a perinatal mortality rate of 15 to 30%.

The anesthetic management of patients with hypertensive disorders of pregnancy is controversial. Regional anesthesia, particularly lumbar epidural block, and general anesthesia have been recommended for both vaginal delivery and cesarean section. If general anesthesia is selected, endotracheal intubation should be performed and neuromuscular blocking drugs are likely to be used. In these patients, a common drug interaction is that between magnesium and neuromuscular blocking drugs, as illustrated in the following case report from the literature.[27]

CASE REPORT

A 24-year-old woman with preeclampsia was treated with phenobarbital, hydralazine, and magnesium sulfate (60 gm intramuscularly in divided doses over 14 hours). Three hours after the last injection of magnesium sulfate, anesthesia for cesarean section was induced with thiopental, succinylcholine (50 mg), nitrous oxide, and oxygen, followed by 30 mg of d-tubocurarine to control respiration. At the end of the operation, despite the usual measures, the neuromuscular block could not be reversed. Ten milliliters of calcium gluconate, 10%, caused some improvement, but the patient required artificial ventilation for eight hours.

Pharmacology of magnesium sulfate

The mainstay of the management of patients with toxemia remains magnesium sulfate by parenteral administration. A common approach is to inject 20 ml of magnesium sulfate, 20% (4 gm), intravenously over three minutes, followed immediately by 10 ml of 50% solution (5 gm), injected deeply intramuscularly into each buttock, and every four hours thereafter, if the patellar reflex is present, if urine flow has been at least 100 ml in the previous four hours, and if respiration is not depressed.[28] If convulsions persist, sodium amobarbital is administered, up to 0.25 gm, in small intravenous increments. If the patient's diastolic blood pressure remains over 110 torr, hydralazine is administered intravenously in divided doses up to a total of 5 to 20 mg until the diastolic pressure falls to about 100 torr. No maternal deaths occurred in the 154 patients with eclampsia who were so treated. Seventy-seven per cent of the patients were delivered vaginally and 23% by cesarean section. All fetuses survived who were alive when treatment was started and who weighed at least 1,800 gm (4 pounds) when delivered.

The magnesium ion is normally present in plasma in a concentration of 1.5 to 2.2 meq/L. When its concentration exceeds 4 to 5 meq/L, following parenteral administration, deep tendon reflexes diminish. They disappear at concentrations of approximately 10 meq/L. At 12 to 15 meq/L, respiratory paralysis may ensue as well as electrocardiographic changes such as heart block.

Magnesium salts were at one time thought to be central nervous system depressants capable of producing general anesthesia. In 1916, Peck and Meltzer described three operations in patients who received no drugs other than magnesium sulfate.[29] In 1966, Somjen and co-workers disproved this notion by administering magnesium sulfate to two human volunteers sufficient to achieve blood levels of 14.6 and 15.3 meq/L.[30] Both subjects were profoundly paralyzed and appeared anesthetized but remained conscious, in contact with their surroundings, sensitive to painful stimuli, and showed no evidence of depression of the central nervous system. The observations of Peck and Meltzer remain unexplained.

The major effect of excess magnesium ion is the suppression of peripheral neuromuscular function by a decrease in the amount of acetylcholine released from motor nerve terminals in response to nerve impulses.[31] Magnesium also decreases the sensitivity of the end-plate to applied acetylcholine as well as the direct excitability of muscle fibers themselves. Experimentally, increasing the concentration of calcium antagonizes the action of magnesium at nerve terminals and restores neuromuscular transmission. In addition, from the point of view of fetal well-being, studies in monkeys have shown that magnesium decreases mean arterial blood pressure and increases uterine blood flow.[32]

Neuromuscular blockers and magnesium

The anesthetic implications of magnesium therapy in the obstetric patient were first described by Morris and Giesecke in 1968. They noted a decreased requirement for succinylcholine in a group of patients undergoing cesarean section after magnesium sulfate therapy for toxemia.[33]

In a subsequent study in cats, Giesecke et al. reported that, although only 1/1,000 as potent as d-tubocurarine at the neuromuscular junction, magnesium sulfate enhanced the neuromuscular blockade from both d-tubocurarine and succinylcholine.[34] Ghoneim and Long reported similar findings in the rat, except that d-tubocurarine and decamethonium were enhanced approximately fourfold and succinylcholine only twofold.[27] The lesser degree of potentiation of succinylcholine may be the result of its more rapid destruction in the presence of elevated magnesium concentrations since cholinesterase activity is enhanced by magnesium.[35] (See Chapter 17.)

In spite of a possible prolonged block in patients treated with magnesium, muscle relaxants are too useful to be avoided. I believe that the dangers of induction by inhalation anesthesia in these seriously ill obstetric patients outweigh the hazards posed by the potentiation of neuromuscular blockade. It is probably safer to avoid or to reduce the dose of the long-acting nondepolarizing relaxants. Certainly the 30 mg of d-tubocurarine described in the case report was excessive. Succinylcholine should be given at roughly half the usual dose and with careful monitoring of neuromuscular function with a nerve stimulator. Although experimentally, magnesium-induced neuromuscular block can be antagonized by calcium, this is not so clinically.[31] The administration of calcium gluconate to two patients under these circumstances was ineffective.[27] The inability of calcium to antagonize completely a magnesium-induced neuromuscular block probably relates to the multiple actions of magnesium at the neuromuscular junction. At any rate, ventilatory support is required until the patient recovers spontaneously.

Other effects of magnesium

Magnesium, given intravenously, but not intramuscularly, may induce hypocalcemia in the mother and in the neonate.[36,37] In a study by Lipsitz, infants born after maternal intravenous therapy for 12 to 24 hours commonly showed signs associated with hypermagnesemia: flaccidity and hyporeflexia, respiratory depression, and a weak or absent cry.[38] The most severely affected infants required resuscitation and ventilatory support for 24 to 36 hours. In a large series of cases, Stone and Pritchard failed to find significant fetal or neonatal effects after the intramuscular regimen described above.[39] This probably means that central nervous system and blood levels were lower when magnesium was given intramuscularly instead of intravenously.

Finally, Alexander and co-workers reported no cardiovascular problems in the anesthetic management of 14 eclamptic patients who underwent cesarean section after large doses of reserpine and/or hydralazine.[40] The interaction between antihypertensive agents and anesthesia is covered in detail elsewhere in this volume.

INTERACTIONS IN THE FETUS AND NEONATE

Fetal pharmacology is a new area of investigation, especially in the human fetus. Anesthesiologists have long recognized that most drugs used for obstetric analgesia and anesthesia cross the placental barrier. Despite a better understanding of the pharmacokinetics of maternal-fetal drug transfer and increased sophistication in the measurement of fetal drug effects, no instances of drug interaction have been noted. One expects that such interactions will be detected eventually.

In the past, more concern has been voiced over the effect of maternally administered drugs on the newborn, who must make the major homeostatic adjustments required for the transition from intrauterine to extrauterine life. At the same time, the neonate is deprived of the umbilical connection to his mother and must cope with whatever drug load he has "inherited" during parturition.

Transplacentally acquired drugs may influence the neonate's physiologic adaptations, particularly respiration, circulation, and thermoregulation; conversely, these major functional changes may themselves influence drug distribution and effects in the newborn. As pointed out in recent reviews,[41-48] our knowledge of drug disposition in the newborn is limited but it suggests that there are profound differences from older children and adults, so much so that the neonate has been termed a "unique drug recipient."[47] Some of the factors that account for these differences are listed in Table 21–1.

All of the factors listed in Table 21–1 may account for drug effects that may be both quantitatively and qualitatively different in the neonate from those effects in older children and adults. Several drug interactions of interest to the anesthesiologist have been described.

Of particular significance in the newborn is the ability to handle an important endogenous substrate, bilirubin.[49,50] Drugs may interfere with the disposition of bilirubin in

two ways: either by competing for binding sites on neonatal plasma protein or by altering hepatic enzyme systems responsible for bilirubin metabolism.

Bilirubin is transported in neonatal blood in two forms, conjugated and unconjugated. Unconjugated, lipid soluble bilirubin is 99% bound to plasma albumin, hence limiting its access to the brain. Unbound unconjugated bilirubin is able to penetrate the brain; if sufficient concentration is achieved in the brain, bilirubin encephalopathy or kernicterus results. Any factor that decreases the binding of unconjugated bilirubin to its albumin binding sites increases the risk of encephalopathy. Clinically, this is more likely to be important in infants who are premature or who are faced with abnormally high bilirubin loads after delivery.[50]

Some drugs compete with bilirubin for plasma protein binding sites in the newborn.[51] Perhaps the best-known example is sulfisoxazole (Gantrisin), whose administration to the neonate is associated with an increased frequency of kernicterus in both

Table 21–1
Factors affecting drug disposition in the neonate

1. Developmental age and state of maturation
   a. organ development
   b. sensitivity of drug receptors

2. Reduced esterase activity

3. Plasma protein binding
   a. reduced protein concentration
   b. qualitatively different albumin
   c. high concentrations of bilirubin and free fatty acids
   d. lower blood pH
   e. competition for binding sites by both endogenous and
      exogenous substrates
   f. increased apparent volume of drug distribution

4. Drug distribution
   a. changing pattern of regional blood flows
   b. relatively greater brain and liver mass
   c. lower myelin content of brain
   d. higher total body water and extra/intracellular water
      content ratio
   e. scanty adipose tissue

5. Biotransformation
   a. immaturity of certain hepatic enzyme systems
   b. enzyme induction or inhibition

6. Reduced renal function

animals and human beings. Of particular concern to the anesthesiologist is parenteral diazepam (Valium). Schiff and co-workers in 1971 demonstrated *in vitro* that injectable diazepam was a potent displacer of bilirubin from plasma proteins. However, sodium benzoate in the buffer preservative was found to be the displacer, rather than diazepam.[52] This finding correlated well with previous observations of the displacing activity of caffeine sodium benzoate, an analeptic drug formerly used as a respiratory stimulant in the newborn with depressed respiration. Recently, another component of drug mixtures, methylparaben, frequently used as a preservative in local anesthetic solutions, in injectable saline, and in bacteriostatic water, has also been shown to have similar displacing activity.[53]

Since injectable diazepam is frequently used as an adjunct during labor, concern was expressed about bilirubin displacement in both the fetus and the neonate. However, Adoni and co-workers in 1973 demonstrated no alterations in bilirubin binding capacity of cord blood from infants whose mothers received diazepam during labor.[54] Benzoate probably either is unable to cross the placenta or is so rapidly metabolized by the maternal liver that significant concentrations are not achieved in the fetus. However, injectable diazepam must be used with caution in the neonate with hyperbilirubinemia. The ability of other analgesics and anesthetics to modify bilirubin-albumin binding in the neonate has not been systematically studied.

A second area of concern is that of drug-induced alterations in fetal and neonatal metabolism of various substrates, including bilirubin. The best-known example is the prenatal administration of phenobarbital to the mother with resultant accelerated conjugation of bilirubin through induction of the hepatic enzyme, glucuronyltransferase. Under these conditions, lower bilirubin levels in the neonate have been demonstrated.[44] Since over 200 enzyme inducers

have been identified, the metabolism of exogenous substrates and drugs may be affected.

Clinically, Morselli and his associates have documented the effects of both phenobarbital administration to the mother and maturity of the newborn on the latter's ability to clear diazepam from the blood stream.[55] The plasma half-life of diazepam was 18 ± 3 (SE) hours in children aged four to eight years and 75 ± 37 hours with a range of 38 to 120 hours in four prematurely born infants (28 to 34 weeks). In a group of full-term newborns whose mothers had received diazepam within 24 hours of delivery, the plasma half-life averaged 31 ± 2 hours. The most striking finding was an average half-life of diazepam of 16 ± 2.5 hours in three term newborns whose mothers received phenobarbital for at least eight days before delivery and diazepam within 24 hours of delivery. The researchers infer that the phenobarbital treatment of the mothers accelerated the disposition of diazepam in these term newborns to the level observed in the older children.

Treatment of pregnant rats and rabbits with phenobarbital during the last week of pregnancy results in accelerated metabolism of both pentobarbital and meperidine in the newborn.[56] Although not studied during pregnancy, the treatment of calves with phenobarbital resulted in a faster disappearance of thiopental from their blood stream and a decrease in the duration of post-anesthetic depression.[57] Further examples of enzyme induction of specific clinical significance to obstetric anesthesia will undoubtedly appear.

Finally, Drew and Kitchen reported the influence of some 20 different maternally administered drugs on total bilirubin levels in over 1,000 infants at 48 and 72 hours of age.[58] They found that maternal administration of meperidine was associated with lower bilirubin levels in the newborn. Maternal diazepam administration was associated with slightly higher levels; various phenothiazine derivatives, regional anesthesia, and general anesthesia had no effect. In general, the magnitude of the changes was not great and their clinical significance was doubtful, except perhaps in infants at risk for hyperbilirubinemia.

Despite the hypothetically fertile physiologic grounds for drug interactions in the fetus and neonate as the result of maternally administered analgesics and anesthetics, reactions of clinical significance have not been described. One may, however, infer that as perinatal pharmacology develops further, such interactions will most likely be identified, especially in infants at risk.

REFERENCES

1. Hill, R. M.: Drugs ingested by pregnant women. Clin. Pharmacol. Ther., *14*:654, 1973.
2. Munsick, R. A.: The pharmacology and clinical application of various oxytocic drugs. Am. J. Obstet. Gynecol., *93*:442, 1965.
3. Pauerstein, C. J.: Ecbolic agents. Clin. Anesth., *10*:299, 1973.
4. Brazeau, P.: Oxytocics. *In* The Pharmacologic Basis of Therapeutics. 5th edition. Edited by L. S. Goodman and A. Gilman. New York, Macmillan, 1975.
5. Brenner, W. E.: The oxytocics: actions and clinical indications. Contemp. OB/GYN, 7:125, 1976.
6. Greene, B. A., and Barcham, J.: Cerebral complications resulting from hypertension caused by vasopressor drugs in obstetrics. N.Y. State J. Med., *49*:1424, 1949.
7. Casady, G. N., Moore, D. C., and Bridenbaugh, D. L.: Postpartum hypertension after use of vasoconstrictor and oxytocic drugs. J.A.M.A., *172*:1011, 1960.
8. Munson, W. M.: The pressor effect of various vasopressor-oxytocic combinations: a laboratory study and a review. Anesth. Analg. (Cleve.), *44*:114, 1965.
9. Lloyd, S., and Pickford, M.: The action of posterior pituitary hormones and oestrogens on the vascular system of the rat. J. Physiol., *155*:161, 1961.
10. Lipton, B., Hershey, S. G., and Baez, S.: Compatibility of oxytocics with anesthetic agents. J.A.M.A., *179*:410, 1962.
11. Nakano, J., and Fisher, R. D.: Studies on the cardiovascular effects of synthetic oxytocin. J. Pharmacol., *142*:206, 1963.
12. Andersen, T. W., et al.: Cardiovascular effects of rapid intravenous injection of synthetic oxytocin during elective cesarean section. Clin. Pharmacol. Ther., *6*:345, 1965.
13. Hendricks, C. H., and Brenner, W. E.: Cardiovascular effects of oxytocic drugs used post partum. Am. J. Obstet. Gynecol., *108*:751, 1970.
14. Weis, F. R., and Peak, J.: Effects of oxytocin on blood pressure during anesthesia. Anesthesiology, *40*:189, 1974.
15. Weis, F. R., et al.: Cardiovascular effects of oxytocin. Obstet. Gynecol., *46*:211, 1975.
16. Gombos, G. M., Howitt, D., and Chen, S.: Bilateral retinal detachment occurring in the immediate postpartum period after methylergonovine and oxytocin administration. Eye Ear Nose Throat Mon., *48*:680, 1969.
17. Abouleish, E.: Postpartum hypertension and convulsion after oxytocic drugs. Anesth. Analg. (Cleve.), *55*:813, 1976.
18. Moodie, J. E., and Moir, D. D.: Ergometrine, oxytocin and extradural analgesia. Br. J. Anaesth., *48*:571, 1976.
19. Davies, D. P., et al.: Neonatal jaundice and maternal oxytocin infusion. Br. Med. J., *2*:476, 1973.
20. Ohrlander, S., Gennser, G., and Eneroth, P.: Plasma cortisol levels in human fetus during parturition. Obstet. Gynecol., *48*:381, 1976.
21. Buchan, P. C., Milne, M. K., and Browning, M. C. K.: The effect of continuous epidural blockade on plasma 11-hydroxycorticosteroid concentrations in labour. J. Obstet. Gynaecol. Br. Commonw., *80*:974, 1973.
22. Hodges, R. J. H., et al.: Effects of oxytocin on the response to suxamethonium. Br. Med. J., *1*:413, 1959.
23. Keil, A. M.: Effects of oxytocin on the response to suxamethonium in rabbits, sheep, and pigs. Br. J. Anaesth., *34*:306, 1962.
24. Ichiyanagi, K., Ito, Y., and Aoki, E.: Effects of oxytocin on the response to suxamethonium and d-tubocurarine in man. Br. J. Anaesth., *35*:611, 1963.
25. Pritchard, J. A., and MacDonald, P. C.: Williams Obstetrics. 15th Edition. New York, Appleton-Century-Crofts, 1976.
26. Speroff, L.: Toxemia of pregnancy: mechanism and therapeutic management. Am. J. Cardiol., *32*:582, 1973.
27. Ghoneim, M. M., and Long, J. P.: The interaction between magnesium and other neuromuscular blocking agents. Anesthesiology, *32*:23, 1970.
28. Pritchard, J. A., and Pritchard, S. A.: Standardized treatment of 154 consecutive cases of eclampsia. Am. J. Obstet. Gynecol., *123*:543, 1975.
29. Peck, C. H., and Meltzer, S. J.: Anesthesia in human beings by intravenous injection of magnesium sulphate. J.A.M.A., *67*:1131, 1916.
30. Somjen, G., Hilmy, M., and Stephen, C. R.: Failure to anesthetize human subjects by intravenous administration of magnesium sulfate. J. Pharmacol., *154*:652, 1966.
31. del Castillo, J., and Engbaek, L.: The nature of the neuromuscular block produced by magnesium. J. Physiol., *124*:370, 1954.
32. Harbert, G. M., Cornell, G. W., and Thornton, W. N.: Effect of toxemia therapy on uterine dynamics. Am. J. Obstet. Gynecol., *105*:94, 1969.
33. Morris, R., and Giesecke, A. H.: Magnesium sul-

fate therapy in toxemia of pregnancy. South. Med. J., *61*:25, 1968.

34. Giesecke, A. H., et al.: Of magnesium, muscle relaxants, toxemic parturients and cats. Anesth. Analg. (Cleve.), *47*:689, 1968.

35. Nachmanson, D.: Action of ions on cholinesterase. Nature, *145*:513, 1940.

36. Monif, G. R. G., and Savory, J.: Iatrogenic maternal hypocalcemia following magnesium sulfate therapy. J.A.M.A., *219*:1469, 1972.

37. Savory, J., and Monif, G. R. G.: Serum calcium levels in cord sera of the progeny of mothers treated with magnesium sulfate for toxemia of pregnancy. Am. J. Obstet. Gynecol., *110*:556, 1971.

38. Lipsitz, P. J.: The clinical and biochemical effects of excess magnesium in the newborn. Pediatrics, *47*:501, 1971.

39. Stone, S. R., and Pritchard, J. A.: Effect of maternally administered magnesium sulfate on the neonate. Obstet. Gynecol., *35*:574, 1970.

40. Alexander, J. A., et al.: Cesarean section in the eclamptic patient on antihypertensive therapy: a review of fourteen cases. South. Med. J., *57*:1282, 1964.

41. Yaffe, S. J., ed.: Symposium on pediatric pharmacology. Pediatr. Clin. North Am., *19*:1, 1972.

42. Ecobichon, D. J., and Stephens, D. S.: Perinatal development of human blood esterases. Clin. Pharmacol. Ther., *14*:41, 1973.

43. Dancis, J., and Hwang, J. C.: Perinatal Pharmacology: Problems and Priorities. New York, Raven Press, 1974.

44. Eriksson, M., and Yaffe, S. J.: Drug metabolism in the newborn. Annu. Rev. Med., *24*:29, 1973.

45. Yaffe, S. J., and Juchau, M.: Perinatal pharmacology. Annu. Rev. Pharmacol., *14*:219, 1974.

46. Gillette, J. R., and Stripp, B.: Pre- and postnatal enzyme capacity for drug metabolite production. Fed. Proc., *34*:172, 1975.

47. Morselli, P. L.: Clinical pharmacokinetics in the neonate. Clin. Pharmacokinetics, *1*:81, 1976.

48. Yaffe, S. J.: Developmental factors influencing interactions of drugs. Ann. N.Y. Acad. Sci., *281*:90, 1976.

49. Odell, G. B.: The distribution and toxicity of bilirubin. Pediatrics, *46*:16, 1970.

50. Dodson, W. E.: Neonatal metabolic encephalopathies, hypoglycemia, hypocalcemia, hypomagnesemia, and hyperbilirubinemia. Clin. Perinatol., *4*:131, 1977.

51. Stern, L.: Drug interactions—Part II. Drugs, the newborn infant, and the binding of bilirubin to albumin. Pediatrics, *49*:916, 1972.

52. Schiff, D., Chan, G., and Stern, L.: Fixed drug combinations and the displacement of bilirubin from albumin. Pediatrics, *48*:139, 1971.

53. Rasmussen, L. F., Ahlfors, C. E., and Wennberg, R. P.: The effect of paraben preservatives on albumin binding of bilirubin. J. Pediatr., *89*:475, 1976.

54. Adoni, A., et al.: Effect of maternal administration of diazepam on the bilirubin-binding capacity of cord blood serum. Am. J. Obstet. Gynecol., *115*:577, 1973.

55. Morselli, P. L., et al.: Drug interactions in the human fetus and newborn infant. *In* Drug Interactions. Edited by P. L. Morselli, S. N. Cohen, and S. Garattini. New York, Raven Press, 1974.

56. Pantuck, E., Conney, A. H., and Kuntzman, R.: Effect of phenobarbital on the metabolism of pentobarbital and meperidine in fetal rabbits and rats. Biochem. Pharmacol., *17*:1441, 1968.

57. Sharma, R. P., Stowe, C. M., and Good, A. L.: Alteration of thiopental metabolism in phenobarbital-treated calves. Toxicol. Appl. Pharmacol., *17*:400, 1970.

58. Drew, J. H., and Kitchen, W. H.: The effect of maternally administered drugs on bilirubin concentrations in the newborn infant. J. Pediatr., *89*:657, 1976.

Index

Page numbers that appear in italics indicate illustrations; page numbers followed by ''t'' indicate tables.